PAEDIATRIC NURSING IN AUSTRALIA AND NEW ZEALAND

Third edition

The health of babies, children and young people is fundamentally different from that of adults, so their healthcare must reflect their unique needs and respectfully engage their parents, family members and communities. *Paediatric Nursing in Australia and New Zealand* introduces nursing students to the care of infants, young children, children, young people and their families in a range of clinical and community settings across Australasia.

This third edition has been expanded to include content on paediatric nursing in New Zealand and includes an increased focus on families. New chapters in this edition cover the health services available for Aboriginal, Torres Strait Islander and Māori children, the transition to parenthood for new families, children's sleep patterns and behaviours, and paediatric health in school settings. Case studies and reflective questions throughout the book introduce students to scenarios they will encounter throughout their careers and encourage them to develop their critical thinking and problem-solving skills.

Written by an expert team of nurses and nursing academics, *Paediatric Nursing in Australia and New Zealand* is an essential resource that equips future nurses with the knowledge and skills to provide evidence-based care to babies, children and their families.

Jennifer Fraser is a Registered Nurse and Associate Professor in the Faculty of Medicine and Health at the University of Sydney.

Donna Waters is a Registered Nurse and Professor in the Faculty of Medicine and Health at the University of Sydney.

Elizabeth Forster is a Registered Nurse and Senior Lecturer in the School of Nursing and Midwifery at Griffith University.

Nicola Brown is a Registered Nurse and Director of Education, Professional Practice and Innovation at Tresillian Family Care Centres, Australia.

Cambridge University Press acknowledges the Australian Aboriginal and Torres Strait Islander peoples of this nation. We acknowledge the traditional custodians of the lands on which our company is located and where we conduct our business. We pay our respects to ancestors and Elders, past and present. Cambridge University Press is committed to honouring Australian Aboriginal and Torres Strait Islander peoples' unique cultural and spiritual relationships to the land, waters and seas and their rich contribution to society.

Cambridge University Press acknowledges the Māori people as *tangata whenua* of Aotearoa New Zealand. We pay our respects to the First Nation Elders of New Zealand, past, present and emerging.

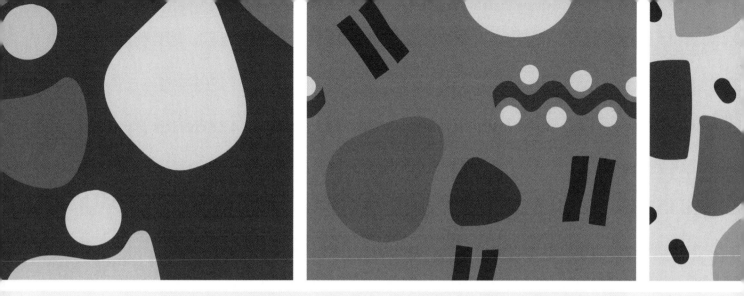

PAEDIATRIC NURSING IN AUSTRALIA AND NEW ZEALAND

Third edition

EDITED BY

Jennifer Fraser
Donna Waters
Elizabeth Forster
Nicola Brown

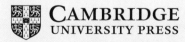

CAMBRIDGE
UNIVERSITY PRESS

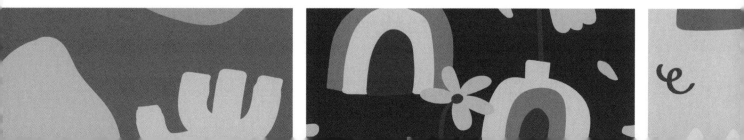

CAMBRIDGE
UNIVERSITY PRESS

University Printing House, Cambridge CB2 8BS, United Kingdom

One Liberty Plaza, 20th Floor, New York, NY 10006, USA

477 Williamstown Road, Port Melbourne, VIC 3207, Australia

314–321, 3rd Floor, Plot 3, Splendor Forum, Jasola District Centre, New Delhi – 110025, India

103 Penang Road, #05–06/07, Visioncrest Commercial, Singapore 238467

Cambridge University Press is part of the University of Cambridge.

It furthers the University's mission by disseminating knowledge in the pursuit of
education, learning and research at the highest international levels of excellence.

www.cambridge.org
Information on this title: www.cambridge.org/highereducation/isbn/9781108984652

© Cambridge University Press 2014, 2017, 2022

First published 2014
Second edition 2017
Third edition 2022

Cover designed by Carolina Kerr
Typeset by Straive
Printed in Singapore by Markono Print Media Pte Ltd, October 2021

A catalogue record for this publication is available from the British Library

A catalogue record for this book is available from the National Library of Australia

ISBN 978-1-108-98465-2 Paperback

Additional resources for this publication at www.cambridge.org/highereducation/isbn/9781108984652

Contents

Part C   Nursing children and young people

Contributors

Editors

Nicola Brown is a Registered Nurse and Director of Education, Professional Practice and Innovation at Tresillian Family Care Centres, Australia.

Elizabeth Forster is a Registered Nurse and Senior Lecturer in the School of Nursing and Midwifery at Griffith University.

Jennifer Fraser is a Registered Nurse and Associate Professor in the Faculty of Medicine and Health at the University of Sydney.

Donna Waters is a Registered Nurse and Professor in the Faculty of Medicine and Health at the University of Sydney.

Chapter authors

Melissa Carey (Ngāti Raukawa, Ngāti Huri) is a Senior Lecturer in Nursing and a Māori Health Research Fellow. She has been a Registered Nurse for over 23 years and has extensive experience working in the acute clinical setting in regional areas.

Liesa Clague is a descendant of the Yaegl, Bundjalung and Gumbayniggir peoples from the North Coast of New South Wales on her mother's side and on her father's side has Manx heritage from the Isle of Man. Liesa has worked in the Aboriginal sector for Aboriginal Medical Services, the Aboriginal Health & Medical Research Council of NSW and in the non-government and government sectors in healthcare as a nurse, midwife and educator. Liesa completed her PhD in education at Macquarie University, on *Gan;na: Listening to the perspectives of Primary School Students on their School-Based Garden.* For the last 15 years, she has worked in roles within universities, embedding Aboriginal and Torres Strait Islander knowledge.

Tara Flemington is a paediatric clinical nurse consultant in the Mid-North Coast Local Health District and adjunct senior lecturer at the University of Sydney. Her areas of research expertise include child protection, the cultural safety for Aboriginal children and their families, and translational research incorporating quantitative and qualitative methodologies.

Lisa Hutchinson is the policy manager for a large disability organisation. Prior to this, she worked for Queensland Health, managing a statewide primary school nursing program, coordinating practice development for statewide secondary school nurses and providing clinical nursing services within both primary and secondary school health settings. Lisa has postgraduate qualifications in child and adolescent health nursing, and community and primary healthcare.

Fleur Magick Dennis is a Wiradyuri and Ngemba/Wayilwan woman. She is the chief executive officer of Milan Dhiiyaan, a 100 per cent Aboriginal-owned and run company that provides Aboriginal cultural and spiritual health education and consulting. Fleur holds a Master of Indigenous Studies (Wellbeing) and a Bachelor of Arts in Adult Education and Community Management.

Laurance Magick Dennis is a Wayilwan and Yuin man. He is a community leader and senior cultural educator with Milan Dhiiyaan. A highly regarded craftsman and artist, he hosts workshops about health through art and craft, and spiritual ceremony.

Amy E Mitchell is a Registered Nurse and a lecturer in the School of Nursing and Midwifery at Griffith University, Queensland. She has clinical and research expertise in family-centred care for children with chronic health conditions and interventions to promote child health and development.

Lee O'Malley is a lecturer at the University of Southern Queensland. She is completing her PhD in nursing care and management of paediatric presentations to emergency departments in the rural setting. She has worked globally as a paediatric nurse and paediatric educator for almost 30 years, and has expertise in paediatric intensive care and paediatric and neonatal emergency transport.

Ibi Patane is a lecturer who coordinates the undergraduate paediatric subjects at Queensland University of Technology. She is a nationally accredited paediatric specialist nurse and has vast evidence-based clinical practice, policy development and managerial experience in the acute paediatric setting.

Robyn Rosina is an academic within the School of Nursing and Midwifery at the University of Newcastle, New South Wales.

Loretta Scaini-Clarke is a paediatric intensive care nurse educator, with over 30 years' experience as a critical care nurse. She is a faculty member in a number of paediatric training courses, and was instrumental in the development of paediatric intensive care unit (PICU) education programs for Queensland Health.

Lindsay Smith is a lecturer in the School of Nursing at the University of Tasmania. He developed the Australian Family Strengths Nursing Assessment (AFSNA) and was elected to the board of directors for the International Family Nursing Association in 2019.

Helen Stasa is a researcher with a focus on nursing and healthcare.

Julia Taylor is a Registered Nurse and clinical lecturer at the University of Tasmania.

Preface

This third edition of *Paediatric Nursing in Australia and New Zealand* expands the focus and content of the two previous editions. This was driven by an understanding of the substantial developments that have occurred not just in paediatric nursing, but also in child health nursing. The book now includes New Zealand content as well as Australian acute care and community health content. A number of broad changes have been made in working with infants, children, families and young people throughout Australian and New Zealand paediatric and child healthcare contexts. The most significant and exciting addition is an emphasis on health services for New Zealand Māori and Australian Aboriginal and Torres Strait Islander children and young people. Cultural safety is fundamental to the nursing care provided across paediatric and child health settings. A new chapter has been created and written by New Zealand Māori and Aboriginal and Torres Strait Islander authors to contribute to building the capacity of our discipline to enable all practitioners to understand and respect the importance of cultural safety in providing equitable healthcare.

This third edition has been written in three parts: Part A examines the contexts of nursing care in Australia and New Zealand; Part B explores nursing infants, young children and their families; and Part C focuses on nursing children and young people. We welcome a number of new authors, including the Māori and Aboriginal and Torres Strait Islander writers who are so committed to the discourse of cultural safety in paediatric and child healthcare. We are most grateful for the ongoing contribution of previous contributors and the improvements they have made in response to feedback and review.

We thank Cambridge University Press for continuing to support us and for publishing this expanded edition of the book. We would also like to particularly thank those who gave their time so generously to provide feedback, reviews and copy editing. The COVID-19 pandemic presented many challenges throughout 2020 as we adapted to new ways of living and working. Completing this edition of the textbook at this time, in its expanded form, with authors from across Australia and New Zealand, could not have been possible without the dedication and strong commitment of all those who contributed. We are very pleased to present this third edition.

Jennifer Fraser, Donna Waters, Elizabeth Forster and Nicola Brown

Acknowledgements

The authors and Cambridge University Press would like to thank the following for permission to reproduce material in this book.

Figures 3.1, 3.2: Courtesy of SNAICC – National Voice for our Children, Design by Mazart Communications. Reproduced with permission. For more information go to: www .familymatters.org.au; **6.1**: Reprinted by permission from Springer Nature from A Morawska & AE Mitchell (2018), Children's health, physical activity, and nutrition, in *Handbook of Parenting and Child Development Across the Lifespan* by Matthew R. Sanders & Alina Morawska (eds) © 2018; **6.2**: adapted from material © Heldref Publications and © Wiley; **8.2, 8.3**: © ARACY 2021. Reproduced with permission; **10.1**: © Getty Images/decade3d; **11.1**: adapted with permission from Wolters Kluwer Health, Inc.: Ronald Dieckmann, Dena Brownstein & Marianne Gausche-Hill, 'The pediatric assessment triangle: A novel approach for the rapid evaluation of children', *Pediatric Emergency Care*, 26(4), pp. 312–15, https://doi .org/10.1097/PEC.0b013e3181d6db37; **11.7**: © 2011 Elsevier Ltd. All rights reserved. Reprinted from Pauline M. Cullen, 'Intraosseous cannulation in children', *Anaesthesia & Intensive Care Medicine*, 13(1), pp. 28–30. Copyright 2011, with permission from Elsevier; **13.1**: republished with modifications with permission of Future Medicine Ltd, from Julia Downing, Satbir Singh Jassal, Lulu Mathews, Hanneke Brits & Stefan J Friedrichsdorf (2015). 'Pediatric pain management in palliative care', *Pain Management*, 5(1), pp. 23–35; permission conveyed through Copyright Clearance Center, Inc.

Table 1.1: adapted from material © Australian Institute of Health and Welfare 2014 and material © New Zealand Child and Youth Epidemiology Service; **3.1**: © Ministry of Health. Reproduced under Creative Commons Attribution 4.0 International Licence (https:// creativecommons.org/licenses/by/4.0/); **6.1**: adapted from material © The Royal Children's Hospital Melbourne. Reproduced with permission; **6.3**: adapted from material © Common-wealth of Australia 2016. Licenced under Creative Commons Attribution 4.0 International licence (https://creativecommons.org/licenses/by/4.0/); **9.1**: adapted from material © Sage Publishing; **10.2**: © 2012 Blackwell Publishing Ltd. Reproduced with minor modifications from APAGBI (2012) with permission of John Wiley and Sons; **10.4**: reproduced by permission, NSW Health © 2011;

Box 3.1: reproduced from material © Crown Copyright. Licenced from the Ministry of Justice for use under the creative commons attribution licence (BY) 4.0; **5.1**: © World Health Organization 2015; **5.2**: adapted from material © Commonwealth of Australia 2016. Licenced under Creative Commons Attribution 4.0 International Licence (https://creativecommons .org/licenses/by/4.0/).

Every effort has been made to trace and acknowledge copyright. The publisher apologises for any accidental infringement and welcomes information that would redress this situation.

Acronyms
and abbreviations

ABS	Australian Bureau of Statistics
ACAMS	Australian Congenital Anomalies Monitoring System
ACARA	Australian Curriculum, Assessment and Reporting Authority
ACCHS	Aboriginal Community Controlled Health Service
ACCYPN	Australian College of Children and Young People's Nurses
ACHS	Australian Council on Healthcare Standards
ACI	Agency for Clinical Innovation
ADHD	Attention Deficit Hyperactivity Disorder
AEDI	Australian Early Development Index
AFSNA	Australian Family Strengths Nursing Assessment
AHPRA	Australian Health Practitioner Regulation Agency
AHRC	Australian Human Rights Commission
AHRQ	Agency for Healthcare Research and Quality (US)
AIDA	Australian Indigenous Doctors' Association
AIFS	Australian Institute of Family Studies
AIHW	Australian Institute of Health and Welfare
AITSL	Australian Institute for Teaching and School Leadership
AMS	Aboriginal Medical Service
AN	Anorexia Nervosa
ANMF	Australian Nursing and Midwifery Federation
ANZCOR	Australian and New Zealand Committee on Resuscitation
AOM	acute otitis media
APA	American Psychiatric Association
APAGBI	Association of Paediatric Anaesthetists of Great Britain and Ireland
APREGN	Australian Paediatric Research Ethics and Governance Network
ARACY	Australian Research Alliance for Children & Youth
ARC	Australian Research Council
AVPU	alert, verbal, responding to pain or unconscious
AWCH	Association for the Wellbeing of Children in Healthcare
BFHI	Baby-Friendly Health Initiative
BiPAP	bilevel positive airway pressure
BMI	body mass index
BN	Bulimia Nervosa
BP	blood pressure
BZP	benzylpiperazine
CCHEWS	Cardiac Children's Hospital Early Warning Score
CD	Conduct Disorder
CDCP	Centers for Disease Control and Prevention
CEWT	Children's Early Warning Assessment Tool

CHA	Children's Hospitals Australasia
CHI	Children's Headline Indicators
CHQ	Children's Health Queensland
CIOMS	Council for International Organizations of Medical Sciences
CNC	clinical nurse consultant
CNS	central nervous system
COAG	Council of Australian Governments
CP	cerebral palsy
CPAP	continuous positive airway pressure
CPG	clinical practice guidelines
CT	computerised tomography
CTZ	chemoreceptor trigger zone
CVAD	central venous access device
CYFS	Child, Youth and Family Services
CYMC	Child and Youth Mortality Review Committee
DHB	District Health Board
DSM-5	Diagnostic and Statistical Manual of Mental Disorders, 5th edition
EBM	evidence-based medicine
EBP	evidence-based practice
EBPG	evidence-based practice guidelines
ED	emergence delirium
EPDS	Edinburgh Postnatal Depression Scale
EU	European Union
FLACC	Face Legs Arms Cry Consolability
FPS–R	Faces Pain Scale – Revised
GCS	Glasgow Coma Scale
GENCA	Gastroenterological Nurses College of Australia
GI	gastrointestinal
GRADE	Grading of Recommendations, Assessment, Development and Evaluations
HDEC	Health and Disability Ethics Committees
HFNC	high-flow nasal cannula
HIB	Haemophilus influenza type B
HIV	human immunodeficiency virus
HPS	Health Promoting Schools
HPE	Health and Physical Education
HPV	human papilloma virus
HRC	Health Research Council (NZ)
HREC	Human Research Ethics Committee
KTA	Knowledge to Action
LASC	Longitudinal Study of Australian Children
LMP	last menstrual period
LSIC	Longitudinal Study of Indigenous Children
MCEECDYA	Ministerial Council for Education, Early Childhood Development and Youth Affairs
MET	Medical Emergency Team

MMR	measles, mumps and rubella
MSD	Ministry of Social Development
MVA	motor vehicle accident
NACCHO	National Aboriginal Community Controlled Health Organisation
NASN	National Association of School Nurses
NEAC	National Ethics Advisory Committee
NHMRC	National Health and Medical Research Council
NICE	National Institute for Health and Care Excellence
NICU	neonatal intensive-care unit
NP	nasopharyngeal
NPMDC	National Perinatal Mortality Data Collection
NRS	numerical rating scores
NSAID	non-steroidal anti-inflammatory drug
NSCDC	National Scientific Council on the Developing Child
NYAS	National Youth Affairs Scheme
NZDPMC	New Zealand Department of the Prime Minister and Cabinet
NZHQSC	New Zealand Health Quality and Safety Commission
NZMHC	New Zealand Mental Health Commission
NZMoH	New Zealand Ministry of Health
NZMYD	New Zealand Ministry of Youth Development
NZNO	New Zealand Nurses Organisation
ODD	Oppositional Defiant Disorder
OECD	Organisation for Economic Cooperation and Development
ORT	oral rehydration therapy
PACU	post anaesthesia care unit
PARIHS	Promoting Action on Research Implementation in Health Services
PCA	patient-controlled analgesia
PEDS	Parents' Evaluation of Developmental Screening
PEWS	Paediatric Early Warning Score
PHAA	Public Health Association of Australia
PICU	paediatric intensive care unit
PKU	phenylketonuria
PREDIC	Paediatric Research in Emergency Departments International Collaborative
PSNZ	Paediatric Society of New Zealand
QFCC	Queensland Family and Child Commission
RACGP	Royal Australian College of General Practitioners
RACP	Royal Australasian College of Physicians
RANZCP	Royal Australian & New Zealand College of Psychiatrists
RSV	Respiratory Syncytial Virus
SCAN	Suspected Child Abuse and Neglect
SDQ	Strengths and Difficulties Questionnaire
SIDS	Sudden Infant Death Syndrome
SMA	Spinal Muscular Atrophy
SPOC	Standard Paediatric Observation Chart
SUDI	Sudden Unexpected Death in Infancy

UNOHCHR   United Nations Office of the High Commissioner of Human Rights
URTI   upper respiratory tract infection
VARK   visual, aural, read/write and kinaesthetic
VAS   visual analogue scales
VICTOR   Victorian Children's Tool for Observation and Response
WHO   World Health Organization
WMA   World Medical Assembly

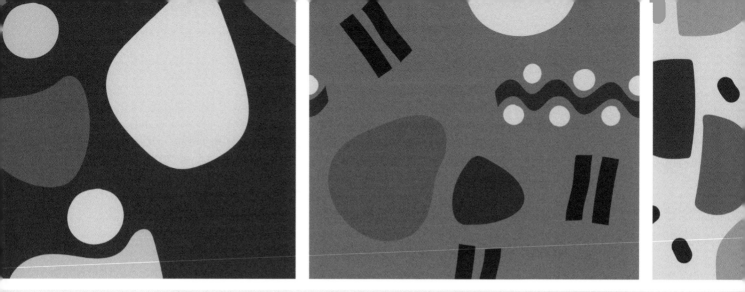

PART A

Contexts of nursing care

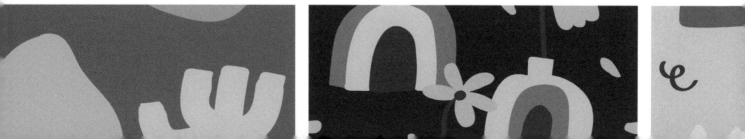

Children and young people of Australia and New Zealand

Donna Waters and Tara Flemington

LEARNING OBJECTIVES

In this chapter you will:

- Be introduced to some of the common measures used to monitor children and young people's health and wellbeing
- Gain an overview of the health and wellbeing of children and young people living in Australia and New Zealand
- Consider social and other determinants of optimal health and wellbeing for children and young people growing up in New Zealand and Australia
- Reflect on emerging health opportunities and challenges for children and young people and ways to work with children, young people and their families to promote their healthy future

Introduction

This introductory chapter examines the health and wellbeing of children and young people growing up in Australia and New Zealand. We will look at the population characteristics of future generations, facilitators and challenges to healthy growth and development, and emerging health and social trends. We invite you to consider the health and wellbeing of children and young people as situated within their individual developmental journey. Whether born in New Zealand or Australia, or arriving as a child or young person, growth will be nested within the social and cultural traditions of family during times of rapid social and environmental change.

As a health professional, accessing global, national and local reports on the health and wellbeing of children and young people enables you to gain an excellent overview of what it is like to grow up in New Zealand and Australia. In your role, you will be challenged to consider the social and other determinants contributing to the optimal health and wellbeing of the families with which you work. An important part of your role is to be informed about the ways in which you can work with children, young people and their families to promote their healthiest future.

We begin this chapter by reviewing some of the common demographic and statistical indicator measures used to monitor the health and wellbeing of children and young people across the world. Being aware of the many different ways that age and other measures are used to describe the health of children and young people can support our best use of the international evidence. We will then explore how these principles can be applied to key conditions and societal constructs relevant to the health and wellbeing of children and young people growing up in Australia and New Zealand.

Monitoring health and wellbeing

Government agencies in Australia and New Zealand routinely collect data on the health and wellbeing of their populations. The best known of these agencies are the Australian Bureau of Statistics (ABS) and Australian Institute of Health and Welfare (AIHW), Stats NZ (Tatauranga Aotearoa) and the New Zealand Ministry of Health (Manatu Hauora). In addition to conducting a national census of population and dwellings/housing every five years (since 1851 in New Zealand and 1911 in Australia), the ABS and Stats NZ collect a wide range of other demographic and statistical data to inform future planning.

Advances in data-capture technologies have enabled health agencies to significantly increase the accuracy and transparency of data recording. Accessibility to organised and standardised sets of health outcome measures, called health *indicators*, is now easier than ever. The use of common terminology and units of measurement enables consistent tracking of health indicators and the comparison of global data over time and between countries. However, it is important to be aware that the use of age and other descriptors to present data about children and young people is not entirely consistent. The ABS, for example, defines children as those aged under 15 years of age and young people as being 15–24 years of age. Legal adulthood is established at 18 years of age in Australia and 20 years in New Zealand.

In this chapter, we refer to infants, children, adolescents and young people approaching adulthood as collectively constituting the group defined as Australia and New Zealand's children and **young people**. We will use the age range 0–1 year to describe the period of **infancy**, 1–4 years as **early childhood**, 5–12 years as **childhood** and 13–18 years as **adolescence**.

Indicator measurement

The populations of New Zealand and Australia are fortunate to have full and free access to a range of excellent data on the past, current and future state of the health of children and young people. In addition to the routine collection of Australian and New Zealand health data, health indicators also enable us to compare the health and wellbeing of Australian and New Zealand children and young people with those of other children growing up in countries similar to ours.

For example, government health reports commonly compare statistics for Australia and New Zealand against those of countries who share membership of the **Organisation for Economic Cooperation and Development (OECD)**. Often, data for an individual country are compared against the combined or average indicator for all OECD countries.

As noted above, however, national indicator development is not perfect and is heavily influenced by the historical and societal contexts of governments and policy-makers. For example, the First Nations peoples of Australia and New Zealand hold broader definitions of health that refer to the community rather than the individual, and that include spiritual and cultural wellbeing (see Chapter 3). National indicators that do not reflect these broader definitions may therefore be contributing to an inequitable allocation of resources and increased disparities in health outcomes across groups.

There also remain large gaps in indicator measurement – both due to a lack of data and from a data quality perspective. In both New Zealand and Australia, there is either limited or no information collected about children with disability, children's cultural, racial and gender identities, or their interactions with the child health and justice systems (AIHW, 2020a; NZDPMC, 2019). These gaps contribute to biases in indicator measurement.

With these important limitations in mind, standardised internationally recognised indicators of health and wellbeing can:

- offer a snapshot of the health of a community or group at a single point in time
- enable long-term tracking of the health of specific populations or groups
- monitor upward and/or downward movements or trends over time
- measure the impact of specific health interventions such as health-promotion strategies
- use past information to predict (or model) what might happen in the future
- facilitate international comparisons (benchmarking).

While **rate**-based statistics are commonly used to describe population-level data, various *clinical indicators* are also used in Australian and New Zealand healthcare

Young people (or youth) – People aged 15–24 years.

Infancy – The period from birth to 1 year of age.

Early childhood – The period from 1 year to the fifth birthday.

Childhood – The period from 5 years to the 13th birthday.

Adolescence – The period from 13 to 18 years of age.

Organisation for Economic Cooperation and Development (OECD) – A group of member countries that for the past 50 years have shared the mission of improving the economic and social wellbeing of people around the world. Starting with developed countries in Europe, the United States and Canada, there are now 37 member countries spanning the globe, including Australia and New Zealand. Various common indicators are collected across the OECD countries.

Rates – Describe health trends over time – for example, a mortality (or death rate) is often presented as the number of deaths per 1000 population and is a ratio measure of the number of deaths from a particular cause (the numerator) presented as a proportion of all deaths from any cause (the denominator) over a defined period of time (usually one year).

settings to measure trends and variations in the quality and safety of healthcare (ACHS, 2019).

Table 1.1 defines some common key indicator measures (sometimes called *head-line indicators*) for the health, development, wellbeing and welfare of children and young people around the world.

Table 1.1   Example of national health indicators for children and young people

Outcome	Indicator	How it is measured (per year)
Mortality	Infant mortality: Number of deaths of infants less than 1 year of age in a given year	Rate per 1000 live births
	Sudden Unexpected Death in Infancy (SUDI) including Sudden Infant Death Syndrome (SIDS)	Rate per 100 000 live births
	Death rate for children 1–14 years	Rate per 100 000 children
Morbidity	Proportion of all children (0–14 years) diagnosed with asthma	Percentage of all children with asthma 0–14 years
	New cases of type 1 diabetes among children 0–14 years	Rate per 100 000 children
	New cases of cancer among children 0–14 years	Rate per 100 000 children
Disability	Proportion of children aged 0–14 years with severe or profound core activity limitations	Percentage of all children 0–14 years
Injuries	Age-specific death rates from all injuries for children 0–14 years	Rate per 100 000 children
Overweight and obesity	Proportion of children whose BMI is above international cut-off point for 'overweight' or 'obese', adjusted for age and sex	Percentage of all children in population of interest

Source: Adapted from AIHW (2017) and Craig, Jackson & Han (2007).

Note that this table illustrates further examples of how different definitions and descriptors are used for reporting on health trends within age groups. Indicator reports will generally outline the following: a rationale for the choice of a unit of measurement (for example, average over one year); definitions of numerators and denominators for rate-based calculations; and reporting of centiles, summary statistics (mean and median) and measures of spread or variation (standard deviation) to facilitate comparison with other data.

It is also important to note that different health indicators are important at different stages of the lifespan. For example, infant mortality (see Table 1.1) is an internationally recognised indicator of health and wellbeing in infancy. This is because a child's risk of death is greatest at the time of birth and during the first year of life (AIHW, 2020a) usually relates to outcomes from perinatal conditions and congenital anomalies. Similarly, birth weight, breastfeeding and immunisation rates are indicators of a healthy early childhood (0–4 years).

As children grow, injury and chronic diseases pose more serious risks, and as children enter adolescence (13–18 years), indicators of mental and physical health are likely to include overweight and obesity, sleep disorders and/or mental health problems (AIHW, 2020a; NZMoH, 2019a).

CASE STUDY 1.1 INJURY PREVENTION: THE VALUE OF MONITORING AND SURVEILLANCE

Childhood injury is a leading cause of death and hospitalisation across the globe. In Australia and New Zealand, injury prevention has been a key public health priority since the 1980s, with successful prevention campaigns that include mass marketing – such as Red Nose Day for Sudden Unexpected Deaths in Infancy (SUDI) – product regulations – such as product safety standards (e.g. household cots; children's toys) – and motor vehicle legislation regulating the use of seatbelts, car restraints and blood alcohol concentration. Despite this, child injury death rates in both Australia and New Zealand rank poorly when compared with other wealthy nations.

Successful injury prevention is grounded in rigorous monitoring and surveillance. Our lack of understanding of injury mechanisms and burden is inhibiting progress on reducing morbidity and mortality. For example, injury prevention and safety initiatives in Victoria, Australia are largely informed by detailed emergency presentation data in the Victorian Emergency Minimum Dataset. However, this dataset includes only children who are treated for injury at hospitals in larger metropolitan centres. This results in a surveillance deficit of up to 35 per cent in this cohort (Peck, Terry & Kloot, 2020).

The impact of research

In 2018, the first comprehensive longitudinal examination of child injury and survival in Australia was published. This nationwide data-linkage study found an age-standardised injury hospitalisation rate of 1489 per 100 000 population (95 per cent confidence interval 1485.3 to 1492.4), with no significant decreases over time. Hospital-related costs per annum totalled approximately A\$212 million, or A\$3119 per child. Fall-related and transport-related injuries were the most costly, and mortality risk was highest for younger children, children living in regional/remote Australia and those with a thorax or head injury (Mitchell, Curtis & Foster, 2018).

This seminal work led to the first National Strategy for Injury Prevention since 2014, and strengthened the case for the establishment of a national injury surveillance network. Evidence-informed national strategies drive consistent and collaborative approaches to public health and health promotion among and between state health departments, facilitate data linkage for monitoring and surveillance, and also facilitate prioritisation of research funding to reducing child injury.

Our children and young people

Following European colonisation, the previously thriving Indigenous populations of Australia and New Zealand declined significantly due to the impacts of racism, dispossession from lands and cultures, the Australian government policy of the Stolen Generations, and profound social and economic disadvantage and exclusion

(Duthie et al., 2019). The estimated New Zealand Māori population of 90 000 at the time of European contact in 1769 had fallen to 42 000 by the 1890s (Moewaka Barnes & McCreanor, 2019). In Australia, the estimated pre-colonisation population of 320 000 Aboriginal and Torres Strait Islander people had decreased to approximately 80 000 by the 1930s (AIHW, 2015).

Despite an increase in the overall number of children born in Australia and New Zealand after World War II, as well as high levels of migration of young couples with children, the proportion of children living in Australia decreased from 36 per cent of the total population in 1925 to 22 per cent in 1990. Another small increase in fertility was observed between the mid-1980s and mid-1990s, when the Baby Boomer generation reached child-bearing age. Since then, fertility rates have generally been below the level required to replace the Australian and New Zealand populations. As in many developed countries, recent population trends show the proportion of people aged 65 years and over to be increasing, with the proportion of Australian and New Zealand children projected to decline. We are yet to fully realise the impact of the recent global COVID-19 pandemic on population trends, but the effects of reduced migration are immediately apparent.

In 2018, 4.7 million children under 15 years of age lived in Australia, comprising 19 per cent of the total population (AIHW, 2020a). The total population of Aboriginal and Torres Strait Islander people was 798 400 (ABS, 2018), with Aboriginal and Torres Strait Islander children comprising 5.9 per cent of all Australian children (AIHW, 2020a).

In 2017, the 920 461 children under 15 years living in New Zealand made up a similar proportion of the total population, at 20 per cent (Duncanson et al., 2019a). Today, more than 740 000 Māori live in New Zealand (Stats NZ, 2018), and Māori children make up almost 30 per cent of all New Zealand children (Duncanson et al., 2019a). While the overall number of children and young people living in New Zealand is projected to stay relatively stable, a doubling of the number of people over 65 years of age, combined with fewer children being born, is expected to reduce the number of children as a proportion of the entire population (NZDPMC, 2019).

Health and wellbeing

Since the early 2000s, New Zealand and Australia have conducted detailed longitudinal cohort studies of their children and young people as they grow. These are respectively called *Growing Up in New Zealand* (University of Auckland, n.d.) and *Growing Up in Australia* (ADSS, n.d.). Such studies are extremely important for health and social policy setting, and for identifying opportunities for early intervention and health promotion. While Australian and New Zealand children are generally healthy and well, health indicators continue to demonstrate large variations between children living in remote and metropolitan areas, between Indigenous and non-Indigenous children, and between regions classified by social and economic advantage and those experiencing disadvantage.

Many other sources of indicator data are available. For example, the AIHW *Australia's Children* report (AIHW, 2020a) describes results for 12 indicators of health and wellbeing for children aged 0–12 years. The AIHW and the New Zealand Child and Youth Epidemiology Service (Te Ratonga Matai Tahumaero Taitamariki o Aotearoa) also offer dynamic online tools for viewing headline indicators by demographic characteristics such as age, cultural background and family type. The New Zealand Child and Youth Epidemiology Service report *Health and Wellbeing of Under-15 Year Olds in Aotearoa 2018* also summarises routinely collected national indicators of health and wellbeing for children and young people living in New Zealand (Duncanson et al., 2019a). However, as we have previously cautioned, it is important to look at the characteristics of groups included in each data set before attempting to compare indicator results across groups, and to regularly review government reports that are continuously updated. For example, 'children' have variously been defined as those aged 0–20 years (AIHW, 2008); 0–14 years (AIHW, 2012); and 0–5 years of age (Duncanson et al., 2019b).

Chronic conditions

Australian and New Zealand governments identify a range of health conditions and priorities that are of specific relevance to their populations because of the **burden** these conditions place on the daily lives of families and communities, and their potential impact on the economic sustainability of the country (NZ Government, 2016; Parliament of Australia, 2000). In particular, chronic ill-health in childhood has the potential to interrupt expected growth and development, and to generate immediate and possible long-term effects on physical, emotional and social wellbeing. The consequences of chronic illness and the effects of treatment are frequently overlooked in children and young people.

Considering that 43 per cent of Australia's and New Zealand's children and young people (0–15 years of age) were experiencing at least one long-term (non-communicable) condition as they approached adult life during the last decade, you can see why the management of **chronic conditions** of childhood is an important determinant of a healthy adult future (AIHW, 2020a; NZMoH, 2020).

The *Australia's Children* report (AIHW, 2020a) identified that up to 14 years of age, the four leading chronic conditions burdening the lives of children in Australia are asthma, hay fever/allergy, anxiety-related conditions and problems with psychological development. Mental health and asthma are two of the nine National Health Priority Areas for Australia – the others being cancer control, cardiovascular health, injury prevention and control, diabetes, arthritis and musculoskeletal conditions, obesity and dementia (AIHW, 2018a).

Interestingly, the fifth most commonly reported condition of Australian children, as measured by a 350 per cent increase in hospital admissions between 1994 and 2005, was food allergy or food-related immune disorders (AIHW, 2020a). Hospitalisation rates (or **hospital separation rates**) are often used to indicate the burden of illness experienced by children and young people with a chronic condition.

The leading causes of health loss from chronic conditions in New Zealand children are similar. The *Longer, Healthier Lives* report (NZMoH, 2020) identifies the main contributor to health loss in infancy as neonatal conditions and birth defects. Up to 15 years of age, the four leading chronic conditions impacting young people's lives in New Zealand are asthma, dermatitis, injury (mostly from falls) and anxiety disorders.

Burden – The impact of disease, illness or injury on a population. Measured by estimating years of life lost due to living with chronic ill-health and injury or dying prematurely.

Chronic condition – Any ongoing physical or mental impairment that causes a functional limitation (or health burden) or necessitates the use of a service or care beyond that which is regarded as routine. A chronic condition is usually defined as one that has lasted, or will last, for six months or more. Chronic conditions are also described as non-communicable diseases – to differentiate them from short-term communicable conditions such as infections.

Hospital separation rate – An episode of care in a hospital – usually the period from admission to discharge (by transfer or death).

The longer-term consequences of neonatal conditions on health and wellbeing are also among the leading causes of burden (NZMoH, 2020). In both countries, the burden of illness is higher for males than for females.

Whereas Australia has specified the prevention of certain diseases and conditions through national health priorities, New Zealand's health and disability strategy (NZ Government, 2016) takes a very different approach. This focuses on five interconnected priority areas for person-centred, smarter and more efficient systems that enable integrated care for health service delivery closer to home. While every health priority is relevant to the current and future lives of children and young people, increasing physical activity, improving nutrition and oral health, reducing violence in families and communities and ensuring access to appropriate child health services are of direct and immediate importance as determinants of a healthy future.

REFLECTION POINTS 1.1

- While many internationally accepted indicators are used to measure health and wellbeing in infants, children and young people, many indicators remain non-evidence based, non-standardised and inherently biased. What effects do you think international and national variances in indicator measurement and reporting might produce and how might these be improved?
- Thirty per cent of Australians and 27 per cent of New Zealanders are born overseas. What was your experience like growing up in Australia or New Zealand? What was your experience if you moved to Australia or New Zealand as a child? What are some of the benefits of working as a paediatric nurse in a culturally and linguistically diverse country?
- The monitoring of hospitalisation rates determines future health service planning needs such as projecting training numbers for specialists in nursing, allied health, medicine and surgery; estimating demand for hospital, operating and intensive care beds; and growth for primary health, virtual health and home care. Where do you see digital and virtual solutions being of most value in planning healthcare and services for children and young people?

Healthy development

The economic and social circumstances of the families and communities in which children and young people grow up are important determinants of their future health. Access to clean water, healthy food, education, an inclusive social environment and family financial and housing security are important determinants of successful physical and mental growth and healthy development. Childhood safety and security (including protection from injury, child abuse and neglect, and children as victims of violence and crime) sit alongside education as equally important determinants. Access to early childhood education, literacy and numeracy rates, and youth participation in university education or work are indicators of wellbeing for children and young people.

Children's mental and physical growth and development are constantly challenged by transitions that occur both within their family and community, and through increasingly broader engagement with their social world through school, sport and social activities – including social media. Indeed, challenge and change are important for transcending many of the normal developmental stages of personhood.

Within this section we will look at some of the common health opportunities and challenges presented to children and young people as they grow, and some emerging priorities for their health and wellbeing into the future. We continue to emphasise the importance of accessing the most relevant and recent national data sets, supported by evidence from systematic reviews and primary research. These sources offer health professionals the tools they need to deliver holistic person- and-family-centred care. However, as we have highlighted previously, it is important to remain aware that, currently, health indicator measures and other data presented in these reports are often not standardised.

Homes and families

New Zealand and Australia use slightly different definitions of 'family' and 'household' within their national censuses; however, both broadly determine that a family is a group of two or more persons living in the same household. As discussed above, it is important to consider how the indicator is measured. For example, some definitions of family exclude parents and children who live in different households, and there is also a distinction between dependant and non-dependant children. The ABS (2016) defines a child within a family as being less than 15 years of age, whereas Stats NZ specifies that a child living in a family can be of any age (Stats NZ, 2020).

A recent report on the family structure and wellbeing of *tamariki Māori* (Māori children and youth) reinforces the strong evidence for families as important determinants of children's health and wellbeing, and the role of families in reducing the transmission of intergenerational trauma and inequities (NZMoSD, 2020a). A range of publications from the Longitudinal Study of Australian Children: Growing Up in Australia project also confirm the important role of family in supporting warm and consistent parenting and a safe home environment for the social and emotional development and wellbeing of children and young people (ADSS, n.d.; Rioseco, Warren & Daraganova, 2020).

You can search more recent data from the 2018 NZ Census of Population and Dwelling; however, the 2013 census shows that the proportion of couple-families and one-parent families had remained relatively stable since the previous New Zealand census in 2006. In 2013, 78.4 per cent of families included at least one dependant child (under the age of 18 years and not employed full time). The average household size of 2.7 people had also not changed since 2006 (Stats NZ, 2014a).

The Australian Institute of Family Studies' *Families Then and Now* series (AIFS, 2020a) has been reporting demographic changes in Australian families since 1980. In 2016, 37 per cent of couple-families had children living at home (AIFS, 2020b). Some of the more significant trends in Australia have been an increase in multicultural households, a decline in couple-families with children and an increase in one-parent families – contributing to an overall reduction in family size over time (the average family was 4.5 people in 1911 and 2.6 in 2016). The majority of Australians are highly satisfied with their family relationships, and satisfaction with relationships with children was the highest (expressed by 82 per cent of parents) (AIFS, 2020c).

Mothers and babies

Parental health and wellbeing are important to establishing a supportive family environment for the developing foetus and growing infant. For example, a mother with healthy eating habits who maintains a healthy weight during pregnancy and is able to breastfeed her infant can reduce her child's lifetime risk of obesity (NZMoH, 2017a). It is also important to acknowledge that patterns for healthy eating are laid down from the very beginnings of life.

According to the *World Data Atlas* (Knoema, n.d.), if you were born after 2018, you were one of 12.7 (Australian) and 12.5 (New Zealand) births per 1000 people. With few **neonatal** deaths per year (2.3 per 1000 in Australia and 2.7 per 1000 live births in New Zealand), and a stable maternal mortality rate of six (Australia) and nine (NZ) deaths per 100 000 per year, it is expected that, in the majority, you will have access to nutritious food, will grow steadily, will be healthy, will attend school and will live a long life (an average of 82.7 years in Australia and 81.9 years in New Zealand).

Neonatal – The period from birth to 28 days of age.

Living in a culturally diverse, stable and democratic society, you will be contributing to an annual population growth rate of 1.5 per cent in Australia and 1 per cent in New Zealand. Further, as a baby born in Australia or New Zealand, the following trends are likely to be the case (AIHW, 2020b; NZMoH, 2019c):

- Around 40 per cent of mothers were within a healthy weight range at their first antenatal visit, and a further one-quarter (New Zealand) or one-fifth (Australia) were classified as having a body weight in the obese range.
- In New Zealand, 87 per cent of you and your mothers would have received care from a midwife throughout the ante- and post-natal period.
- Your mother was around 30 years of age when you were born and for 40 per cent, you were her first baby.
- More than half of all babies born in New Zealand and around 20 per cent of those born in Australia were born to mothers living in areas classified as socioeconomically deprived.
- You were delivered vaginally in a hospital following a spontaneous labour, although 26 per cent (New Zealand) and 35 per cent (Australia) of babies were born following a caesarean section.
- You weighed an average of 3.3–3.4 kilograms at birth, although 6.7 per cent (Australia) and 6.1 per cent (New Zealand) of babies weighed less than 2500 grams and were considered to be of low birth weight.
- More than 80 per cent of you were exclusively breastfed at two weeks after birth. In Australia, this is measured again at 4 months of age, when 57 per cent of you were still being exclusively breastfed.
- You were one of the 94 per cent (Australian) and 93 per cent of New Zealand infants fully immunised at 1 year of age.

Interestingly, rates of stillbirth in Australia and New Zealand remain among the highest reported for high-income countries. Also called foetal or perinatal death, stillbirth accounts for more than half of all perinatal deaths in Australia (AIHW, 2019b). Defined as the birth of a baby without signs of life after 20 weeks' gestation, gestational age and birth weight remain the most common predictors of a stillbirth (others are perinatal complications related to the mother, the placenta, cord or membranes). Each year more than 2200 Australian and almost 300 New Zealand families will experience a stillbirth (AIHW, 2019b; NZHQSC, 2019). Congenital anomalies and malformations remain the second most common cause of perinatal death for Australian and New Zealand babies (AIHW, 2020b; NZMoH, 2019b).

Infants

As defined above, infancy is the period from birth to 1 year of age. A number of factors have contributed to Australia and New Zealand's progress in significantly reducing infant mortality, particularly over the past 30 years. These include improved effectiveness of and participation in maternal antenatal care, better nutrition, public education for safe infant sleeping and the advantageous economic and environmental climate enjoyed by the majority of Australians and New Zealanders. In 2018, infant mortality was 3.1 per 1000 live births in Australia and 3.8 per 1000 live births in New Zealand (OECD, 2020).

More than two-thirds of infant deaths in Australia and New Zealand occur during the neonatal period, the first 28 days after birth, and almost half of these occur on the day the baby is born. The AIHW has established a separate National Perinatal Mortality Data Collection (NPMDC) to capture complete information on these deaths. However, it is important to note that stillbirth and **neonatal death**, as defined by the NPMDC differs from standard definitions used by the World Health Organization (WHO) for international comparisons.

Neonatal death – Death of a liveborn baby less than 28 days, of at least 400 grams birth weight and at least 20 weeks' duration (AIHW, 2020c).

Infant mortality rates are strongly associated with economic advantage and vary across populations. For example, in remote and very remote areas of Australia, the infant mortality rate of 5.9 per 1000 live births is almost twice that of babies born in major cities. In 2017, infant mortality was 4.2 per 1000 in the lower socioeconomic areas of Australia, compared with 2.3 in those areas designated by the ABS as of higher socioeconomic wealth. While death rates for Aboriginal and Torres Strait Islander infants have decreased by 14 per cent over the past 10 years (to 6.2 deaths per 1000 live births in 2017), the priority target set by the Council of Australian Governments (COAG) to halve the death rate between Indigenous and non-Indigenous children (0–4 years of age) by 2018 was not met (AIHW, 2020a). A comparison of infant mortality in OECD countries in 2019 (OECD, 2020) revealed that infant mortality was highest in India (29.9 deaths per 1000 live births) and lowest in Estonia (1.6 deaths per 1000 live births), with Australian and New Zealand infant mortality rates equivalent to the OECD average.

Neonatal intensive-care units (NICUs), with their associated specialised technology and staff, combined with improved communications and emergency flight retrieval systems, have contributed significantly to reducing neonatal deaths. Beyond birth, increasing awareness of national immunisation schedules and prevention strategies to reduce the risk of Sudden Unexpected Death in Infancy (SUDI) and Sudden Infant Death Syndrome (SIDS) through national health-promotion campaigns has contributed to reductions in vaccine-preventable diseases in infants and reduced the rate of sudden and unexpected death in infants less than 1 year of age during sleep.

Rates for SUDI and SIDS continue to decline. In New Zealand, SUDI declined from 1.4 per 1000 live births in 2000, to 0.7 per 1000 live births in 2016, although rates for babies in Māori and Pacific Islander families remain higher than those for babies born into Asian, European and other ethnic families living in New Zealand (NZMoH, 2019b). In Australia, SIDS accounted for 3 per cent of all infant deaths in 2017 – declining from 28 per 100 000 live births in 2007 to 6 per 100 000 in 2017 (AIHW, 2020a). However, rates for SUDI/SIDS remain higher for babies born to younger mothers (less than 25 years), within families from areas of deprivation and for babies born earlier than 36 weeks' gestation and of lower birth weight.

The most common non-life-threatening congenital anomaly presenting at birth is hypospadias (a defect of the male urethra) (Abeywardana & Sullivan, 2008). Conditions of the heart and circulatory system are also common (9 per 1000 live births) and are more likely to cause death. Congenital heart disease accounted for 6.9 per cent of all infant deaths in 2017 (AIHW, 2019a), but significant advances in paediatric cardiac surgery have led to many more infants living into adulthood with congenital heart conditions. Since the mandatory introduction of folic acid fortification in bread and cereals in Australia in 2009 (AIHW, 2016), congenital neural tube defects such as anencephaly and spina bifida have decreased by 14.4 per cent.

Children

Despite being relatively safe, economically wealthy countries, Australia and New Zealand ranked poorly (32nd and 34th, respectively) on the most recent global comparison of children's health, education and social outcomes across 41 high-income countries of the OECD and European Union (EU). The *Worlds of Influence* report (UNICEF Innocenti, 2020) identifies that nearly half of the 41 wealthy countries included in the report recorded more than one in five children living in poverty. Bullying by peers is also reported as a serious problem, with many children living in high-income countries identifying a lack of opportunity to be part of decision-making at home and at school.

In New Zealand and Australia, injury and chronic conditions – including asthma and allergies, obesity and neurological diseases – pose the most serious health risks to children. However, different risks are present at different ages. The death rate for children aged 1–4 years remains almost twice that of older children due to higher rates of serious injury and **comorbidities** associated with congenital conditions affecting this age group. Clearly, the above report also raises questions about how well we are doing with supporting **mental wellbeing**, health and life satisfaction among our children.

Comorbidity – The presence of one or more additional disorders (or diseases) co-occurring with a primary disease or disorder.

Mental wellbeing – Not simply the absence of mental ill-health. Mental wellbeing encompasses a broad sense of positive functioning including feeling happy, feeling satisfied and flourishing in life (UNICEF Innocenti, 2020).

Childhood injury

Injuries not only contribute to mortality in children, but account for a significant number of admissions to hospital and longer-term effects on children's physical and emotional wellbeing. For example, in Australia, injuries were responsible for 563 deaths in children aged 0–14 years during 2015–17 (4.1 per 100 000 children). For infants, up to 30 per cent of traumatic injuries are inflicted (child physical abuse). For older children, the most common cause of death from injury is land transport accidents, followed by drowning and assault (homicide) (AIHW, 2020a). The next most common causes of death in Australian children were cancer and neurological conditions (AIHW, 2020a).

CASE STUDY 1.2 TECHNOLOGY AND INNOVATION IN THE MANAGEMENT OF ASTHMA

Asthma is the leading chronic condition requiring paediatric healthcare in Australia and New Zealand, with around 10 per cent of children and adolescents diagnosed with this condition. For most, exacerbations can be controlled by following an individualised asthma action plan, which includes directions for preventer and reliever medication usage, and avoiding or controlling trigger factors. Poor treatment adherence can impact on symptom control, leading to an increase in hospital presentations and an impact on the child's activities of daily living and quality of life.

Adolescence is a period of development associated with increased participation in decision-making, including decisions about health. The child with asthma transitions from being a (largely) compliant recipient of medical care to an adolescent with ownership of self-management accompanied by caregiver support. Given the widespread use of smartphones among adolescents, mobile phone apps have become an important adjunct in supporting this transition.

A systematic review of eight studies assessed the 'feasibility and effectiveness of mobile phone apps in improving asthma self-management' and outcome measures among children and adolescents (Alquran et al., 2018). Apps have the potential functionalities of medication reminders, tracking symptoms and triggers, and sharing data with healthcare providers. Results found that such apps were very positively received by the adolescents using them, had high levels of participant satisfaction and were effective in improving asthma control and medication adherence (Alquran et al., 2018). While the small sample sizes in these studies limit the generalisability of findings, they do herald an exciting new era of mobilising technology for innovative approaches that engage with patients and improve health outcomes.

Leading causes of accidental death in New Zealand children (under 4 years of age) were suffocation (with possible associations to SUDI/SIDS) and drowning (Safekids, 2015). Older children are more likely to die from land transport accidents, including as cyclists. Higher injury death rates are also observed with geographical remoteness (in Australia), and between socioeconomic, ethnic and cultural groups. In New Zealand, hospital separations data indicate that nine in every 100 000 children under 14 years will suffer a fatal unintentional injury (Safekids, 2015).

As children move into adolescence, the variety and risks of injuries become greater as the propensity for developmental risk-taking behaviours increases. Falls, from playground equipment, skates, skis and skateboards, remain the most common reason for injury hospitalisations in Australia (1445 per 100 000 children in 2016–17) and in New Zealand (18 636 per 100 000 children in 2008–12). Injury rates are consistently 1.5 times higher in boys than girls.

Different reporting practices across jurisdictions make confirmation of childhood suicide rates difficult to interpret. *Australia's Children* (AIHW, 2020a) reports a suicide rate of 0.4 per 100 000 children under 14 years, with little change in this rate over the past 10 years. However, rates of intentional self-harm more than doubled between 2007–08 and 2012–13. In 2016–17, rates of self-harm in girls increased to 87.0 per 100 000 among those aged 0–14 years in Australia. In 2016, age-standardised rates for serious injury from self-harm in New Zealand (girls and boys) were 2.5 per 100 000 children aged 0–14 years (Stats NZ, 2019).

Chronic diseases of childhood

Around 7 per cent of Australian and 11 per cent of New Zealand children aged 0–14 years have a disability of some kind. Most commonly, these are intellectual or sensory, and speech deficits, leading to learning difficulties (AIHW, 2020a; Stats NZ, 2014b). Severe disability – defined as sometimes or always needing help with self-care, mobility or communication – is present in 4 per cent of Australian children in this age group. For almost half of all children living with a disability, this has resulted from a condition that existed at birth (Stats NZ, 2014b) – for example, congenital anomalies such as spina bifida and neural tube defects, cardiac conditions such as transposition of vessels, Tetralogy of Fallot and gastrointestinal, renal and limb deficits. Genetic conditions (trisomy 13, 18 and 21, phenylketonuria and cystic fibrosis) also constitute an important ongoing burden for Australia and New Zealand's children and young people, despite dramatic reductions in the incidence of these conditions through pre-natal and newborn screening.

Asthma and allergy-related disorders remain the most common chronic conditions affecting children in Australia and New Zealand, but chronic psychological and anxiety-related conditions are significant and emerging (AIHW, 2020a; NZMoH, 2020). Other emerging health issues impacting on the complex interaction of factors contributing to children's overall wellbeing are obesity and poor sleep quality. For example, while energy intake (from food) is a key factor in overweight and obesity, parental health and wellbeing, eating patterns laid down during infancy, socioeconomic, and cultural and environmental influences (such as the effects of climate change on our physical, social, economic and political world) all play a part. Physical activity is important for cognition, school performance and healthy growth and development. Physical activity is also inversely linked to screen use (electronic devices) and sleep quality. Similarly, childhood obesity is known to be associated with other chronic conditions of childhood, such as asthma, sleep apnoea, musculoskeletal and psychological problems – all with potential to contribute to higher risk of poor self-esteem and body image, anxiety and depression (NZMoH, 2017a).

Body mass index (BMI)–
Calculated as follows: BMI = weight in kilograms (kg) divided by the square of height in metres (m^2).

Body mass index (BMI) is the most common indicator measure of overweight or obesity. While BMI is not a direct measure like height or weight, international cut-off points based on age and sex are used to determine the number of children who are overweight or obese in any given population. BMI is also used to compare (benchmark) across child populations. As an indicator (but not a direct measure), the widespread use of BMI as a singular measure of overweight in childhood is of limited value. As such, health professionals should consider BMI as just one component of a comprehensive clinical assessment of a child's health and wellbeing.

The AIHW recently compared overweight and obesity between two birth cohorts (2007–08 and 2017–18). While more than 20 per cent of children aged 5–14 years were classified as **overweight** or **obese**, it appears that public health messaging about healthy food choices and physical activity may be reaching our families. The 5–14-year-olds were one of few age groups who were not significantly more likely to be overweight or obese than those born 10 years earlier (AIHW, 2020d). The *New Zealand Health Survey* conducted in 2018–19 (NZMoH, 2019a) found that approximately 11 per cent of children aged 2–14 years were obese, with no significant change since the previous 2011–12 survey.

There is considerable potential to reduce the adult health burden by preventing children from becoming overweight or obese, and the importance of establishing healthy eating, sleeping and exercise habits and behaviours in children should not be under-estimated. The New Zealand Ministry of Social Development (NZMoSD, 2020b) recently reported, for example, that up to 30 per cent of 2-year-olds and 20 per cent of 45-month-old children have a high probability of inappropriate sleep duration. Approximately half of these children will also have a high probability of ongoing compromised sleep quality.

Overweight – defined as a body mass index $\geq 25\,kg/m^2$.

Obesity – defined as a body mass index $\geq 30\,kg/m^2$. The World Health Organization identifies three categories of obesity with the most extreme (class III) describing a BMI of $\geq 40\,kg/m^2$.

CASE STUDY 1.3 WORKING WITH CHILDREN AND THEIR FAMILIES: WEIGHT AND BODY IMAGE

Claire is a 4-year-old girl admitted to the children's ward post-operatively following a tonsillectomy and adenoidectomy for obstructive sleep apnoea. During routine height and weight measurement, Claire's height is noted to be in the 50th percentile and weight above the 95th percentile for her age. The treating team uses the height and weight chart to initiate a conversation with Claire's parents about weight, nutrition and physical activity. Claire's parents seem relieved that the topic has been brought up and discuss their own concerns about Claire's physical and psychological wellbeing.

Early life overweight and obesity have a high likelihood of persisting into adulthood, and place children at greater risk of associated long-term health complications. However, disordered eating, depressive symptoms and body dissatisfaction have wide-ranging and serious health and psychological consequences, such as reduced self-esteem, depression, drug and alcohol use, unsafe sexual behaviours, earlier smoking onset, reduced physical activity, and overweight and obesity. This interconnectedness of body dissatisfaction, disordered eating and overweight highlights the value of a balanced public health approach that emphasises physical and mental health and wellness, rather than weight loss or muscle building (Bray et al., 2018).

Claire's discharge planning includes multidisciplinary referrals to the community child and family health nurse, the hospital dietitian and a children's healthy lifestyle program run by the local health promotion department. The family is also provided with health information that includes examples of supportive language and actions that can be taken by Claire's parents and older siblings, who can be key influencers of Claire's development of a positive body image and long-term wellbeing.

Social and emotional health in childhood

Social and emotional wellbeing refers to the way children feel about themselves and others, including how they adapt to and cope with daily challenges (resilience and coping skills). Social and emotional wellbeing is one of 19 Children's Headline Indicators (CHI) for Australia, focusing on the strengths of families and communities to positively influence the child's environment (AIHW, 2018b).

While yet to establish nationally reproducible indicators, data from the Young Minds Matter survey of 2013–14 suggested that difficulties with social and emotional health increase over time as children grow (Telethon Kids Institute, 2015). The Strengths and Difficulties Questionnaire (SDQ), answered by both parents and children, indicates that socioeconomic conditions and family composition (e.g. step- and blended families) are associated with higher rates of difficulty in children 4–12 years of age. Interestingly, overseas-born children have lower rates of difficulty with social and emotional wellbeing (6.2 per cent) than Australian children (11 per cent). It is disturbing that the *Australia's Children* report (AIHW, 2020a) identified around 19 000 children aged 0–14 years as being homeless on the night of the 2016 census.

REFLECTION POINTS 1.2

- The definitions of household and family are broad, and are unique to each individual. Think about your interactions with families. What have you learned from these interactions? How can you support families through stressful life events such as economic downturns and the effects of climate change?
- The proportion of children and young people in the Australian and New Zealand population is declining while the proportion of adults over 65 years is increasing. What impact might this have on future health funding? What are the physical, emotional and social implications for Australia's and New Zealand's children of the future?
- Consider disparities in the burden of illness among children from different cultural backgrounds and families. To what extent is equity, as opposed to equality, a critical factor in improving health outcomes?

Prevalence – A term used to describe the existence of a condition or problem in any defined sector of the population at any given point in time.

The *New Zealand Health Survey* uses the same questionnaire (SDQ) to measure children's social and emotional strengths and difficulties, with parental responses indicating that approximately 8 per cent of New Zealand children (3–14 years) have significant levels of difficulty (NZMoH, 2018). Similar to Australian children, emotional, peer and conduct difficulties are more likely in older primary and high school children in New Zealand. Socioeconomic factors, gender and culture are similarly indicators of the **prevalence** of difficulties (NZMoH, 2018). In general, however, children in Australia and New Zealand are doing well and growing up without substantial social, emotional and behavioural problems.

Based on 2017 population estimates, attention deficit hyperactivity disorder (ADHD) was the most common behavioural disorder experienced by 7.4 per cent of Australian children and adolescents (4–17 years), closely followed by anxiety disorders

(6.9 per cent). ADHD affects approximately 5 per cent of all New Zealand children (2–14 years). Four per cent of boys and 3 per cent of girls were diagnosed with anxiety disorder in New Zealand in 2019 (AIHW, 2020e; NZMoH, 2019d).

Young people

The independence of adolescence introduces a whole new set of opportunities and challenges for the health and wellbeing of young people aged 13–18 years. Physical and mental health are highly valued by young people (Carlisle et al., 2018) and are important for achieving educational and other outcomes supporting the transition to adult life. The AIHW *Health of Young People* report (following the United Nations) defines young people or youth as those aged 15–24 years (AIHW, 2020e). In 2019, there were an estimated 3.3 million young people living in Australia, representing 13 per cent of the total population. Data from the 2013 New Zealand census shows that those aged 15–24 years account for approximately 16 per cent of the total New Zealand population (Stats NZ, 2015).

The most serious health risks to the youth population are overweight and obesity, substance use, social and emotional wellbeing, and sexual and reproductive health; however, these risks rarely exist as single entities. The largest total health burden arises from suicide and self-harm (in males) and anxiety disorders (in females) (AIHW, 2020e; NZMoH, 2014). The UNICEF Innocenti (2020) *Worlds of Influence Report* states that suicide is the most common cause of death for those aged 15–19 years across all 41 countries included. The report quotes suicide rates for New Zealand at 14.9 per 100 000 and for Australia, 9.7 per 100 000 (based on a three-year average). Unintentional injuries from on- or off-road traffic or workplace accidents, and the harmful effects of substance use are the other main causes of death in young people (AIHW, 2020f).

As more is discovered about the important role of sleep for health, young people have emerged as a group of interest. While eight to 10 hours of sleep is recommended for adolescents (14–17 years), the *Growing Up in Australia* study reveals that up to 26 per cent of 14–15-year-olds and more than half of 16–17-year-olds are not meeting the recommended minimum on school nights (ADSS, n.d.). When asked, more than three-quarters of those not meeting recommended sleep guidelines felt they were getting enough sleep.

Sleep quality and quantity have been linked to both physical health (overweight and obesity) and mental wellbeing in young people. Of the 10 000 young people aged 12–17 years in the *Growing Up in Australia* cohort, those not meeting minimum sleep recommendations were more likely to report not being happy and to show signs of depression and anxiety (ADSS, n.d.). The profile of a young person who is not getting enough sleep (compared with national guidelines) is:

- more likely to be female and aged between 12 and 15 years of age
- more likely to be the youngest in the family
- less likely to have parents who regularly enforce sleep hygiene practices, such as a regular bedtime.

Delayed sleep onset and poor-quality sleep are also associated with the use of electronic devices, particularly when a child is able to access the internet in the bedroom (ADSS, n.d.). However, better access to quality health information through technology has been a positive development for improving health literacy among young people. As an example, the sixth National Survey of Australian Secondary School Students and Sexual Health (AIHW, 2020e) found that in 2018, 79 per cent of students had accessed the internet to find answers to questions relating to their sexual health. Young people are also having more conversations prior to engaging in sexual activity – either online or in person – about protecting their sexual health and avoiding pregnancy. Other positive developments in young people's health are that in Australia in 2017, 80 per cent of girls and 76 per cent of boys had received vaccination against the Human Papilloma Virus (HPV) before turning 15 years of age. Similarly, New Zealand has achieved 70 per cent HPV immunisation of those young people born before 2003 (NZMoH, 2017b).

Youth overweight and obesity

National health surveys identify rates of obesity among 15–24-year-olds living in New Zealand as 19 per cent in males and 22 per cent in females, for the years 2011–13 (NZMoH, 2015). In Australia, 47 per cent of males and 36 per cent of females aged 15–24 were overweight or obese in the 2017–18 ABS survey, accounting for 8.4 per cent of Australia's total (non-fatal) burden of disease (AIHW, 2020e). The significance of this health risk lies in established associations between being overweight or obese and increased risk of other diseases and chronic conditions, including poor self-esteem, sleep disturbances and obesity in adulthood.

Youth injury

The teenage years mark a point of transition from the injury patterns of childhood. In trying to adjust to individual variations in physical and emotional development, adolescents (13–18 years) are more likely to engage in risk-taking behaviours. The highest rates of serious, non-fatal injuries requiring hospitalisation among New Zealand 15–29-year-olds are the result of intentional self-harm (27.8 per 100 000) (Stats NZ, 2019). Similarly, Australian adolescents (15–17 years) have the highest rate of intentional self-harm in the Australian population (320 per 100 000) (AIHW, 2020e), with girls harming at more than four-times the rate of boys.

New risk exposures, such as driving and commencing work, are also now present. Australian males in the 18–24 years age group contributed more than 40 per cent of all male injury cases in 2011–12, with road transport and assault injuries being more common in this age group (Pointer, 2014). Serious injury during youth poses significant risk to future prospects for employment and quality of life, and may lead to permanent disability.

Youth substance use

The developing independence of the adolescent also coincides with a growing interest in experimentation and the opinions of peers, such as through Instagram followers. It is gratifying that rates of smoking have decreased among young people living in New Zealand and Australia; however, abuse of alcohol and other drugs continues to expose young people to health risks, including those related to injury and accident.

Results from the New Zealand Alcohol and Drug Use Survey were last published in 2010 (NZMoH, 2010). The report showed that young adults (16–24 years), were more likely to use recreational drugs than people of any other age. At this time in New Zealand, cannabis (14.6 per cent) and the party drug benzylpiperazine (BZP) (5.6 per cent) were the most commonly used recreational drugs in the previous 12 months; however, the past 10 years has seen a steady rise in the use of methamphetamines (MDMA or ecstasy).

The Australian National Drug Strategy Household Survey (AIHW, 2020g) reports that the proportion of 14–17-year-olds who were daily smokers had decreased from 11 per cent in 2001 to just 1.9 per cent in 2019. However, one in five current smokers in the 18–24 years age group has also tried e-cigarettes (or vapes) (AIHW, 2020g). High-risk alcohol use is relatively stable in Australia, with a trend for young people to consume alcohol in a less harmful manner; however, for the first time in 10 years, males in their twenties are reporting increased illicit drug use. This trend is largely driven by increases in cocaine and ecstasy use (AIHW, 2020g).

Youth social and emotional health

Maintaining the mental, social and emotional wellbeing of young people is a national priority for both Australia and New Zealand (ADH, 2020; NZDPMC, 2019); however, the process of conceptualising the multidimensional and complex nature of 'wellbeing' in order to define meaningful indicators remains a challenge. In the absence of agreed national indicators (and therefore data) on the social and emotional wellbeing of Australia's and New Zealand's children and young people, measures such as hospitalisation rates for mental ill-health offer a very poor estimate of prevalence.

The causes of mental and behavioural disorders in young people are complex and may be related to any combination of family, community, environmental, cultural, genetic, sexual or societal factors experienced by the young person over the course of their life. Other equally important – though perhaps less obvious – determinants of the mental health of Australia's and New Zealand's young people include health literacy, parental mental illness, school and peer stress and bullying, teenage pregnancy and birth, poverty, crime and the misuse of drugs and alcohol, including a range of increasingly sophisticated and easily available psychedelic and hallucinogenic agents.

The Australian Child and Adolescent Survey of Mental Health and Wellbeing – also known as the Young Minds Matter survey, as referred to earlier in the chapter (Telethon Kids Institute, 2015), was last conducted in 2013–14 and found that almost one in seven (14 per cent) of Australian 4–17-year-olds were assessed as having one or more mental disorders in the previous 12 months. Anxiety disorders were the most prevalent, but depending on how age and gender data are considered, ADHD or conduct disorders can be viewed as the most common. For example, ADHD is more common among young men (10 per cent in those aged 12–17 years), while anxiety or major depressive disorders are more common in young women (AIHW, 2020e). Disturbingly, the Young Minds Matter survey (Telethon Kids Institute, 2015) also reported that almost one-third of respondents diagnosed with a mental disorder had two or more conditions at the same time, equating to 4.2 per cent of all 4–17-year-old Australians. In essence, 14 per cent of 12–17-year-old Australians have experienced a mental health condition of some type (AIHW, 2020e).

CASE STUDY 1.4 SOCIAL MEDIA AS THE NEW FRONTIER OF GENDERED VIOLENCE

In one of the largest global studies of social media interaction, 14 071 young women across 22 countries participated in the Free to Be Online study (Plan International, 2020). The most common type of online violence experienced by survey respondents was abusive or insulting language (59 per cent). Deliberate embarrassment (41 per cent), threats of sexual violence (39 per cent) and body shaming (39 per cent) were also common.

Of 1000 young women aged 15–25 years living in Australia who took part in the survey, 99 per cent were social media users (Facebook, Instagram, WhatsApp, Snapchat, Twitter and TikTok), with 75 per cent describing themselves as frequent users. Two-thirds (65 per cent) of the young women surveyed in Australia had been exposed to some type of online bullying or violent interaction, with most having first experienced harassment on social media between the ages of 12 and 16 years. The most frequent perpetrators of online harassment were identified as people from school or work, but more than one-third also chose to remain anonymous online.

For almost 50 per cent of young Australian's identifying as LGBTIQ+, online harassment was directed towards their sexual or gender identity. Another 60 per cent reported online harassment targeting their cultural or ethnic background.

In total, 71 per cent of Australian respondents reported negative effects from being harassed on social media, including a lowering of self-esteem, mental or emotional distress and loss of confidence. One in five respondents experienced feeling physically unsafe. With half of all survey respondents (7000 young women across the world) reporting mental and emotional distress as a result of online threats, Plan International (a charity for girls' equality) proposes social media as the new 'frontier for gendered violence'.

The mental wellbeing of young New Zealanders presents a similar profile. In 2011, the New Zealand Mental Health Commission estimated that 29 per cent of young people (aged 16–24 years) had a mental disorder in the previous 12 months (NZMHC, 2011). Compared with adults (over 25 years of age), young people in New Zealand were more likely to demonstrate a higher 12-month prevalence of anxiety (17 per cent), mood (13 per cent) and substance use (9 per cent) disorders, including alcohol abuse and drug dependence. A survey of more than 9000 secondary school students in New Zealand in 2007 showed that approximately 11 per cent of students had mood disorders (depression or bipolar disorder), with young women (especially those aged between 14 and 16 years) being more than twice as likely as their male peers to have significant depressive symptoms for longer periods of time (NZMHC, 2011). The prevalence of anxiety disorder in this student cohort was around 3 per cent.

As we have already discussed, more males than females will die by suicide, but young women are more likely to be hospitalised for intentional self-harm. In 2016–17, hospitalisations for intentional self-harm by males aged 15–19 years was 180 per 100 000 population. At the same time, the rate of hospitalised injury for intentional self-harm by young women of the same age was 686 per 100 000 (AIHW, 2020e). In 2008, hospitalisation rates for intentional self-harm among 15–19-year-olds were significantly lower at 179 per 100 000 population for young women and 60 per 100 000 among young men (NZMHC, 2011).

More than 80 per cent of young people in New Zealand report interaction with a primary care provider – most commonly a general practitioner (GP) in the past 12 months, and in 2011, approximately 5 per cent of those aged 15–24 years reported seeing a psychologist, counsellor or social worker (NZMHC, 2011). Seventeen per cent of young people aged 4–17 years had accessed similar services in Australia (including those of a paediatrician) for emotional or behavioural problems in the previous 12 months (AIHW, 2020e). As we so often see, young people living in remote or disadvantaged areas, who are Indigenous or from non-dominant ethnic backgrounds, are less likely to access mental health services. Sometimes this is simply due to a lack of mental health services in their community.

REFLECTION POINTS 1.3

- Approximately one-quarter of children and young people in Australia and New Zealand are overweight or obese. The potential to intervene and prevent overweight or obesity is greatest in early childhood. Do you think current preventative health strategies in New Zealand and Australia are adequately addressing this potential for change?
- Serious intentional, non-fatal injury rates have risen steadily in young people over the past five years. What factors do you think may have contributed to this rise? What is the role of health professionals in reporting injury resulting from self-harm?
- The association between dental health and the development of future chronic disease is currently being investigated. What impact do you think ongoing disparities in dental health across Australia and New Zealand might have on the current and future health and wellbeing of children and young people?
- Upwards of 90 per cent of adolescents in Australia and New Zealand have their own smartphone or other device. To what extent might these devices and their associated applications be of benefit to young people's health and wellbeing? What are some potential negative implications?

More than 20 years ago, the New Zealand Ministry of Health established benchmarks to ensure access to public mental health services for at least 3 per cent of their population with serious mental health problems. This health initiative has seen more service delivered to the 15–19 years age group than any other age, and similarly, this age group has had the highest rate of access (NZMHC, 2011). The Australian survey of children and young people's mental health and wellbeing conducted in 2013–14

(Telethon Kids Institute, 2015) also showed that the proportion of youth accessing mental health services increased from one-third in the first survey in 1998 to two-thirds accessing health services in 2013.

Partnering with children and young people

In this chapter, we have taken a closer look at some of the many influences on the health and wellbeing of children and young people in Australia and New Zealand. We have encouraged you to think about the wider context of family and community, and other social, environmental and cultural influences experienced by children and young people as they grow. While there are many positives to growing up in comparatively wealthy countries like New Zealand and Australia, our countries do not present a 'level playing field' of opportunity for access to safe water, food, shelter and supportive healthcare.

Responsive and respectful practice in working with children and young people relies on an understanding of the impacts of social and environmental determinants on their health. We encourage you to read the following chapters of this book with this broader vision in mind, and to keep your understanding of the complex interactions that impact the lives of children and young people present in your work. Monitoring trends in health, estimating the effects of emerging infections or threats, and improving your knowledge of the many cultural, environmental or global factors that impact on your care of families, children and young people provide a context for practice that will not come from your reading of any single text, research paper or systematic review.

The governments of both Australia and New Zealand provide a range of excellent resources to help you keep track of the health and wellbeing of children and young people living in Australia and New Zealand. These publications should become as much a part of your evidence base for practice as any emerging research (see Further Reading section). However, as with all evidence, it is important to develop a critical lens for your reading of these frequently published reports. You need to remain aware of differences in units of measurement, age groups and denominators reported, and think carefully about the demographic characteristics of the groups you are aiming to compare. You have already seen in this chapter how many different age ranges are used to report on various health indicators and how the lack of quality data from sectors of the Australian and New Zealand populations can impact upon the integrity and accuracy of reported statistics. You may also have identified that significant inequalities within population groups can be masked by looking only at nationally aggregated population statistics and not at the specific sub-group or region in which children and young people live.

Throughout this text, we will refer to the global context in which Australian and New Zealand children and young people are growing up. The somewhat rosy social and economic pictures Australia and New Zealand present to the world will some-times conflict with the impoverished or disturbing history of the infant for whom you may be caring, the child or young person in detention or experiencing abuse, or the angry young person struggling to make sense of themselves and their place in the world. We already have evidence of our failure to maintain global wellbeing indices compared with other similar countries. Looking at 'the bigger picture' is something a health professional invited into the life of a child, young person and their family must be able to do. And, as in all nursing care, the person in front of you – no matter how young or how old – is only ever one part of a much larger story, which belongs only to them.

SUMMARY

- Australian and New Zealand government data collections are an extremely useful and important resource for recording and monitoring the demographic profile of children and young people living in Australia and New Zealand.
- Government data collections define a range of national indicators to describe the health and wellbeing of different age groups; they focus on a particular condition of interest and capture trends over periods of time. National health indicators are developed to be consistent with international indicators in order to facilitate benchmarking or comparisons.
- The health of Australia and New Zealand's children and young people is good overall, but there are differences within and between socioeconomic, geographic and cultural sub-populations. It is sometimes difficult to navigate the breadth and complexity of sub-population data to get a clear picture of what is happening to a particular group of children and young people living in a particular place at any point in time.
- Being overweight or obese, having suffered an injury – either as a congenital anomaly present at birth or by accident – and social and emotional wellbeing (of which mental health and wellbeing is a component) are responsible for the majority of the health burden experienced by Australia and New Zealand's children and young people.
- Asthma remains the most common chronic condition affecting children in Australia and New Zealand. Neurodevelopmental conditions (such as ADHD) have become increasingly more common, partly due to improved diagnostic and assessment techniques.
- Social and emotional health are related to many factors, including how the child or young person feels about themselves, which in turn may be related to their experiences of exercise, nutrition, sleep, peers, culture, intergenerational trauma and tolerance for risk-taking. Depression, anxiety, self-harm and suicide rates among Australian and New Zealand youth are rising. This is a result of a complex interplay of many social, emotional and environmental stressors.
- Current and past influences on the health and wellbeing of children and young people in Australia and New Zealand constitute a broad contextual framework. It is fundamental to the holistic and person-and-family-centred approach of the paediatric nurse to consider the complex interactions between these influences when caring for children, young people and their families.

LEARNING ACTIVITIES

1.1 Search the World Health Organization Statistical Information System (WHOSIS) website at www.who.int/whosis/en (data are also published in May each year in the *World Health Statistics Report*). Here you can search among more than 70 health indicators collected for WHO member countries. Answer the following questions:

- Choose two indicators measuring an aspect of health or wellbeing in children or youth. Describe three or more major differences between the results of these indicators in developed and developing countries.
- What have been some major successes or failures in terms of healthcare interventions for children and young people in these countries or regions – for example, child obesity strategies, immunisation?

1.2 Conduct an online search for reports or data that publish indicators of major health trends for the children and young people in your own health district or region. You may wish to limit your search to children or youth within a particular age range, or look for information about those with a specific health challenge. Answer the following questions:

- What upward or downward trends (if any) are identified in the health indicators of interest?
- Can you identify possible reasons for positive or negative trends emerging over the past five or 10 years?
- What level of data are reported – for example, death rates, specific diseases, age groups – and do these measures enable you to directly compare data over time?

FURTHER READING

The Australian and New Zealand governments provide a range of excellent resources to help you keep track of the health and wellbeing of their children, young people, families and communities. These are constantly updated and freely accessible through online searching. A range of useful resources can be found at:

- Australian Bureau of Statistics (ABS), www.abs.gov.au
- Australian Institute of Health and Welfare (AIHW), www.aihw.gov.au
- Australian Government Department of Health, www.health.gov.au
- New Zealand Ministry of Health, www.health.govt.nz
- Statistics New Zealand (Stats NZ), www.stats.govt.nz

REFERENCES

Abeywardana S & Sullivan EA 2008, *Congenital anomalies in Australia 2002–2003*, AIHW National Perinatal Statistics Unit, Sydney, viewed 27 September 2020, www.aihw .gov.au/getmedia/fe8e4da8-3983-4d1c-8af5-e0d9a3bef956/Congenital% 20anomalies%20in%20Australia%202002-2003.pdf.aspx?inline=true

Alquran A, Lambert KA, Farouque A, Holland A, Davies J, Lampugnani ER & Erbas B 2018, Smartphone applications for encouraging asthma self-management in adolescents:

A systematic review, *International Journal of Environmental Research and Public Health,* 15(11), p. 2403.

Australian Bureau of Statistics (ABS) 2016, *Census of population and housing: Census dictionary, Australia 2016*, cat. no. 2901.0, ABS, Canberra, viewed 23 September 2020, www.abs.gov.au/ausstats/abs@.nsf/Lookup/2901.0Chapter32102016#:~:text=A%20family%20is%20defined%20by,resident%20in%20the%20same%20household.

—— 2018, *Estimates of Aboriginal and Torres Strait Islander Australians*, ABS, Canberra, viewed 9 October 2020, www.abs.gov.au/statistics/people/aboriginal-and-torres-strait-islander-peoples/estimates-aboriginal-and-torres-strait-islander-australians/latest-release#data-download

Australian Council on Healthcare Standards (ACHS) 2019, *Australasian clinical indicator report: 2011–2018*, 20th ed., ACHS, Sydney.

Australian Department of Health (ADH) 2020, *National Action Plan for the Health of Children and Young People: 2020–2030,* viewed 16 January 2021, www1.health.gov.au/internet/main/publishing.nsf/Content/4815673E283EC1B6CA2584000082EA7D/$File/National%20Action%20Plan%20for%20the%20Health%20of%20Children%20and%20Young%20People.docx

Australian Department of Social Services (ADSS) n.d., in collaboration with the Australian Institute of Family Studies (AIFS) and Australian Bureau of Statistics (ABS). *Growing up in Australia: The longitudinal study of Australian children (LASC)*, viewed 12 September 2020, https://growingupinaustralia.gov.au/about-study

Australian Institute of Family Studies (AIFS) 2020a, *Families then and now*, AIFS, Canberra.

—— 2020b, *Families then and now: Households and families*, AIFS, Canberra, viewed 23 September 2020, https://aifs.gov.au/publications/households-and-families

—— 2020c, *Families then and now: Having children*, AIFS, Canberra, viewed 23 September 2020, https://aifs.gov.au/publications/having-children

Australian Institute of Health and Welfare (AIHW) 2008, *Making progress: The health, development and wellbeing of Australia's children and young people*, AIHW, Canberra, viewed 11 October 2020, www.aihw.gov.au/reports/children-youth/making-progress-the-health-development-and-wellb/contents/table-of-contents

—— 2012, *A picture of Australia's children 2012*, AIHW, Canberra, viewed 11 October 2020, www.aihw.gov.au/reports/children-youth/a-picture-of-australias-children-2012/contents/table-of-contents

—— 2015, *The health and welfare of Australia's Aboriginal and Torres Strait Islander peoples 2015*, AIHW, Canberra, viewed 11 October 2020, www.aihw.gov.au/reports/indigenous-health-welfare/indigenous-health-welfare-2015/contents/table-of-contents

—— 2016, *Monitoring the health impacts of mandatory folic acid and iodine fortification 2016*, AIHW, Canberra, viewed 11 October 2020, www.aihw.gov.au/reports/food-nutrition/monitoring-health-impacts-of-mandatory-folic-acid/contents/table-of-contents

—— 2017, *Key national indicators of children's health, development and wellbeing 2004 (updated 2017)*, AIHW, Canberra, viewed 8 October 2020, www.aihw.gov.au/reports/children-youth/indicators-childrens-health-development-wellbeing/contents/table-of-contents

—— 2018a, *Improving Australia's burden of disease*, AIHW, Canberra, viewed 11 October 2020, www.aihw.gov.au/getmedia/28c917f3-cb00-44dd-ba86-c13e764dea6b/Improving-Australia-s-burden-of-disease-9-01-2019.pdf.aspx

—— 2018b, *Children's Headline Indicators*. AIHW, Canberra, viewed 5 October 2020, www.aihw.gov.au/reports/children-youth/childrens-headline-indicators/contents/overview

—— 2019a, *Congenital heart disease in Australia*, AIHW, Canberra, viewed 12 September 2020, www.aihw.gov.au/reports/heart-stroke-vascular-diseases/congenital-heart-disease-in-australia/contents/summary

—— 2019b, *Stillbirths and neonatal deaths in Australia 2015 and 2016*, AIHW, Canberra, viewed 10 October 2020, www.aihw.gov.au/reports/mothers-babies/stillbirths-neonatal-deaths-australia-2015-2016/contents/overview-of-stillbirths-and-neonatal-deaths

—— 2020a, *Australia's children*, AIHW, Canberra, viewed 12 September 2020, www.aihw.gov.au/getmedia/6af928d6-692e-4449-b915-cf2ca946982f/aihw-cws-69-print-report.pdf.aspx?inline=true2019

—— 2020b, *Australia's mothers and babies*, AIHW, Canberra, viewed 12 September 2020, www.aihw.gov.au/reports/mothers-babies/australias-mothers-and-babies-2018-in-brief/contents/table-of-contents

—— 2020c, *National Perinatal Data Collection (NPDC)*, AIHW, Canberra, viewed 12 September 2020, www.aihw.gov.au/about-our-data/our-data-collections/national-perinatal-data-collection

—— 2020d, *Overweight and obesity in Australia: an updated birth cohort analysis*, AIHW, Canberra, viewed 4 October 2020, www.aihw.gov.au/reports/overweight-obesity/overweight-obesity-updated-birth-cohort-analysis/contents/differences-between-birth-cohorts

—— 2020e, *Health of young people*, AIHW, Canberra, viewed 5 October 2020, www.aihw.gov.au/reports/australias-health/health-of-young-people

—— 2020f, *Deaths in Australia*, AIHW, Canberra, viewed 5 October 2020, www.aihw.gov.au/reports/life-expectancy-death/deaths-in-australia/contents/leading-causes-of-death

—— 2020g, *National Drug Strategy Household Survey 2019*, AIHW, Canberra, viewed 5 October 2020, www.aihw.gov.au/reports/illicit-use-of-drugs/national-drug-strategy-household-survey-2019/contents/table-of-contents

Bray, I, Slater, A, Lewis-Smith, H, Bird, E & Sabev, A 2018, Promoting positive body image and tackling overweight/obesity in children and adolescents: A combined health psychology and public health approach, *Preventive Medicine,* 116, pp. 219–21.

Carlisle, E, Fildes, J, Hall, S, Hicking, V, Perrens, B & Plummer, J 2018, *Mission Australia's 2018 Youth Survey report*, Mission Australia, Sydney, viewed 11 October 2020, www.missionaustralia.com.au/publications/youth-survey/823-mission-australia-youth-survey-report-2018/file

Craig, E, Jackson, C & Han, DY for the NZCYES Steering Committee 2007, *Monitoring the health of New Zealand Children and Young People: Indicator handbook*, Paediatric Society of New Zealand, New Zealand Child and Youth Epidemiology Service, Auckland, viewed 8 October 2020, www.otago.ac.nz/nzcyes/otago086469.pdf

Duncanson, M, Oben, G, Adams, J, Richardson, G, Wicken, A & Pierson, M 2019a, *Health and wellbeing of under-15 year olds in Aotearoa 2018*, New Zealand Child and Youth Epidemiology Service, University of Otago, Dunedin, viewed 4 October 2020, www.otago.ac.nz/nzcyes

Duncanson, M, Oben, G, Adams, J, Wicken, A, Morris, S, Richardson, G & McGee, MA 2019b, *Health and wellbeing of under-five year olds in New Zealand 2017 (National)*, New Zealand Child and Youth Epidemiology Service, University of Otago, Dunedin, viewed 3 October 2020, http://hdl.handle.net/10523/8795

Duthie, D, Steinhauer, S, Twinn, C, Steinhauer, V & Lonne, B 2019, Understanding trauma and child maltreatment experienced in Indigenous communities, in B Lonne, D Scott, D Higgins & TI Herrenkohl (eds), *Re-visioning public health approaches for protecting children*, Springer, Cham, pp. 327–47.

Knoema, n.d., *World data atlas*, viewed 3 October 2020, https://knoema.com/ATLAS

Mitchell, RJ, Curtis, K & Foster, KA 2018, 10-year review of child injury hospitalisations, health outcomes and treatment costs in Australia, *Injury Prevention*, 24, pp. 344–50.

Moewaka Barnes, H & McCreanor, T 2019, Colonisation, *hauora* and *whenua* in Aotearoa, *Journal of the Royal Society of New Zealand*, 49, Supp 1, 19–33.

New Zealand Department of the Prime Minister and Cabinet (NZDPMC) 2019, *Child and youth wellbeing strategy*, NZDPMC, Wellington, viewed 11 September 2020, https://childyouthwellbeing.govt.nz/resources/child-and-youth-wellbeing-strategy

New Zealand Government 2016, *New Zealand Health Strategy: Future direction*, New Zealand Government, Wellington, viewed 20 September 2020, www.health.govt.nz/system/files/documents/publications/new-zealand-health-strategy-futuredirection-2016-apr16.pdf

New Zealand Health Quality and Safety Commission (NZHQSC) 2019, *Thirteenth annual report of the Perinatal and Maternal Mortality Review Committee*, Health Quality & Safety Commission, Wellington, viewed 10 October 2020, www.hqsc.govt.nz/our-programmes/mrc/pmmrc

New Zealand Mental Health Commission (NZMHC) 2011, *Child and youth mental health and addiction*, NZMHC, Wellington, viewed 10 October 2020, www.mentalhealth.org.nz/assets/ResourceFinder/Child-and-youth-mental-health-and-addiction-2011-MHC.pdf

New Zealand Ministry of Health (NZMoH) 2010, *Drug use in New Zealand: Key results of the 2007/08 New Zealand Alcohol and Drug Use Survey*, NZMoH, Wellington, viewed 20 September 2020, www.health.govt.nz/system/files/documents/publications/drug-use-in-nz-v2-jan2010.pdf

—— 2014, *Annual update of key results 2013/14: New Zealand Health Survey*, NZMoH, Wellington, viewed 12 September 2020, www.moh.govt.nz/notebook/nbbooks.nsf/0/997AF4E3AAE9A767CC257F4C007DDD84/$file/annual-update-key-results-nzhs-2013-14-dec14.pdf

—— 2015, *Understanding excess body weight: New Zealand Health Survey*, NZMoH, Wellington, viewed 4 October 2020, www.health.govt.nz/system/files/documents/publications/understanding-excess-body-weight-nzhs-apr15-v2.pdf

—— 2017a, *Children and young people living well and staying well: New Zealand Childhood Obesity Programme baseline report 2016/17*, NZMoH, Wellington, viewed 4 October 2020, www.health.govt.nz/system/files/documents/publications/children-young-people-living-well-staying-well-childhood-obesity-programme-baseline-report-2016-17-jun17.pdf

—— 2017b, *Final dose HPV immunisation coverage all district health boards*, NZMoH, Wellington, viewed 11 October 2020, www.health.govt.nz/system/files/documents/pages/hpv_-selected_cohorts_-all_dhbs_-31_dec_2017_0.pdf

—— 2018, *Social, emotional and behavioural difficulties in New Zealand children: Technical report*, NZMoH, Wellington, viewed 5 October 2020, www.health.govt.nz/system/files/documents/publications/social-emotional-behavioural-difficulties-nz-children-technical-report-may18.pdf

—— 2019a, *Annual update of key results 2018/19: New Zealand Health Survey*, NZMoH, Wellington, viewed 12 September 2020, www.health.govt.nz/publication/annual-update-key-results-2018-19-new-zealand-health-survey

—— 2019b, *Fetal and infant deaths 2016*, NZMoH, Wellington, viewed 27 September 2020, www.health.govt.nz/publication/fetal-and-infant-deaths-2016

—— 2019c, *Report on maternity 2017*, NZMoH, Wellington, viewed 12 September 2020, www.health.govt.nz/publication/report-maternity-2017

—— 2019d, *New Zealand Health Survey: Prevalence datasets 2019*, NZMoH, Wellington, viewed 10 October 2020, https://minhealthnz.shinyapps.io/nz-health-survey-2018-19-annual-data-explorer/_w_fca0c755/_w_8ba7f72d/#!/download-data-sets

—— 2020, *Longer, healthier lives: New Zealand's health 1990–2017*, NZMoH, Wellington, viewed 20 September 2020, www.health.govt.nz/system/files/documents/publications/longer-healthier-lives-new-zealands-health-1990-2017.pdf

New Zealand Ministry of Social Development (NZMoSD) 2020a, *Poipoia te kākano kia puawai Family structure, family change and the wellbeing of tamariki Māori*, NZMoH, Wellington, viewed 20 September 2020, www.msd.govt.nz/about-msd-and-our-work/publications-resources/research/family-structure-change-and-the-wellbeing-of-tamariki-maori/index.html

—— 2020b, *Are New Zealand children meeting the Ministry of Health guidelines for sleep?* NZMoH, Wellington, viewed 20 September 2020, www.msd.govt.nz/documents/about-msd-and-our-work/publications-resources/research/are-nz-children-meeting-the-moh-guidelines-for-sleep/are-nz-children-meeting-the-moh-guidelines-for-sleep-final-21august.pdf

Organisation for Economic Co-operation and Development (OECD) 2020, *Infant mortality rates (indicator)*, OECD, New York, viewed 27 September 2020, https://data.oecd.org/healthstat/infant-mortality-rates.htm

Parliament of Australia 2000, *The National Health Priority Areas Initiative.* Australian Parliamentary Library, Canberra, viewed 11 October 2020, www.aph.gov.au/About_Parliament/Parliamentary_Departments/Parliamentary_Library/Publications_Archive/CIB/cib9900/2000CIB18#...

Peck, B, Terry, DR & Kloot, K 2020, Understanding childhood injuries in rural areas: Using Rural Acute Hospital Data Register to address previous data deficiencies, *Emergency Medicine Australasia*, 32(4), pp. 646–9.

Plan International 2020, *Free to be online*, viewed 10 October 2020, www.plan.org.au/media-centre/social-media-new-frontier-for-gendered-violence-as

Pointer, S 2014, *Hospitalised injury in children and young people 2011–12*, AIHW, Canberra, viewed 6 October 2020, www.aihw.gov.au/getmedia/0bf3dcfe-f3b6-4857-9116-f28bfc2649c8/17903.pdf.aspx?inline=true

Rioseco, P, Warren, D & Daraganova, G 2020, *Children's social-emotional wellbeing: The role of parenting, parents' mental health and health behaviours*, AIFS, Canberra, viewed 23 September 2020, https://aifs.gov.au/sites/default/files/publication-documents/2003_childrens_social-emotional_wellbeing_paper.pdf

Safekids 2015, *Child unintentional deaths and injuries in New Zealand, and prevention strategies*, Safekids Aotearoa, Auckland, viewed 30 September 2020, www.moh

.govt.nz/notebook/nbbooks.nsf/0/05ED778EE1B2C6D6CC257F4C007A779C/$file/
Safekids%20Aotearoa%20Databook%20CIP%20NZ%20and%20Prevention%
20Strategies.pdf

Statistics New Zealand (Stats NZ) 2014a, *2013 Census QuickStats about families and
households*, Stats NZ Tatauranga Aotearoa, Wellington, viewed 23 September
2020, www.stats.govt.nz

—— 2014b, *2013 New Zealand Disability Survey*, Stats NZ Tatauranga Aotearoa,
Wellington, viewed 23 September 2020, http://archive.stats.govt.nz/browse_for_
stats/health/disabilities/other-versions-disability-survey-2013.aspx#gsc.tab=0

—— 2015, *2013 Census profile and summary reports*, Stats NZ Tatauranga Aotearoa,
Wellington, viewed 5 October 2020, http://archive.stats.govt.nz/Census/2013-
census/profile-and-summary-reports.aspx#gsc.tab=0

—— 2018, *Māori population estimates: At 30 June 2018*, Stats NZ Tatauranga Aotearoa,
Wellington, viewed 9 October 2020, www.stats.govt.nz/information-releases/
maori-population-estimates-at-30-june-2018#:~:text=At 30 June 2018%3A,males
and 381%2C000 Māori females

—— 2019, *Increase in life-threating injuries from self-harm*, Stats NZ Tatauranga Aotearoa,
Wellington, viewed 30 September 2020, www.stats.govt.nz/news/increase-in-life-
threatening-injuries-from-self-harm#:~:text=Serious%20non%2Dfatal%20injuries
%20from%20self%2Dharm%20in%202018%20occurred,people%2C%20from%
203.5%20in%202013.

—— 2020, *Families and households in the 2018 census: Data sources, family coding, and
data quality*, Stats NZ Tatauranga Aotearoa, Wellington, viewed 23 September
2020, www.stats.govt.nz

Telethon Kids Institute 2015, *Young Minds Matter: The second Australian Child and
Adolescent Survey of Mental Health and Wellbeing, survey user's guide*, Centre for
Child Health Research, University of Western Australia, Perth, viewed 11 October
2020, https://youngmindsmatter.telethonkids.org.au/siteassets/media-docs—
young-minds-matter/ymmoverview.pdf

UNICEF Innocenti 2020, *Worlds of Influence: Understanding what shapes child well-being
in rich countries*, Innocenti Report Card 16, UNICEF Office of Research, Florence,
viewed 29 September 2020, www.unicef.org.au/Upload/UNICEF/Media/
Documents/Innocenti-Report-Card-16-Worlds-of-Influence.pdf

University of Auckland n.d., *Growing up in New Zealand*, Auckland UniServices on behalf of
the NZMoSD, Auckland, viewed 12 September 2020, www.growingup.co.nz

2

Child rights in Australia and New Zealand

Jennifer Fraser and Helen Stasa

LEARNING OBJECTIVES

In this chapter you will:

- Become familiar with the United Nations Convention on the Rights of the Child
- Develop an understanding of how these rights translate into paediatric care settings through charters and standards for practice
- Develop an understanding of Australian and New Zealand age of majority legislation
- Learn about the particular health challenges facing vulnerable groups of children and young people and their families in Australia and New Zealand
- Consider your professional priorities in relation to children's rights and the duty to report child protection concerns to child protection authorities

Introduction

This chapter builds on the information in Chapter 1 about the context of paediatric nursing in Australia and New Zealand. It provides a basis for students of nursing to understand the ways in which the rights of children and young people are upheld in these two countries, particularly within the healthcare system. This extends to child protection, including nurses' legal and moral responsibility to report child abuse and neglect.

As a nurse working with children, young people and their parents, you will consider many important issues regarding their involvement as active participants in their healthcare decisions. In your practice, you will explain which treatments or interventions are necessary and decide whether the child or young person has the capacity to understand the importance and consequences of the choices that you make in collaboration with them and their family. Your assumptions about childhood and the role of parents, families and caregivers will underpin the way you approach the child or young person, and their family. These assumptions need to be evaluated critically. They demand scrutiny and review so you can provide the best possible care within a variety of contexts. This can sometimes be challenging. The power in the relationships between the child or young person, you and the family needs to be acknowledged and addressed.

The purpose of this chapter is to provide insight into the ways in which human rights, and particularly child rights, inform paediatric nursing policy and practice in both Australia and New Zealand. The chapter explains how current Australian and New Zealand legislation attempts to ensure that child rights are protected within healthcare systems, particularly for Māori and Aboriginal and Torres Strait Islander children and other vulnerable groups. It begins by looking at the international agreements and covenants regarding the protection of child rights that have been endorsed by Australia and New Zealand before moving on to examine the national legislation and the implications for health and social support systems. The second part of the chapter looks at some of the ethical challenges regarding child and family rights that you will have to consider as a paediatric nurse in Australia and New Zealand. In particular, we look at issues surrounding access to family, advocacy and consent to treatment of specific diseases in some situations. The chapter also provides a basis for understanding the ways in which children and young people's rights – including the right to be protected from all forms of violence and neglect – are upheld in Australia and New Zealand, particularly within the health and welfare systems.

REFLECTION POINTS 2.1

Rights are often discussed in law, philosophy and healthcare. They are based on shared values such as dignity, equality and respect. But what does it mean to 'have rights'?

- Can you think of some examples of rights? Why are they important? And how are they protected?

International convention

In November 1989, the United Nations Convention on the Rights of the Child (UN, 1989a) was drawn up to provide a reference for the way in which the dignity, wellbeing and human rights of children, young people and their families are respected globally.

The Convention sets out the standards of rights that are required to ensure that children and young people can live a minimally decent life. It was adopted by the United Nations in 1989 and then ratified in Australia in 1991 and New Zealand in 1993 (UN, 1989b). The convention does not just serve as a mechanism of protection for human rights; it also ensures the welfare status of the child. Children are also valued as individuals with human rights, and they are viewed as active participants in promoting and protecting their own rights – that is, they are not considered passive agents of human rights. The Convention is based around four general principles: non-discrimination; life, survival and development; the best interests of the child; and respect for the child's preferences and viewpoints. These underlie its specific Articles.

The role of the United Nations Committee on the Rights of the Child is to monitor the implementation of the Convention on the Rights of the Child. The UN Committee on the Rights of the Child meets to hear from governments, civil society organisations, and children and young people to consider the actions that are needed to uphold the rights that are enshrined in the Convention. The committee makes important recommendations (called 'concluding observations') to governments about what they need to do better for children and young people. In 2019, the committee noted its main concerns for Australian children. These were: (1) violence, including sexual violence, abuse and neglect; (2) children deprived of a family environment; (3) mental health; (4) the impact of climate change on child rights; (5) asylum-seeking, refugee and migrant children; and (f) administration of child justice (UN, 2019). Australia was urged to consider the extent to which children are included in the design and implementation of policies and programs aimed at achieving the 17 Sustainable Development Goals in relation to children and young people.

Regarding healthcare, the Convention explicitly states that the child 'shall be entitled to grow and develop in health … [and] shall have the right to adequate nutrition, housing, recreation and medical services' (UN, 1989b).

Other relevant international human rights laws applicable to the health of children and young people in the Australian and New Zealand context include Article 3 of the Universal Declaration of Human Rights, which states that 'everyone has a right to life' (and the treatment required to sustain life). Additionally, Article 12(1) of the UN International Covenant on Economic, Social and Cultural Rights recognises 'the right of everyone (of which children and young people are one group) to the enjoyment of the highest attainable standard of physical and mental health' (UN, 1966). This Article is especially notable, as it makes specific reference to the fact that health encompasses both physical and mental aspects, rather than just focusing on the physical aspects of health. Article 19 of the UN Convention on the Rights of the Child (UN, 1989a) expands upon this Covenant, and obligates state parties to take action and intervene to 'protect the child from all forms of physical and mental violence, injury or abuse, neglect or negligent treatment'. Australian and New Zealand children are legally protected from harm through a number of **child protection** Acts aimed at shielding them from abuse and neglect in all their forms. These vary between states and territories in Australia. Australia's *Family Law Act 1975* does serve to protect children and have decisions made in the child's best interests; however, child protection proceedings come under state and territory laws. This can become complicated in cases where there are child-protection concerns and parenting matters in the Family Court of Australia. In New Zealand, the *Children, Young Persons and Their Families Act 1989* (NZ) governs child protection. It is administered by the Ministry of Social Welfare (the Ministry).

The rights of the child or young person to make their own decisions about treatment or non-treatment are enshrined in Article 13(1), which provides:

> The child shall have the right to freedom of expression; this right shall include the freedom to seek, receive and impart information and ideas of all kinds, regardless of frontiers . . . (UN, 1989a)

Clearly, at younger ages and in cases of cognitive impairment, a child may not have formed considered preferences regarding their medical care. In such situations, the healthcare staff may need to rely on parents or caregivers to provide information about the child's treatment. However, in some situations the parents' preferences may conflict with what is thought to be in the best healthcare interests of the child. In such circumstances, nursing staff have an important role to play in advocating for the child and consulting with relevant experts to ensure that the child's rights are protected, while also acknowledging the rights of parents to have their views heard.

Child protection – Not limited to the prevention of physical and mental abuse; also includes the prevention and surmounting of disadvantageous conditions in children's lives. According to the Convention, these rights include, but are not limited to, the right to be protected from all kinds of abuse and discrimination (UNICEF, 2004).

REFLECTION POINTS 2.2

Moral and ethical nursing practice is based on an ethos of lawful scope of practice and ethical standards. We acknowledge Article 13(1) of the UN Convention on the Rights of the Child:

> The child shall have the right to freedom of expression; this right shall include the freedom to seek, receive and impart information and ideas of all kind. (UN, 1989a)

- List specific groups of children and young people within Australian and New Zealand society who you believe need special safeguarding and care, as well as legal protection.
- Identify ways in which Australian and New Zealand paediatric nurses can apply children's rights and healthcare decision-making frameworks, ethical decision-making and informed consent for two of these highly vulnerable groups.

Australian and New Zealand legislation, charters and standards

The Australian and New Zealand legislation surrounding the protection of **child rights** is based on the international charters outlined above. Implementation of international

Child rights – Political, economic, civil, cultural and social human rights are afforded to children with consideration for their vulnerability and potential for exploitation as they grow and develop. These rights are protected in Australian and New Zealand law.

rights of the child occurs through enacting child-specific treaties such as distinctive national policies, protocols and legislation.

Protecting children and their rights in the context of healthcare in Australian paediatric settings requires that the principles of family unity and kinship groups are recognised. This ensures that children and their families are not separated by hospital policy or discriminated against for any reason. Moreover, it ensures that they have access to appropriate services and service providers, and that children's agency is respected. One of the greatest challenges lies in developing and maintaining a model of care that is child focused and that prioritises children's inclusion. Children themselves must be at the forefront of stating how they wish to be cared for, and by whom (Coyne, Hallstrom & Soderback, 2016).

Key documents that take a human rights-based approach to the care of children and young people in the Australian healthcare system include:

- the *Charter on the Rights of Children and Young People in Healthcare Services in Australia* (CHA & AWCH, 2010)
- the *Standards for the Care of Children and Adolescents in Health Services* (RACP, 2008), and
- the *Standards of Practice for Children and Young People's Nurses* (ACCYPN, 2016).

First, *A Charter on the Rights of Children and Young People in Healthcare Services*, developed by Children's Hospitals Australasia (CHA) in collaboration with the Paediatric Society of New Zealand (PSNZ) and the Association for the Wellbeing of Children in Healthcare (AWCH), has both Australian (CHA & AWCH, 2010) and New Zealand (CHA & PSNZ, 2020) versions. These documents stipulate 11 key rights that children and young people have as healthcare consumers. These include the right to information in a form that is understandable to them and to participate in health decision-making; the right to privacy; the right to be kept safe from all forms of harm; and the right to continuity of care. The Charter specifically acknowledges some of the distinct challenges that both Aboriginal and Torres Strait Islander children and young people, and Māori children and young people (*tamariki* and *rangatahi*), may encounter when accessing healthcare services.

In Australia, a range of resources have been developed to promote the uptake of the charter, including child and youth-friendly posters and videos (AWCH, 2020). Second, the Royal Australasian College of Physicians (RACP) publishes *Standards for the Care of Children and Adolescents in Health Services* (RACP, 2008). The RACP document was developed with input from physicians from both Australia and New Zealand, and the same document is applicable to both countries. These articulate guidelines for high-quality healthcare that is safe and appropriate for the child or adolescent. The Standards aims 'to ensure that quality care is provided in an environment that is safe and appropriate for the age and stage of development of the child or adolescent' (2008, p. 3). The Standards emphasise that psychosocial and medical needs of children and young people differ greatly from those of adults, and state that it is important for health services to be designed to accommodate these diverse needs. The Standards aim to ensure that the rights of children and young people are respected, that the facilities in which they receive care are appropriate for their developmental age, and that specially qualified staff are responsible for their care. The Standards advocate for separate facilities for children and adolescents in all areas of the health service where they are cared for.

The third key Australian document related to the care of children and young people is a position statement entitled *Standards of Practice for Children and Young People's Nurses*, published by the Australian College of Children and Young People's Nurses (ACCYPN, 2016). This statement emphasises the engagement of all relevant stakeholders (such as the child or young person, their family, nursing and medical staff, allied health professionals and others) in the planning and delivery of care. It details the knowledge expected of nurses working with children and young people, and elucidates the expectations surrounding communication, family involvement and advocacy.

For nurses working in paediatric settings across Australia, these documents are important references for the provision of high-quality care that, together with the international documents (such as the UN Conventions), provide a mechanism for attempting to ensure that the rights of children, young people and their families are protected by the healthcare system.

In New Zealand, Kids Health – a joint initiative between the Starship Foundation and the Paediatric Society, funded by the Ministry of Health – has published *Principles Guiding Provision Of Health & Disability Services* (Kids Health, 2018). The principles are intended to outline how healthcare providers should meet the needs of children and young people, and their families at each stage of the wellness/illness journey. They emphasise, among other things, the importance of holistic, family-centred care, putting children's and young people's needs first, and the need for care to be culturally appropriate.

REFLECTION POINTS 2.3

- List ways in which nurses can protect children's rights in hospital. Identify potential barriers to such protection and consider how these barriers may be addressed.
- Talk to a child or young person about a recent experience of illness. How did they feel about the care they received? Did they receive information in a form that was understandable to them and did they participate in treatment decisions? Were they listened to by their parents/caregivers and health agency staff?

Practice implications

Having briefly outlined the key international and Australian and New Zealand national declarations regarding children, young people and their families, and their applicability to the healthcare setting, it is important to examine practical situations where, as a paediatric nurse, you may be required to make decisions that require a clear understanding of child rights and your associated responsibilities. In this section, we will examine some of the challenging situations that paediatric nurses may face regarding access to family, consent to treatment and advocacy for children at risk of abuse or neglect.

Access to family

Paediatric nursing care in Australia and New Zealand emphasises the importance of family-centred care. Family-centred care emerged as best practice in children's health settings due to widespread interest in patient advocacy, with hospital visiting rights for parents one outcome of the advocacy movement. Within paediatric healthcare settings, the term 'family-centred care' is used to describe an approach to nursing care that focuses on issues such the active involvement of parents in the care of the child; consideration of the child's perspectives and views; and increasing children's involvement in their treatment and decision-making about their treatment (Kuo et al., 2012). Family-centred care designed around 'kinship' is particularly important for children and young people who belong to the Aboriginal and Torres Strait Islander communities, while the notion of *whānau*-centred care, which focuses on the family and community context of care, is frequently mentioned in Māori health.

CASE STUDY 2.1 TIA

Tia Waaka is a 5-year-old girl living in Auckland, New Zealand, who comes from a Māori family. Tia arrives at the hospital emergency department in a state of semi-consciousness, accompanied by her parents, Tama and Aroha. Upon questioning, Tama notes that over the past few days, Tia has been extremely thirsty, has constantly asked to use the toilet and is always tired and irritable. The staff at the hospital run some tests and diagnose that Tia has type 1 diabetes.

Initially, the Waakas are referred to an endocrinologist and a diabetes educator for practical advice on managing Tia's condition. However, after the first two visits, Aroha calls the hospital and cancels all further appointments. She explains that the family is overwhelmed by the amount of information that they are receiving, that Tia is frightened by the atmosphere in the hospital and that she and her husband feel extremely stressed and isolated. In particular, Aroha notes that she feels helpless and detached from the decision-making process: 'I'm her mum, but it's like I don't matter at all,' she says.

Case study resolution

The hospital staff suggest that Tia and her family may benefit from visiting a Māori health centre, which takes a *whānau ora* approach. *Whānau ora* emphasises the importance of family, and aims to empower individuals within the community rather than the institutional context. The Waakas are referred to Mateo, a paediatric nurse practitioner with a special interest in diabetes. Mateo is able to connect with the Waakas through their shared Māori culture, and he offers practical, holistic advice to the entire family, covering topics such as diabetes management, healthy eating and psychological strategies for managing chronic illness. Aroha, Tama and Tia feel more supported, knowing they can consult Mateo for help in monitoring Tia's condition.

As a paediatric nurse, you may need to rely on the child's parents or guardians to make healthcare decisions on the child's behalf, particularly if the child is very young or has a condition that prevents them from exercising their autonomous choice. It is assumed that the parents will make decisions based on the *child's* best interests. It is therefore fundamental to consider models of family-centred care. These models emphasise training of parents to assume responsibility for care and decision-making, and that move towards truly collaborative relationships between children, their families and nurses.

The ways in which children's choices can best be acknowledged within the Australian and New Zealand paediatric healthcare system are supported by a broad literature devoted to the topic. Much of this relies on well-executed qualitative research that provides key insights into the ways in which nurses negotiate and coordinate the views and decisions of children and their parents. Unfortunately, it seems that there is still a long way to go before we can be confident that children are not marginalised in the healthcare system, and therefore guarantee that their needs are not overlooked.

In summary, using a developmental approach, children become increasingly involved in their own healthcare decisions as health literacy develops. In line with a child rights perspective, children with the necessary capacity and capability should be involved despite their age. That is, rather than suggesting a particular age at which decision-making is encouraged, children are deemed to be capable of making their own decisions and ought to be involved and consulted. In Australia and New Zealand, children must assent (voluntarily agree) to treatment before legal autonomy; however, it is their parents who must give formal consent (YouthLaw Aotearoa, 2020).

Vulnerable populations

Generally, most Australian and New Zealand children have good health outcomes and access to healthcare. However, some groups of children and young people are vulnerable. They are at greater risk of poorer health outcomes due to factors including locational disadvantage, health literacy, culture, and social and economic circumstances and need additional support to achieve equitable health outcomes (AHRC, 2019).

Vulnerable and marginalised groups include children and young people who are Aboriginal and Torres Strait Islander, Māori, in contact with the criminal justice system, refugees and asylum seekers, sexuality and gender diverse, experiencing homelessness, living with a disability and young parents, and who have experienced trauma and/or have a parent with a mental disorder.

From a child rights perspective, these groups of children and young people deserve particular attention to safeguard their wellbeing and achieve optimal health. Some of the issues that vulnerable families face when accessing care include structural barriers such as transport, cost, and opening hours. Attitudinal barriers include stigma, discrimination, and a lack of welcoming and non-judgmental services (Robards et al., 2019a).

Vulnerable families may need assistance to understand and navigate healthcare and social support systems (Robards et al., 2019b). For example, vulnerable migrant families (recently arrived from a non-English speaking background) can lack English

CASE STUDY 2.2 TAMICA

Tamica is a 15-year-old young woman from a rural area who has moved to Sydney to escape family violence. Tamica is moving between houses of friends and people she recently met (also known as 'couch surfing'). She does not own her own Medicare card and has limited financial support. She is not able to cook so mainly purchases takeaway food. Tamica smokes and says she is 'feeling a bit down'. She says she always has a cough and sometimes finds it hard to breathe. She doesn't have a regular GP.

Case study resolution

Tamica has a right to be to be protected from harm and to access healthcare that is planned and supported. She also has the right to be respected in her values, beliefs and culture. She should be fully informed, able to express her views and involved in decisions that affect her.

After exploring a range of concerns, Tamica says her persistent cough is her biggest worry. The nurse suggests that Tamica should see a doctor and explains that doctors can help with a range of health problems, including physical and mental health concerns. The nurse suggests that Tamica find a GP she can trust, who can be her 'regular GP'. Together they search for a GP who is convenient, and after checking that the GP will bulk bill, they make an appointment. The nurse informs Tamica that as she is aged 15, she is eligible for her own Medicare card. Due to having low access to financial support, Tamica is also eligible for a healthcare card to access medications at reduced cost.

The nurse recognises that Tamica is homeless because her accommodation is not secure. The nurse informs Tamica that she must contact child protection services due to concerns about her safety.

With Tamica's agreement, the nurse also contacts the youth homelessness advice line to find out about refuge supported accommodation where young people can live safely. The refuge support staff help Tamica learn how to cook, help her find work and/ or educational opportunities and assist her to apply for a Medicare and healthcare card.

When Tamica visits the GP, they do a holistic psychosocial assessment exploring the strengths and concerns across important life areas (this is also known as the HEEADSSS assessment, which explores home environment, education and employment, eating, activities, drugs, sexuality, suicide/depression and safety (Goldenring & Rosen, 2004). The GP identifies that Tamica may have asthma, and discusses the risks of smoking. The GP also feels she could benefit from the support of a counsellor. Together they make a treatment plan to which Tamica agrees. With Tamica's permission, the GP communicates the treatment plan to her support workers at the refuge, who agree to help Tamica access medications and attend appointments with the counsellor.

Taking time to engage early with Tamica to help her access the help she needs may greatly assist her wellbeing and prevent lifelong harm. As Tamica is homeless, the support of health and refuge workers has been essential for her to have her rights realised.

language skills and health system knowledge. Young people in the family may have better English language skills, resulting in them supporting their family to access healthcare, and providing English language interpretation. Healthcare services should always use interpreter services when needed rather than asking children and young people to act as interpreters. In contrast, homeless young people frequently lack the support of their families, so youth and health workers become important supports to help them contact and engage with services.

Many groups of vulnerable young people highly value services that are welcoming and non-judgemental. 'Welcoming signals', such as Indigenous and rainbow flags, are important ways in which services can communicate that they welcome patients from diverse backgrounds. Gender diverse children and young people (for example, those who are transgender) appreciate being asked about their preferred name and pronouns (for example, he, she, or they).

To prevent intergenerational trauma, supports should be in place early to prevent family breakdown and child protection concerns. For Aboriginal families, kinship care is important for maintaining a connection to culture. Culturally sensitive and appropriate programs are needed.

It is important to be aware that some children, young people and families belong to multiple vulnerable groups, leading to greater disadvantage. It can be much harder for patients experiencing multiple challenges to access the healthcare they need. For example, if a young person is gender diverse and homeless without family support, it can be much more difficult to access healthcare than for a young person who is gender diverse and has good family supports. Young people who live in rural and remote areas may experience difficult accessing health services. At the same time, refugee young people who live in rural and remote locations may experience greater challenges. Young parents who are in contact with the criminal justice system may find it much harder to access healthcare to support their wellbeing (and that of their own child) than other young parents.

Health professionals, including nurses, should be aware of the sociodemographic background of their patients and also be mindful of how their background impacts the patient's ability to access and engage with healthcare. Professionals need to consider the patient's journey through the health system and provide information and support as needed.

Australian and New Zealand age-of-majority legislation

For most Australian jurisdictions, 18 years is the age of legal autonomy, when the person can give consent for healthcare without parental approval. This does vary, however. Generally, if a young person is under the age of 14 years, the consent for healthcare of the parent or guardian is needed. However, young people aged 14 years and above can consent to healthcare if they can understand the proposed treatment, its consequences and the severity of treatment. It is therefore possible that a child younger than 14 may be competent to consent to treatment. Conversely, a child aged 16 or over may lack competence. In South Australia, a person 16 years of age or older may make decisions about their own medical treatment (*Consent to Medical Treatment and Palliative Care Act 1995*, s 6) (see Box 2.1).

Similarly, in New Zealand, a person over 16 years of age may make their own medical decisions (*Care of Children Act 2004, No. 90*).

BOX 2.1 AGE-OF-MAJORITY LEGISLATION IN AUSTRALIA

Consent to medical treatment

In Australia, the age of consent is 18 years (the general age of majority in Australia); however, in practice the age of consent for making decisions regarding medical treatment is generally considered to be from the age of 14 years, depending on the maturity of the young person (Kang & Sanders, 2014). In South Australia and New Zealand, the age of consent for medical treatment is 16 years.

If a child under 18 does not have the capacity to consent to treatment, a parent may consent on their behalf. A healthcare professional may also seek the consent of parents or guardians, even if a child is competent to consent on their own behalf. Parents may only consent to treatment that is in the best interests of the child.

In all jurisdictions, the consent of the child alone may be sufficient in circumstances where the child has 'sufficient understanding and intelligence to enable him or her to understand fully what is proposed' (*Gillick* test, from the case *Gillick v West Norfolk AHA* (1986); see also Harrison, 1992). In South Australia, this test has been modified by statute to be: where the child consents, as well as where (1) the medical practitioner is satisfied that the child is capable of understanding the nature, consequences and risks of the treatment, and that the treatment is in the best interests of the child's health and wellbeing; and (2) this opinion of the medical practitioner is supported by the written opinion of another medical practitioner who has also examined the child.

Source: Law Library of Congress (2014); AIFS (2013).

As children make the transition to adulthood, they develop the ability to be responsible for their actions. The parents' responsibility for the child gives way to the child's autonomy. In the paediatric hospital setting, the adolescent may make a difficult transition into adult care – especially if they have had multiple hospital admissions and developed close relationships with their caregivers.

One particularly pertinent issue that arises with the transition to adult care concerns the competence of the adolescent to make informed, rational decisions about their care and treatment. Regarding consent to medical treatment, the term '*Gillick* principle' must be understood. A House of Lords ruling in *Gillick v West Norfolk Area Health Authority* (1986) states that if a child under the age of 16 can demonstrate sufficient understanding and intelligence (whether through words or actions) to fully understand the treatment proposed, they can give their consent to treatment in the absence of parental consent (Woolley, 2005, p. 717). This ruling only applies to medical treatment that has clear potential for direct benefit to the health of the child. It is also important to remember that the *Gillick* principle applies only to a decision to receive treatment: it does not apply in cases of refusing treatment. In some cases, treatment may proceed without obtaining parental or patient consent – overriding a young person's decision to refuse treatment if the treatment is urgent (Kang & Sanders, 2014).

CASE STUDY 2.3 ARIEL'S REQUEST

You are working as a practice nurse at a paediatric clinic in Sydney, New South Wales, when you receive a call from Ariel. Ariel is 14 years old, and she and her three older siblings have been patients at the clinic since birth. She is a friendly, confident teenager, but sounds very nervous on the phone, and asks whether it is possible for her to make an appointment to see the doctor without her parents being in attendance.

At the consultation, Ariel mentions that she has become sexually active with her boyfriend, Todd, who is also 14. Ariel has not told her parents about this, as she would prefer to keep it private.

Ariel requests a prescription for birth control pills.

Case study resolution

The doctor considers both consent to healthcare and any child protection concerns, including consent to sex.

The doctor assesses Ariel as having the capacity to consent as a mature minor, and therefore able to make medical decisions. In the consultation, Ariel has clearly displayed that she has the capacity, maturity and understanding to make decisions about her own care. The doctor therefore agrees to prescribe birth control pills to Ariel without seeking permission from her parents.

Second, the doctor considers Ariel's age and laws regarding consent to sex. In New South Wales, the age of consent is 16 years. However, if a young person is aged 14–16 years, they can legally agree to have sex with another person who is less than two years older than them (as long as they both agree to it). The doctor finds out the boyfriend's age is 14 (the same age as Ariel) and that the sex is consensual.

In Australia and New Zealand, the law is clear that a child can give legally informed and effective consent to medical treatment, including contraception, using a *Gillick* assessment (Kang & Sanders, 2014).

The next section of this chapter looks more closely at the relationship between children and their parents, and presents the responsibilities of healthcare professionals, including Registered Nurses, in protecting children from harm.

Priorities in relation to children's rights and child-protection legislation

Child abuse and neglect refer to a wide range of behaviours. These include acts of commission related to physical, sexual, emotional or psychological harm to children, as well as acts of omission related to physical and emotional neglect. The categories of neglect, physical injury, sexual abuse and emotional abuse are widely used for the purposes of child abuse notification, substantiation of child abuse cases and prosecution.

Notwithstanding this, there are variations between Australian states and territories regarding what constitutes child abuse and neglect. Not only do the definitions vary; there are also some differences in what nurses are mandated to report to the child-protection authorities. This is because each state and territory in Australia has separate legislation aimed at protecting children from abuse and neglect. Thus child abuse and neglect notifications are substantiated in accordance with legislation in each jurisdiction. Australia has an estimated child abuse and neglect incidence rate of nine per 1000 children in the age group from birth to 16 years (AIHW, 2020).

The rates of child abuse and neglect in New Zealand are extremely concerning, and are one of the highest in the developed world (UNICEF, n.d.). Each year, Oranga Tamariki (the Ministry for Children) receives around 150 000 reports of concern. In a study using linked data, Rouland and Vaithianathan (2018) report that between the years of 1998 and 2015, almost one in four children (23.5 per cent) had been subject to at least one report to the child protection services at age 17 years. Upon investigation of the reports, it was found that 9.7 per cent of children had been a victim of substantiated abuse or neglect.

Being able to recognise the abuse and neglect of children is the most important first step in being able to provide early intervention and reduce the harm these actions can cause. Prevention is even better, so once a child and family are recognised as needing extra support, there is a chance that risk factors for child abuse and neglect can be reduced. At the same time, it must be recognised that the parent, child and environment transact over time. The scope of child abuse and neglect becomes even more extensive as research reveals the impact of maltreatment on children's development. These issues then further impact other parts of the child's personality and behaviour in a dangerous spiral.

Registered Nurses in Australia play a significant role in recognising, reporting and responding to child abuse and neglect. **Mandatory reporting** of known and suspected child abuse and neglect is well established in all Australian states and territories, and guidelines are available to make reporting efficient and effective.

Mandatory reporting – The legal requirement for people who work in particular professions (such as nurses, doctors or teachers) to report a reasonable belief of child physical, sexual or emotional abuse, or neglect to the relevant child protection authorities.

Registered nurses identify, evaluate and document injuries, and manage the protection of children in their care to intervene early and prevent further harm. Collaboration with law-enforcement bodies, social service agencies, advocacy organisations (where they exist) and the criminal justice system is essential to provide a network of support.

The intent of legislation that mandates reporting to child-protection authorities is to promote early intervention and prevent further violence and abuse. There are no penalties that can be applied to nurses who, in the course of their duty, make a report in good faith. Unfortunately, the penalty for children who are not recognised or reported can be further abuse or neglect. Almost one-third of infants who presented to one of four hospitals with head injuries sustained through acts of child abuse in a North American study of 232 infants could have been identified as being at risk prior to the admission for abusive head trauma (Letson et al., 2016). Had these children's vulnerabilities been recognised in earlier admissions to the hospital or healthcare agency, the chances of prevention of ongoing disability or even death may have increased.

The situation in New Zealand is somewhat different to in Australia, as there is no mandatory reporting for healthcare professionals (New Zealand Nurses Organisation (NZNO), 2018; Ministry of Health, 2018). However, as the NZNO notes, some hospitals and healthcare facilities have their own policies, which make it mandatory for employees to report suspected or actual child abuse and neglect. In addition, according to the *Crimes Amendment Act 1985*, an individual may be held criminally liable if they fail to act in a case of known or suspected child abuse and neglect. Nonetheless, New Zealand nurses are not, by definition, mandated reporters.

The responsibility to report child maltreatment

It must be understood that registered nurses in Australia are mandated by state and territory laws to report to a designated authority any knowledge or suspicion of a child who is experiencing, has experienced or is likely to experience significant harm. Legislation in some jurisdictions is limited to type of abuse and significant harm. Nevertheless, where this is the case – that is, where there is not a legislative duty to report certain forms of abuse – occupational and health service policy requirements exist. This is similar to the situation in New Zealand, where nurses are not mandatory reporters but may nevertheless be subject to employer duties to report.

Yet, despite these legal and policy obligations, just over 10 per cent of all reports to statutory child-protection authorities in Australia came from health professionals, compared with over 20 per cent from police and almost 20 per cent from school personnel in the 2018–19 report (AIHW, 2020). This also occurs in Canada, where 'school personnel, police and social workers report more child abuse and neglect than healthcare professionals do' (Tonmyr et al., 2009). There is growing research interest in determining the underlying reasons for this, given nurses' exposure to children and families across a range of settings. It is important to tease out whether these factors are related to nurses' skills, knowledge and attitudes, or there are more systematic work-place issues creating barriers to reporting. Do nurses in Australia view child protection as part of their role to the same extent as doctors, social workers, police and others? Are nurses conflicted about their role as advocates for families and children, versus their role as advocates for their profession or the healthcare agency? These and other questions have been studied in recent Australian research.

In a study of Queensland nurses, 21.1 per cent of nurses surveyed had never reported maltreatment and 26.6 per cent who had made notifications had failed to report on at least one occasion (Fraser et al., 2010), despite being aware of the legal responsibility to do so. Nurses are not alone in their reluctance to report. Even though 97 per cent of general practitioners surveyed in Queensland were aware of the responsibility to report child abuse and neglect, 26 per cent had decided at least once not to do so (Schweitzer et al., 2006). Alarmingly, one of the reasons they gave for not reporting was that they considered the abuse to be a one-off event and viewed further harm to the child as being very unlikely.

Compliance with legislation to report child abuse and neglect is compromised by a number of individual and contextual factors. At the level of the individual – let's call this a proximal factor – is the ability to recognise past, current and future abuse and neglect. Knowledge of child abuse and neglect recognition is variable, and depends on whether the topic is covered in professional development courses or staff training. There is sufficient evidence to indicate the relationship of injury presentations and physical and sexual abuse, for example, but staff need to have this knowledge. Certain physical injury presentations are more likely to have resulted from maltreatment. All fractures in a pre-ambulatory child should be treated as suspicious. The child-protection registrar, where available, or a senior medical officer must be notified immediately of any such presentation. Fractures of the femur (Leventhal et al., 2011), rib fractures and those caused by twisting forces, skull fractures or a combination of a skull and long bone fracture are associated with abuse (Bandyopadhyay & Yen, 2002). Head injury is the most common cause of fatal inflicted injury in children (King, Kiesel & Simon, 2006). Unfortunately, it is seen in those under 2 years of age due to the increased vulnerability of infants (Berkowitz, 1995; DiScala et al., 2000).

Acceleration–deceleration injuries indicate that the infant has been shaken, and a diagnosis of Shaken Baby Syndrome will be investigated: 'When considering the causes of injury, it is not enough to undertake a physical assessment of injury and risk alone. Shaken baby syndrome often presents with subdural or subarachnoid bleeding, cerebral oedema, long bone and/or rib fractures, retinal bleeding and little or no craniofacial trauma' (Cadzow & Armstrong, 2000; Kairys et al., 2001; Reece & Sege, 2000). Careful documentation is necessary, as the case may not be clear and symptoms can be diverse, such as abdominal pain and loss of consciousness (Jenny et al., 1999; Kairys et al., 2001; Keenan et al., 2004). Detailed recording of the history – that is, the parents' story – is necessary every time it is told. Inconsistencies across time and between the parents' recall are suspicious (Scott, 2013; Scott, Higgins & Franklin, 2012).

Cases of emotional abuse have emerged as the most problematic forms of child maltreatment in Australia, and represent the most common primary type of abuse substantiated for children (54 per cent) (AIHW, 2020). While progress has been made in identifying and reducing both child physical and sexual abuse, substantiated notifications of neglect and emotional abuse are increasing. It is crucial to be able to recognise the risks of abuse and neglect, and to report suspicion. In all cases of reporting, it is the nurse's individual responsibility not to substantiate the suspicion, but rather to detail the seriousness of the harm or potential harm to the child.

CASE STUDY 2.4 A NURSE'S DILEMMA

Chung is an 8-year-old boy born to Chinese parents in Australia. He is often struck by his father with a rod, sometimes for only minor infractions such as being late home from school. Over a period of time, Chung starts to feel sad a lot and loses confidence in himself. He subsequently suffers high levels of anxiety, and withdraws from his friends, which leads him to distance himself from them. His friends do not understand why this is happening and start to tease him. Chung responds to this with physical violence, which gets him in trouble with the teacher at his school and consequently into more trouble with his father.

Chapter 2: Child rights in Australia and New Zealand   47

Wang Li (Lianne) is a registered nurse working in the emergency department of a busy children's hospital in metropolitan Sydney. Wang Li has a legal obligation to report child abuse and neglect to the child-protection authorities, depending on the severity of harm to the child. If the abuse or neglect is deemed to be serious, then she is compelled by legislation and of course hospital policy to make a report. Chung has presented to the hospital where she is working. He is anxious and struggling to breathe. He presents regularly at the hospital, always accompanied by his mother. He has asthma and a strong history of eczema. His mother says both conditions are really playing up at the moment and that Chung is very anxious. He has been doing exams at school and is worried he has not done well.

Using their shared Mandarin language, Wang Li asks Chung's mother whether she knows what might be upsetting him. In Mandarin, Chung's mother discloses the extent to which her husband beats young Chung and makes him spend hours doing homework, even when he is too tired to concentrate. She wants him to stop but is afraid of his reaction if she says anything. She appeals to Wang Li not to mention it to anyone, as she is so ashamed and believes that no other Chinese parent living in Australia would treat their child in this way.

Wang Li is aware of her legal obligation to report the abuse, which she understands to be causing serious harm to Chung's wellbeing. However, she is uncertain about whether reporting the concern would be in the best interests of this family. She too was brought up to believe that if you spare the rod you spoil the child – that is, that harsh punishment of children is necessary for their growth and development. Her father was very stern but loving towards her. She has developed a trusting relationship with Chung's mother and feels that she would betray her trust by making a report. Wang Li is not sure whether she can discuss the report with colleagues and whether her identity would be protected.

The multidisciplinary response to child protection

Concerns expressed by Wang Li in this scenario are known to be barriers to reporting. Approximately one-fifth of the population of nurses surveyed in Australia and overseas (Feng & Levine, 2005; Fraser et al., 2010; Lee, Fraser & Chou, 2007) admit to having not reported their suspicion of abuse or neglect, even when mandated to do so.

Case study resolution

The Registered Nurse is mandated to report the abuse to the appropriate child-protection agency. In most jurisdictions in Australia, this is enabled by the fact that the nurse can confer with other health professionals and follow a protocol. The Registered Nurse in this case is mandated to report any child abuse and neglect that she identifies or suspects in the course of her professional work. Some jurisdictions may have legislation that compels the nurse to report even if it is not part of the professional role. Details of the current legislation for the jurisdiction within which you are working should be well understood and opportunities for training taken.

(cont.)

Wang Li's identity in this case would be protected by Australian law, and she would not be liable for making a report that could not be substantiated if she makes the report in good faith. Depending on the jurisdiction, if she fails to report, a penalty may be incurred. It is important to note that to make a report in Australia, the Registered Nurse does not have to be able to substantiate the abuse or neglect. She makes a report so that an investigation can be commenced.

A Chinese family was presented in the case study to highlight some of the cultural considerations nurses may need to make when reporting. The case study highlights that child abuse and neglect occur across cultures and religions.

Apart from the legal responsibility, the ethical and moral obligation to report abuse to the appropriate child-protection authority should actually enhance the nurse–family relationship because it should allow for the provision of much-needed assistance to families struggling to provide good parenting for their children. Unfortunately, we know that a number of health professionals, doctors and nurses do not share this optimism, and a critical debate remains about further expansion of mandatory reporting laws for child abuse and neglect (Mathews, 2012).

SUMMARY

- This chapter introduced the concept of child rights within the scope of paediatric nursing, and particularly the rights of children and young people experiencing paediatric nursing care in Australia and New Zealand.
- The relationship between the UN Convention on the Rights of the Child, to which Australia and New Zealand are signatories, and policies on the quality of healthcare received by children and young people in Australia and New Zealand were explored.
- The chapter explained the way in which child rights are integrated into Australian and New Zealand policies that determine how children and young people will be cared for in Australian paediatric healthcare settings and outlined the mandatory reporting legislation that promotes nurses as advocates for children.
- It is anticipated that you will consider your professional priorities in relation to children's rights and child-protection legislation.

LEARNING ACTIVITIES

2.1 Describe standards of nursing practice that relate to the care of children in Australia and New Zealand.

2.2 Describe standards of nursing practice related to the care of young people in Australia and New Zealand.

2.3 Discuss professional boundaries in the therapeutic relationship when providing nursing care for children and families.

2.4 Analyse nursing roles and responsibilities with regard to protecting children from harm.

2.5 Do you think it should be the responsibility of nurses to report child abuse and neglect? Discuss.

FURTHER READING

For more detailed information about child maltreatment and the obligation you have as a health professional to recognise and respond to known or suspected cases in your professional role, access the excellent training materials provided by the health authority of the jurisdiction in which you work.

For example, in New South Wales go to www.health.nsw.gov.au/parvan/childprotect/Pages/policies-guidelines.aspx

In Queensland: www.health.qld.gov.au/clinical-practice/guidelines-procedures/patient-safety/duty-of-care/child-protection

In Victoria: https://services.dhhs.vic.gov.au/child-protection

REFERENCES

Association for the Wellbeing of Children in Healthcare (AWCH) 2020, *Promotion Children's Rights*, viewed 12 October 2020, https://awch.org.au/projects/promoting-childrens-rights

Australian College of Children and Young People's Nurses (ACCYPN) 2016, *Standards of practice for children and young people's nurses*, ACCYPN, Brisbane.

Australian Institute of Family Studies (AIFS) 2013, *Age of consent laws*, viewed 1 June 2014, www.aifs.gov.au/cfca/pubs/factsheets/a142090/#table-1

Australian Institute of Health and Welfare (AIHW) 2020. *Child protection Australia 2018–19*, cat. no. CWS 74, AIHW, Canberra.

Australian Human Rights Commission (AHRC) 2019, *Children's rights in Australia: A scorecard*, viewed 12 October 2020, https://humanrights.gov.au/our-work/childrens-rights/publications/childrens-rights-australia-scorecard

Bandyopadhyay, S & Yen, K 2002, Non-accidental fractures in child maltreatment syndrome, *Clinical Pediatric Emergency Medicine*, 3(2), pp. 145–52.

Berkowitz, C 1995, Pediatric abuse, *Emergency Medical Clinics of North America*, 13, pp. 321–42.

Cadzow, SP & Armstrong, KL 2000, Rib fractures in infants: Red alert! The clinical features, investigations and child protection outcomes, *Journal of Paediatrics and Child Health*, 36(4), pp. 322–6.

Children's Hospitals Australasia (CHA) & Association for the Wellbeing of Children in Healthcare 2010, *Charter of Children's and Young People's Rights in Healthcare Services in Australia*, viewed 12 October 2020, https://children.wcha.asn.au/sites/default/files/australian_version_final_210911web.pdf

Children's Hospitals Australasia (CHA) & Paediatric Society of New Zealand 2020, *Charter on The Rights of Tamariki Children & Rangatahi Young People in Healthcare Services in Aotearoa New Zealand: A consensus statement by Children's Hospitals Australasia (CHA) and the Paediatric Society of New Zealand*, viewed 7 August

2020, www.cdhb.health.nz/Hospitals-Services/Child-Health/Documents/Charter-on-the-rights-of-children-New-Zealand.pdf

Coyne, I, Hallstrom, I & Soderback, M 2016, Reframing the focus from a family-centred to a child-centred care approach for children's healthcare, *Journal of Child Healthcare*, 20(4), pp. 494–502.

DiScala, C, Sege, R, Li, G & Reece, RM 2000, Child abuse and unintentional injuries: A 10-year retrospective, *Archives of Pediatric and Adolescent Medicine*, 154(1), pp. 16–22.

Feng, JY & Levine, M 2005, Factors associated with nurses' intention to report child abuse: A national survey of Taiwanese nurses, *Child Abuse and Neglect*, 29(7), pp. 783–95.

Fraser, JA, Mathews, B, Walsh, K, Chen, L & Dunne, M 2010, Factors influencing child abuse and neglect recognition and reporting by nurses: A multivariate analysis, *International Journal of Nursing Studies*, 47(2), pp. 146–53.

Goldenring, JM & Rosen, DS 2004, Getting into adolescent heads: An essential update, *Contemporary Pediatrics*, 21(1), pp. 64–90.

Harrison, M 1992, What's new in family law? Parental authority and its constraints – the case of Marion, *Family Matters*, 32, pp. 10–12, viewed 3 August 2007, www.aifs.gov.au/institute/pubs/fm1/fm32mh.html

Jenny, C, Hymel, KP, Ritzen, A, Reinert, SE & Hay,TC 1999, Analysis of missed cases of abusive head trauma, *JAMA: The Journal of the American Medical Association*, 281 (7), pp. 621–6.

Kairys, S. Alexander, R, Block, R, Everett, D, Hymel, K & Jenny, C 2001, Shaken Baby Syndrome: Rotational cranial injuries – technical report, *Paediatrics*, 108(1), pp. 206–10.

Kang, M & Sanders, J 2014, *Medico-legal issues in youth health resource kit, NSW kids and families*, viewed 12 October 2020, www.health.nsw.gov.au/kidsfamilies/youth/Documents/youth-health-resource-kit/youth-health-resource-kit-sect-3-chap-5.pdf

Keenan, H, Runyan, D, Marshall, S, Nocera, M & Merten, D 2004, A population-based comparison of clinical and outcome characteristics of young children with serious inflicted and non-inflicted traumatic brain injury, *Pediatrics*, 114(3), pp. 633–9.

Kids Health 2018, Introduction to Principles Guiding Provision Of Health & Disability Services, viewed 12 October 2020, https://www.kidshealth.org.nz/introduction-principles-guiding-provision-health-disability-service.

King, W, Kiesel, E & Simon, H 2006, Child abuse fatalities: Are we missing opportunities for intervention?, *Pediatric Emergency Care*, 22(4), pp. 211–14.

Kuo, DZ, Houtrow, AJ, Arango, P, Kuhlthau, KA, Simmons, JM & Neff, JM 2012, Family-centered care: Current applications and future directions in pediatric healthcare, *Maternal and Child Health Journal*, 16(2), pp. 297–305.

Law Library of Congress 2014, *Children's rights: Australia*, viewed 12 March 2014, www.loc.gov/law/help/child-rights/australia.php#f9.

Lee, PY, Fraser, JA & Chou, FH 2007, Nurse reporting of known and suspected child abuse and neglect cases in Taiwan, *Kaohsiung Journal of Medical Sciences*, 23(3), pp. 128–37.

Letson, ML, Cooper, JN, Deans, KJ, Scribano, PV, Makoroff, KL, Feldman, KW & Berger, RP 2016, Prior opportunities to identify abuse in children with abusive head trauma, *Child Abuse & Neglect*, 60, pp. 36–45.

Leventhal, JM et al. 2011, Are abusive fractures in young children becoming less common? Changes over 24 years, *Child Abuse & Neglect*, 35(11), pp. 905–14.

Mathews, BP 2012, Exploring the contested role of mandatory reporting laws in the identification of severe child abuse and neglect, in M Freeman (ed.), *Law and childhood studies*, Oxford University Press, Oxford, pp. 302–38.

Ministry of Health 2018, Family violence questions and answers, viewed 7 August 2020, www.health.govt.nz/our-work/preventative-health-wellness/family-violence/family-violence-questions-and-answers

New Zealand Nurses Organisation (NZNO) 2018, Reporting abuse – actual or suspected: Frequently asked questions, viewed 7 August 2020, www.nzno.org.nz/LinkClick.aspx?fileticket=_BTyMUO5JqE%3D&portalid=0

Reece, RM & Sege, R 2000, Childhood head injuries: Accidental or inflicted?, *Archives of Pediatric and Adolescent Medicine*, 154(1), pp. 11–15.

Robards, F, Kang, M, Luscombe, G, Sanci, L, Steinbeck, K, Jan, S, Hawke, C, Kong, M & Usherwood, T 2019a, Predictors of young people's healthcare access in the digital age, *Australian and New Zealand Journal of Public Health*, 43(6), pp. 582–8.

Robards, F, Kang, M, Steinbeck, K, Hawke, C, Jan, S, Sanci, L, Liew, YY, Kong, M & Usherwood, T 2091b, Healthcare equity and access for marginalised young people: A longitudinal qualitative study exploring health system navigation in Australia, *International Journal for Equity in Health*, 18, Article 41, doi:10.1186/s12939-019-0941-2

Rouland, B & Vaithianathan, R 2018, Cumulative prevalence of maltreatment among New Zealand children, 1998–2015, *American Journal of Public Health*, 108, pp. 511–13.

Royal Australasian College of Physicians (RACP) 2008, *Standards for the care of children and adolescents in health services*, viewed 1 June 2014, www.racp.edu.au/index.cfm?objectid=393E4ADA-CDAA-D1AF-0D543B5DC13C7B46

Schweitzer, R, Buckley, L, Harnett, P & Loxton, N 2006, Predictors of failure by medical practitioners to report suspected child abuse in Queensland, *Australian Health Review*, 30(3), pp. 298–304.

Scott, D 2013, *Meeting children's needs when the family environment isn't always 'good enough': A systems approach*, viewed 20 December 2013, www.aifs.gov.au/cfca/pubs/papers/a144433/cfca14.pdf

Scott, D, Higgins, D & Franklin, R 2012, *The role of supervisory neglect in childhood injury*, viewed 20 December 2013, www.aifs.gov.au/cfca/pubs/papers/a142582

Tonmyr, L, Li, A, Williams, G, Scott, D & Jack, S 2009, Patterns of reporting to child protection services in Canada by healthcare and non-healthcare professionals, *Paediatrics & Child Health*, 15(8), pp. 25–32.

United Nations (UN) 1966, *UN International Covenant on Economic, Social and Cultural Rights*, United Nations, New York.

—— 1989a, *Convention on the Rights of the Child*, United Nations, New York.

—— 1989b, Treaty collection, viewed 1 June 2014, https://treaties.un.org

—— 2019, *Concluding observations on the combined fifth and sixth periodic reports of Australia*, United Nations Committee on the Rights of the Child, New York.

United Nations International Children's Emergency Fund (UNICEF) 2004, *Convention on the rights of the child*, viewed 4 November 2016, www.unicef.org/crc/index_30177.html

—— n.d., *Safe childhood*, viewed 7 August 2020, www.unicef.org.nz/in-new-zealand/safe-childhood

Woolley S 2005, Children of Jehovah's Witnesses and adolescent Jehovah's Witnesses: What are their rights?, *Archives of Disease in Childhood*, 90, pp. 715–19.

YouthLaw Aotearoa 2020, Medical Decisions, viewed 7 August 2020, http://youthlaw.co .nz/rights/health-wellbeing/medical-decisions

Legislation and cases cited

Care of Children Act 2004 (NZ)

Children, Young Persons and Their Families Act 1989 (NZ)

Consent to Medical Treatment and Palliative Care Act 1995 (SA)

Crimes Amendment Act 1985 (NZ)

Family Law Act 1975 (Aus)

Gillick v West Norfolk and Wisbech Area Health Authority [1986] 3 All ER 402 (HL)

Health services for New Zealand Māori and Aboriginal and Torres Strait Islander Australian children and young people

3

Melissa Carey, Liesa Clague, Fleur Magick Dennis and
Laurance Magick Dennis

LEARNING OBJECTIVES

In this chapter you will:

- Develop an understanding of the historical and contemporary contexts of health systems and services for New Zealand and Australian First Peoples (Māori, and Aboriginal and Torres Strait Islander) children and youth
- Develop knowledge about the application of *kawa whakaruruhau* (cultural safety) within New Zealand and Australia around policies and practices in health
- Recognise and acknowledge how the dominance of underlying paradigms and discourses of Western culture and policies impacts health outcomes for Māori and Aboriginal and Torres Strait Islander children, their families and communities regarding health
- Recognise and understand the importance of the establishment of community-led health services within New Zealand and Australia

A note on terminology

Throughout this chapter, we will be using specific terminology to identify groups of First Peoples from Aotearoa New Zealand and Australia. Terms are influenced by our history, stories and politics, and each is interpreted differently by different people. There is not a common understanding, but certain words are more appropriate to use than others (Common Ground, 2021). This section outlines the preferred terminology and the meaning behind the terminology.

Aboriginal: This is a Latin term meaning 'original inhabitants', which is used to refer to the original peoples of mainland Australia, a member of a race of people who were the first peoples to live in their country (lands and water). The First Peoples of the land now called Australia are the Aboriginal Peoples; however, Aboriginal people also refer to each other by Aboriginal English terms and/or their nations or language groups: Goori, Koori, Yungl, Yaegl, Wiradjuri, Wayilwan, Ngemba, Yuin, Nunga and many more.

Torres Strait Islander: A seafaring people, whose traditional countries are in the Torres Strait, off the most northern point of Queensland. The region has 274 islands located north of mainland Australia, in the Torres Strait and is the only part of Australia that borders another country – Papua New Guinea.

Aboriginal and Torres Strait Islander: Used to acknowledge the vast diversity of First Peoples we have in Australia. The term 'Indigenous' will only be referred to if it relates to a reference article. We choose not to use 'Indigenous' as it does not reflect the many nations of First Peoples.

Māori: The First Nations, Indigenous people of New Zealand. There are many Māori tribes, known as *Iwi*, and subtribes, known as *Hapū*. Customs and practices differ across Māori people, *Iwi* and *Hapū* and relate to the complex relationship between people and place.

Te Reo Māori: Māori language is an official language of New Zealand; the language revitalisation movement aims to ensure that all New Zealanders learn to speak and understand Te Reo Māori. This acknowledges the human rights of the Māori people to retain their language.

Aotearoa/New Zealand: New Zealand is often known as Aotearoa, as this is the most widely accepted Māori name for the country. This chapter will use both terms.

Introduction

This chapter covers the government and non-government systems and services aimed at supporting New Zealand Māori children and Australian Aboriginal and/or Torres Strait Islander children, their families and communities in achieving optimal health and wellbeing objectives and outcomes. New Zealand and Australia are separate countries with distinct diverse colonial histories, policies, healthcare systems, practices and ways of life, although their First Peoples may share common experiences of colonisation, invasion, cultural oppression and marginalisation. Contemporary health services in the two countries are also separate and unique, so the content in this chapter is provided in discrete sections for New Zealand and Australia.

Cultural safety

Kawa whakaruruhau (cultural safety) was first explored and developed by Irihapeti Ramsden, a Māori nurse (Papps & Ramsden, 1996), in response to the poor health outcomes experienced by Māori people in Aotearoa, New Zealand. Recognising the need for radical change to health service delivery, cultural safety theory promotes a self-examination approach to nursing education and practice, bringing about a change in the delivery of care, aimed at reducing healthcare inequities. Since its conception, a culturally safe approach has been recommended and adopted across Aotearoa, New Zealand and Australia within registration requirements, governing bodies and service providers.

The Nursing Council of New Zealand (nursingcouncil.org.nz) provides guidelines for Cultural Safety, the Treaty of Waitangi and Māori health for nursing education and practice. Advocacy for cultural safety for Aboriginal and Torres Strait Islander peoples is embedded in the Australian Health Practitioner Regulation Agency (AHPRA) and national boards. In 2018 and 2020, nurses and midwives led the way for safer healthcare with a joint statement about cultural safety as standards of practice and embedded in the code of conduct as well as developing a cultural safety strategy for 2020–25 (AHPRA & National Boards, 2020).

According to the Australian Indigenous Doctors' Association (2018, p. 1), cultural safety in the Australian context is

> the accumulation and application of knowledge of Aboriginal and Torres Strait Islander values, principles and norms . . . overcoming the cultural power imbalances of places, people and policies . . . with cultural awareness being the first step in the learning process and cultural safety being the outcome.

Māori *tamariki* and *rangatahi*

Throughout this chapter, you will be able to identify key concepts related to the delivery of care that is culturally safe for Māori *tamariki* (children) and *rangatahi* (young people). This includes a *whānau* (family) and community approach to health and wellbeing as the *whānau* is central to the wellbeing of the growing Māori child. Te Reo Māori is an official language of New Zealand; it is important to learn key terms and to understand important concepts when working with *whānau* in Aotearoa, New Zealand. This chapter will introduce a few of the most commonly used terms to discuss *tamariki* and *rangatahi*. If you are working in Aotearoa, New Zealand or with Māori *whānau* in Australia (or elsewhere), learning more Te Reo Māori will assist you with providing culturally safe care, as understanding this language helps to build a trusting therapeutic relationship with *whānau* carers (Moeke-Maxwell et al., 2019). There are important *tikanga* (protocols) and *kawa* (knowledge) that surround the health and wellbeing of *tamariki* and *rangatahi* – if you are not sure, you can start by asking the *whānau* and experienced cultural care practitioners. For Māori *whānau*, there are important aspects to holistic wellbeing, which include *mana* (personal and social esteem), *mauri* (life force energy), *wairua* (spirit), *tinana* (body) and *hinengaro* (mind and consciousness). Several Māori health models can be drawn upon to gain greater insight into these aspects of Māori life. However, this chapter will explore the overarching health service elements, concepts, frameworks and guidelines. It will also provide some information about key services provided by health and social care services.

Aboriginal and Torres Strait Islander children and young people

We (Aboriginal and/or Torres Strait Islander peoples) are a diverse peoples made up of many nations (see the Aboriginal and Torres Strait Islander language map in the Further Reading section), each with its own language, culture, lore and Dreaming, customs, geographical differences and child-rearing practices. What is fundamental is that we love our children and we want to introduce some of the ways of knowing, being and doing from the various nations around Australia. Recognising the important diversity of Dreaming, our connection to land underpins our beliefs, practices, responsibilities and relationships. Each region – whether urban, rural or remote – has a different way of relating to the geographical features, and different connections to stories and spirituality.

The authors of this section use a diverse lens and their personal perspectives as Aboriginal people who are working in health and community. They look from both within and outside the health system as parents, aunties, uncles, mothers, fathers, sisters and brothers, and use their cultural lens of knowing, being and doing through Aboriginal ways. They highlight the key challenges in relation to meeting the needs of Aboriginal and Torres Strait Islander children and their connections (family/ies, community/ies and Country). The authors bring to your attention cultural awareness, sensitivity and safety for Aboriginal and Torres Strait Islander children and peoples. Building good practices around these concepts, as well as networking with Aboriginal and Torres Strait Islander peoples in these areas, can achieve better outcomes for Aboriginal and Torres Strait Islander children. The emphasis in this chapter is on recent data, and evidence for strengths-based practice for paediatric and child health nurses working with Aboriginal and Torres Strait Islander children, families and their communities. Underpinning the data is the understanding that healthcare practices are developed with time, respectful engagement, learning from experience, listening and building connections in relationships with Aboriginal and Torres Strait Islander families and communities.

The health status of Māori *tamariki* and *rangatahi*

Māori *tamariki* and *rangatahi* continue to experience health inequities within Aotearoa, New Zealand. In 2017, Te Ohanga Ake, a health status review of Māori *tamariki* and *rangatahi* in Aotearoa, New Zealand, was conducted utilising available epidemiological data. The subsequent report highlighted poor health outcomes related to poverty, poor living conditions, mental health problems and suicide as key areas of concern (Simpson et al., 2017). Hospitalisation rates (per 1000 population) for Māori *tamariki* and *rangatahi* aged 0–14 years are significantly higher when compared with those aged 15–24 years. The causes of these hospitalisations also differ across age groups; in particular, there are differences in the rates of respiratory diseases and injuries (Ministry of Health, 2020a).

There have been some improvements in reducing the gap in Māori *tamariki* and *rangatahi* health compared with non-Māori children and young people, with improvements in sudden infant death, hospitalisations for meningococcal disease and the rates of skin infections (Table 3.1). Despite these improvements Māori infants are still almost twice as likely as non-Māori to die and nearly three times more likely than non-Māori, non-Pacific infants to die during the post-neonatal period. Findings of the Te Ohanga Ake report (Simpson et al., 2017) have clearly identified that the experience of inequities for Māori *tamariki* and *rangatahi* are evident across the key indicators within the report.

Table 3.1 Main categories and potential mechanisms to avoid hospitalisation

Main category	Primary care intervention	Public health intervention	Social policy intervention
Respiratory conditions	✓		✓
Dental conditions	✓	✓	✓
Gastrointestinal diseases	✓	✓	✓
Nutrition deficiency and anaemia	✓	✓	✓
Cardiovascular diseases	✓	✓	✓
Otitis media	✓		✓
Dermatological conditions	✓	✓	✓
Diabetes complications	✓	✓	✓
Kidney, urinary tract infection	✓		
Sexually transmitted infections	✓	✓	
Vaccine-preventable diseases	✓	✓	✓
Meningococcal infection	✓	✓	✓
Epilepsy	✓		
Other non-injury conditions	✓		
Injury and poisoning			
Unintentional injuries		✓	✓
Intentional injuries		✓	✓

Source: Ministry of Health (2020a, p. 3).

A framework of recommendations for mechanisms to reduce the rates of hospital-isations for Māori *tamariki* and *rangatahi* was developed by the Ministry of Health (2020a).

Historical factors and Te Tiriti o Waitangi

Māori people travelled throughout Polynesia, arriving in Aotearoa, New Zealand in canoe migrations over many years. A long history of cultural development took place over that time, including the shifting of land boundaries as *Iwi* (tribes) grew. There were many *Hapū* (sub-tribes) throughout the North (Te Ika-a-Māui) and South (Te Wai Pounamu) Islands, which affiliated with particular *Iwi* through ancestral lines. The understanding of ancestral ties and their significance is known as *whakapapa*. This knowledge of *whakapapa* is significant to understanding not only where Māori people link to, in terms of land and place, but also in terms of physical and personal traits that have been passed through genealogical lines, including spiritual gifts. In 1642, the first documented European colonial ships began to arrive in New Zealand; however, the country did not attract attention as a colonial settlement until the late 1800s. In 1840, a Treaty was negotiated and signed between many, although not all, Māori chiefs and European settlers. This is known as Te Tiriti o Waitangi (the English version is the Treaty of Waitangi). Te Tiriti o Waitangi has two versions, which has caused much debate; while it is not within this chapter's scope to discuss the full extent of the documents and their differences, it is important to note that the Treaty was incorporated into New Zealand law by the *State Owned Enterprises Act 1986* with the provision that the Act does not allow the Crown to act in a manner that is inconsistent with the principles of the Treaty of Waitangi. However, many Tribunals continue to contest the actions of the Crown against Māori rights and sovereignty as outlined within the Te Tiriti o Waitangi.

Māori Health Trends Report

In 2019 the *Wai 2575 Māori Health Trends Report* (Ministry of Health, 2020b) was a result of an inquiry into the Health Services and Outcomes initiated in November 2016. This inquiry was established to 'hear all claims concerning grievances relating to health services and outcomes of national significance for Māori' (Ministry of Health, 2020c). This was a response to dissatisfaction that the New Zealand government, as agents of the Crown, had failed to fulfil its responsibilities under Te Tiriti o Waitangi. Under the Treaty, the government is required to ensure that there is Māori equity in health services, care and outcomes compared with non-Māori citizens. When there are continued disparities in health outcomes for Māori, and in particular for *tamariki* and *rangatahi*, this must be called into question. The 2017 UNICEF Annual Report (UNICEF, 2018) assessed 41 high-income countries against nine of the United Nations' Sustainable Development Goals. Aotearoa, New Zealand was found to be in the bottom three countries for 'ensuring healthy lives' across the lifespan, despite ranking 38 for 'good health and wellbeing'. This was partly due to the number of children living in a jobless household, which was one in seven (Department of the Prime Minister and Cabinet, 2019).

The *Hauora: Report on Stage One of the Health Services and Outcomes Kaupapa Inquiry* (Haurora Report, 2019) exposes the primary healthcare framework and its failure to achieve Māori health equity. The inquiry found that the existing health services in Aotearoa, New Zealand, including legal requirements, strategy and policy, have failed to consistently address the requirements of the Treaty. This ongoing reform will continue over the coming years as the claims are being heard. In 2020, the New Zealand Government requested that the New Zealand Ministry of Health prepare a new set of performance indicators to benefit health outcomes for all New Zealanders.

Recommendations from the reform relate to the amendment of the *New Zealand Public Health and Disability Act 2000* to include a new Treaty of Waitangi clause, and to call the Crown to commit to achieving health equity for Māori people.

He Korowai Oranga (Māori Health Strategy)

He Korowai Oranga is New Zealand's Māori Health Strategy, which sets the overarching framework for the government's approach to health and wellbeing for Māori people in New Zealand. The strategy addresses the New Zealand Health Strategy, the New Zealand Disability Strategy and the *New Zealand Public Health and Disability Act 2000*. This high-level government strategy supports the Ministry of Health and the District Health Boards (DHBs) to work towards enabling improvements in Māori health. The strategy began in 2002 and was last updated in 2013–14 with a vision of Pae Ora (Healthy Futures) in mind. The new refreshed strategy builds upon Whānau Ora (Healthy Families), and now includes Mauri Ora (Healthy Individuals) and Wai Ora (Healthy Environments). An implementation action plan for the strategy was developed by the Ministry of Health in collaboration with health and social care providers. The action plan provides the framework for achieving collaborative ways to address inequity, enabling the delivery of high-quality services that meet the needs and aspirations of Māori people.

District Health Boards

New Zealand healthcare is a complex system that involves the Ministry of Health; however, most of the responsibility for the delivery of healthcare within the system is attributed to the DHBs. This means that they also receive around three-quarters of all funding for health services (Ministry of Health, 2017b). Each DHB is responsible for providing, managing, planning and purchasing health services for the population of its individual district. They must also work together to ensure that there are sufficiently effective health services for all of Aotearoa, New Zealand. The DHBs oversee a range of health services for their communities and districts, such as primary care, public health services, hospital services, aged care services and services provided by other non-government health providers, including Māori and Pacific providers (Ministry of

Health, 2017b). The DHBs are given targets for the health goals of New Zealand by the Ministry of Health; in 2020, these targets were being revised based on the outcomes of the Wai 2575 inquiry. However, in the meantime the DHBs will work towards the existing health targets, which include recommendations for Māori *tamariki* and *rangatahi* healthcare.

BOX 3.1 SYSTEM LEVEL MEASURES 2017–18

System Level Measures, implemented in July 2016, are nationally set measures that focus on helping children, youth and vulnerable populations.

For 2017–18, the measures were:

- reducing hospital admission rates for children aged up to 4 years old
- reducing how long people stay in hospital
- reducing amenable mortality
- improving patient experience of care
- increasing the proportion of babies living in smoke-free homes at six weeks post-birth
- improving youth access to and use of appropriate health services.

Source: Hauora Report (2019, p. 63).

Health Alliances

The Ministry of Health expects that DHBs will work within Health Alliances to meet these targets. These alliances are known as District Health Alliances, and consist of members from primary, hospital and community care providers who work locally within the health district. It is recommended that alliances be made up of healthcare professionals from a variety of disciplines such as nursing, paramedicine, pharmacy and midwives, as well as social care providers such as community youth workers, community mental health providers, Māori health providers and Tamariki Ora providers.

Child and Youth Wellbeing Strategy

Launched on 29 August 2019, the New Zealand Government Child and Youth Wellbeing Strategy (Department of the Prime Minister and Cabinet, 2019) sought to address the requirements of the Te Tiriti o Waitangi (Treaty of Waitangi) as a tool for empowering the strategy to address the needs of Māori *tamariki* who are *tangata whenua* (First Nations people). This strategy hopes to transform systems, policies and services to enable Māori-developed and driven solutions for Māori children and youth. The strategy also aims to empower local communities to make the changes that they need in ways that work for their needs, rather than being driven by an external community agenda.

BOX 3.2 CONCERNS TO BE ADDRESSED

The following are some key concerns outlined in the Child and Youth Wellbeing Strategy 2019:

- Nearly a quarter of New Zealand's children and young people (up to 250 000) are growing up in households considered to be in poverty, when the cost of housing is taken into account.
- It has been estimated that an even greater number of children and young people (nearly 300 000) experience or are exposed to family and sexual violence every year.
- Around 6400 children and young people require the care of the state due to family violence, being abused or neglected, or through youth offending.
- Half of all lifetime cases of mental illness start by age 14 and the number of young people accessing specialist mental health and addiction services has more than doubled in recent years.
- New Zealand has the highest suicide rate for young people aged 15 to 19 years compared with other countries.

Source: Department of the Prime Minister and Cabinet (2019, p. 12).

During the development of the strategy, it became clear that a new way of working was required to ensure the best outcomes for current and future generations of New Zealand children and young people. A shift towards more holistic health goals was identified as the best way to address the social, environmental and economic implications of healthcare decision-making. Aotearoa, New Zealand sought to achieve a similar level of wellbeing for *tamariki* and *rangatahi* as comparable countries. This identified that there is a need to rapidly improve health outcomes currently experienced by the most disadvantaged groups within the country. One important strategy to achieving this is ensuring that the heritage, culture and identities expressed by *tamariki* and *rangatahi* in Aotearoa, New Zealand are celebrated as a strength and encouraged. In terms of measuring the outcomes of success, it was determined that the measures must be implemented in a way that reflects the value of people and the environment, and enables a community strengths-based approach to national prosperity.

Six outcomes were developed in conjunction with a review of existing models and a consultation group. These outcomes make up the framework for the strategy (see Table 3.2). The strategy outcomes will be measured by indicators that are statistically robust and collected regularly. The New Zealand Government has determined that these measures must be strengths based, broadly informative and relevant. They should also be easily understood and applicable to all children and young people. It is important to ensure that the measures are internationally comparable and culturally responsive. Any measure applied should be aligned with the other government indicators and measurement frameworks (Department of the Prime Minister and Cabinet, 2019). The aim of obtaining alignment is to promote consistency and cohesion across government organisations and sectors. The strategy will also take into consideration the voices of children and young people as experts in their own wellbeing and lived experiences. By doing this, it is hoped that the indicators will reflect what children and young people say they need to achieve health and wellbeing.

Table 3.2 Six outcomes for the Child and Youth Wellbeing Strategy

	Outcome	Description
1.	Children and young people are loved, safe and nurtured.	This includes loving homes that are free from violence, having time with family and *whānau*, and being safe from avoidable harm and accidents.
2.	Children and young people have what they need.	This includes income and resources, as well as other important aspects of material wellbeing such as nutritious food and quality housing.
3.	Children and young people are happy and healthy.	This includes physical and mental health, spaces and opportunities to play and healthy environments.
4.	Children and young people are learning and developing.	This includes education to build knowledge, skills and capabilities, and encouragement to achieve potential and navigate life's transitions.
5.	Children and young people are accepted, respected and connected.	This includes feeling a sense of belonging, living free from racism and discrimination, having good relationships and being connected to identity.
6.	Children and young people are involved and empowered.	This includes support to contribute, be listened to, care for others, make healthy choices and develop autonomy.

Source: Adapted from Department of the Prime Minister and Cabinet (2019, p. 30).

The Ministry of Children

The Ministry of Children, known as the Oranga Tamariki, is a New Zealand Government body that aims to support children and young people whose wellbeing is at risk. This service has changed its name over the years, beginning in the Child Welfare Division of the Department of Education. In 1972, the division was merged with the Social Security Department to form the Department of Social Welfare. Child, Youth and Family became a functional unit of the Ministry of Social Development (MSD) after the merge between the Department of Child, Youth and Family Services (CYFS) and MSD in 2006. Oranga Tamariki was established in 2017, and since that time has been focused towards improving the outcomes for Māori *tamariki* and their *whānau*. However, in May 2019 the work processes and practices of Oranga Tamariki were called into question during an attempt to uplift (remove) a newborn baby, *pēpi Māori*, to be taken into care, removing the baby from the breastfeeding mother. This event attracted media attention and there were several complaints and concerns raised about the treatment of Māori mothers and their *tamariki* when they were in contact with Oranga Tamariki. This event triggered a Māori-led inquiry into the way Oranga Tamariki works and the legislation, policies and practices that guide the work it does.

Whānau Ora

Led by prominent Māori figures, the Whānau Ora Commissioning Agency commenced an inquiry into Oranga Tamariki that recognised the need for urgent reform to improve the health outcomes and *whānau* wellbeing for Māori people (Whānau Ora 2019). Whānau Ora is jointly implemented by the Ministry of Health, Te Puni Kōkiri and the Ministry of Social Development. Whānau Ora describes its aim as putting '*whānau* and families in control of the services they need to work together, to build on their strengths and achieve their aspirations' (Te Puni Kōkiri, 2020). Within Whānau Ora, the 'collective strength and capability of *whānau* (Māori families) is recognised as the key to achieving better outcomes in areas such as income levels, health, employment, housing and education' (Te Puni Kōkiri, 2020). Whānau Ora puts *whānau* at the centre of decision-making about their future. Whānau Ora is considered to be a revolutionary approach because it transfers the delivery of services to community-based commissioning agencies, which has never been considered before. The community agencies are tasked with delivering customised support and services that are central to *whānau* wellbeing in collaboration with partners, providers and navigators. The Whānau Ora Outcomes Framework (Te Puni Kōkiri, 2016) was developed and agreed to by the Whānau Ora Partnership Group. It is considered to be the best practice measurement for determining the success of Whānau Ora strategies.

These seven outcomes are:

- self-managing
- living healthy lifestyles
- participating fully in society
- confidently participating in Te Ao Māori (the Māori world)
- economically secure and successfully involved in wealth creation
- cohesive, resilient and nurturing, and
- responsive to living and natural environments (Te Puni Kōkiri, 2016).

Te Puni Kōkiri is an agency that was established under the *Māori Development Act 1991*, with the aim of supporting and promoting Māori growth and achievement in a number of key areas, including health and wellbeing. Te Puni Kōkiri and the Commissioning Agencies are also engaged in the evaluation of the Whānau Ora service delivery model and its outcomes. Most importantly, they are responsible for monitoring and understanding what is actually being achieved for *whānau*.

Research reports are produced relating to the monitoring and evaluation outcomes and effectiveness of Whānau Ora, as this is a new evidence-based model evaluation for improvement and future developments in family-centred care. This will enable growth and development of future activities related to the work of Whānau Ora. Te Puni

Kōkiri publicly releases its reports, which provide valuable insights into the Whānau Ora commissioning agency model (Te Puni Kōkiri, n.d.).

Tamariki and *rangatahi* health and community services

The various frameworks and strategies that have been discussed within this section of the chapter are enacted within the health and community service provision for *tamariki* and *rangatahi*. Starting before birth, there are a range of services for a family expecting a new baby. After a child is born in Aotearoa, New Zealand, the Ministry of Health advises that the family enrol the child with a general practice. Within the general practice setting, visits to a doctor or practice nurse are usually free until the child turns 13, and include prescriptions for medicines. Immunisations begin at the age of 6 weeks via the child's general practice. The New Zealand immunisation schedule includes 'five immunisation visits for babies and children up to age 5 years: the first is at 6 weeks, then at 3 months, 5 months, 15 months and 4 years' (Ministry of Health, 2017a).

The Well Child Tamariki Ora Programme

The Well Child Tamariki Ora Programme is a free service that offers health visits to support all families in Aotearoa, New Zealand with children aged from 6 weeks to 5 years of age. The free Tamariki Ora visits include checks of child growth and development, family health and wellbeing, immunisation information, oral health checks, early childhood education, vision and hearing checks, and health and development checks for learning well at school (Ministry of Health, 2015). The Well Child Tamariki Ora health book supports families to engage with this free service, enabling the family to track their own child's developmental progress.

SmartStart

SmartStart is an online tool, developed and designed through a collaboration with the Department of Internal Affairs, the Ministry of Health, Inland Revenue and the Ministry of Social Development (NZ Digital Government, 2018). It also received feedback from industry experts, the New Zealand College of Midwives and Plunket New Zealand. SmartStart was launched in 2016 and is aimed at parents and caregivers who are preparing to have a baby (NZ Digital Government, 2018). The site provides 'online access to integrated government information', including information and support relevant to each stage of pregnancy as well as the first six months of a child's development (NZ Digital Government, 2018). SmartStart provides a platform where a parent or caregiver can create a profile of personalised timelines, adding key dates that are important to their personal journey. The resources provided include tips for supporting the health and wellbeing of the baby and the parents or caregivers, and contact details for organisations that can assist parents-to-be.

Plunket

Plunket is a national not-for-profit organisation that provides support services for the development, health and wellbeing of *tamariki* and *whānau*. Plunket has three main goals, which are supported by Māori principles: healthy *tamariki*, confident *whānau*, and connected communities. The three *kaupapa* principles of Plunket are: *Mohiotanga*, setting the foundation of knowledge; *Hononga*, building strategic partnerships and a collective approach; and *Raranga*, earning trust. Once these three principles are achieved, a fourth *kaupapa* can be realised: *Mana Taurite*, equitable access and outcomes for Māori *whānau* (Plunket, 2021).

Kids Health NZ

Kids Health aims to deliver reliable information to families, caregivers and parents about the health of their children. It has a wide range of resources and connects parents and caregivers with wider networks including the Ministry of Health Programmes. Included within this site is important information related to disability services, information and support. The A–Z directory enables parents and caregivers to explore questions they may have across the life of their growing child. There are also resources for when unexpected events occur, including injury, accidental death, terminal illness, palliative care and end-of-life support.

CASE STUDY 3.1

It is your first week in a new position at Counties Manukau DHB, at Middlemore Hospital. You attend your orientation and you wonder what you might need to know about caring for the *whānau* in your health district. In your orientation, you learn that Middlemore Hospital has a Kidzfirst Paediatric Inpatient Service and that there are a range of services dedicated to helping Māori children and young people.

Your first shift is in the emergency department, where you meet a 12-year-old girl called Kahurangi, who identifies as being of Māori descent. Kahurangi is attending the department with her female non-kin caregiver after recently collapsing at home. Kahurangi has been in short-term care for three months, and is reported not to have been eating well. Her caregiver is worried that there is something wrong with Kahurangi, and wants to make sure she is okay. She has noticed that Kahurangi has been missing school and doesn't seem to be interested in anything that they try to do as a *whānau*. The caregiving family has three other children for whom they care, who are not related to Kahurangi.

You try to talk to Kahurangi to develop a therapeutic relationship, and to undertake clinical assessments. Kahurangi is reluctant to talk, doesn't make eye contact and shrugs her shoulders when you ask questions. You direct your questions to her caregiver, but she can't answer all of them as she doesn't know Kahurangi's past medical history or much about her life story.

Whānau stories

The Māori Inquiry into Oranga Tamariki was about *whānau* first and foremost. It aimed to hear the stories of pain and trauma experienced by people and their *whānau* when they come into contact with government services, but also to hear about their vision, hopes and aspirations for a better future for *tamariki* and *rangatahi*. The Māori-led team listened to *whānau* stories as a way to learn what had happened and what was continuing to happen. Trauma that had spanned generations of *whānau* was the most common theme emerging throughout the inquiry. Whānau stories included expressions of grief, depression, hopelessness and suicide when they had a *tamariki* uplifted or they had been uplifted themselves (Whānau Ora, 2019).

REFLECTION POINTS 3.1

Many of the experiences of Māori *whānau* who have had interactions with Oranga Tamariki are sharing their stories to demonstrate what has gone wrong with a system that was meant to protect Māori children. Often services think they know what is best, but their decisions can have lifelong impacts.

- What might be some of the contributing factors to Kahurangi not engaging with you as a healthcare professional?
- How might you overcome some of the barriers to effectively caring for Kahurangi?
- As a nurse, what role can you have in supporting children and young people to have the best outcomes from interaction with child services?

Aboriginal and Torres Strait Islander children and young people

In Aboriginal and Torres Strait Islander culture, birthing babies is women's business and, just as babies are born to their mothers, many Aboriginal and Torres Strait Islander children are also born to Mother Earth – or Country as it is referred to in Australia.

In an Aboriginal and Torres Strait Islander worldview, Country is not just dirt or earth. Country is everything in existence: the trees, the plants, the animals, the insects, the weather, the rocks, the mountains, the water, the air and the celestial bodies. Aboriginal babies are born into both a cultural understanding of the interconnectedness of all things in existence, and also into specific cultural relationships:

> Our Elders teach us 'We are this Country', Country is us, we are Country. We breathe Country, we drink Country, we eat Country, we live Country. Country is everything, without Country there is not life. So, we sing Country, we dance Country, we care for Country, we re-energise Country. In so doing, through giving 'thanks' we also re-energise ourselves and everything in existence. (Magick Dennis & Keedle, 2019)

Many Aboriginal women, families and communities have been fighting for the right to birth their babies according to their cultural beliefs and values. The term 'Birthing on Country' has been coined to represent this movement, which is about championing the best start in life for babies, their mothers, families and the whole community. Birthing on Country strives to return birthing decisions to Aboriginal communities, thus enabling the communities to create culturally safe birthing that cares for the **wholistic health** of babies, mothers, families and the wider community. (Note that when we place a 'w' in front of 'holistic' it helps us reflect on what the process, design and collaboration could look like in its entire 'whole approach'.)

Historical journey

In the early days of colonisation, local Aboriginal women were relied upon as a source of midwifery knowledge to assist all women, including non-Aboriginal women, during childbirth (Barber, 1999; Gilmore, 1934). When hospitals were eventually built in townships, Aboriginal women were prohibited from giving birth in those hospitals, as the maternity wards were only for white women 'settlers'. Australia actively practised segregation by disallowing Aboriginal women access to maternity wards and services. Awareness of the breakdown of the cultural knowledge on birthing for some Aboriginal communities meant they needed to access other birthing practices. Aboriginal women were sometimes allowed to give birth under a tree outside the hospital, or on the verandah of the hospital or 'segregated to an iron shed at the back which could be hot or cold' (Jones, 2012, p. 104). In many hospitals, Aboriginal women's linen was marked and washed separately so that the women settlers did not have to use the same linen as the Aboriginal women.

The setting up of a penal colony in Australia by the Europeans was also the invasion of the country. Aboriginal babies and children were stolen from their families and Country (birth place) by the European settlers and the authorities. The process of stealing Aboriginal children was informal in the early days and then became a formal, systematic part of Australian law and policy under the 1915 amendments to the *Aborigines Protection Act 1909*. This meant that the NSW Aborigines Protection Board had the power to remove any Aboriginal and or Torres Strait Islander child at any time and for any reason. This practice became widespread, creating what is now known as the Stolen Generations; it involved thousands of Aboriginal and Torres Strait Islander babies, children and young people.

The unjust and systemic process of removal of our Aboriginal children continues today, and the systems in place continue to cite the reason for removal as being the alleged incapacity of Aboriginal and Torres Strait Islander people to parent our own children to the satisfaction of the Western legal system. The historical conduct of non-Aboriginal people towards Aboriginal children and families has left a legacy of genocide and violence in Australian history. Living through such genocide and violence has caused trans-generational and inter-generational trauma of individuals and their communities. This is a result of the compounding of the historical violence

Wholistic health – An Aboriginal lens for looking at health that is broader than just physical and mental health through a Western lens, including spiritual, emotional, social and cultural wellbeing (identity and the ability to practise culture), health of Country, and its relationship and connection to our health – whether limiting or not.

that has not been able to heal, with living and ongoing systemic racism and traumas that are enacted against Aboriginal children, families and the wider Aboriginal and Torres Strait Islander communities today. This legacy of violence and genocide affects all Australians, not just Aboriginal and Torres Strait Islander Australians and their children.

The historical violence and genocide have been woven into the present-day Dreaming of every Aboriginal and or Torres Strait Islander person. According to Aboriginal beliefs, we all have the power to create new Dreaming for our Aboriginal and Torres Strait Islander children and for all our children in Australia. Aboriginal cultural belief systems also hold a way of looking at the world that could potentially improve all relationships and the conduct of all human beings towards all of existence.

A national survey of Aboriginal families across Australia in 2014 used qualitative research methods to identify strengths of Aboriginal cultural practices that contribute to Aboriginal child and family health (Lohoar, Butera and Kennedy, 2014). Aboriginal family life and child-rearing are enhanced when certain characteristics that are held as integral to Aboriginal family life are featured. These are:

- a collective community focus on child-rearing
- the opportunity for children to explore the world around them
- elderly family members who are valued for their contributions to their family
- a sense of identity based on engagement with spiritual practices (Lohoar, Butera and Kennedy, 2014).

The challenge for health professionals and other service providers lies in having the communication skills and knowledge to be able to assess strengths-based services that are culturally appropriate and safe for Aboriginal and Torres Strait Islander families and to build on community strengths instead of looking at the deficits.

The health status of Aboriginal and Torres Strait Islander children and young people

The historical legacy outlined above continues to impact and influence Aboriginal and Torres Strait Islander people, their families and communities, even to the present day. The disproportionate health outcomes for Aboriginal and Torres Strait Islander children and young people relate to widespread socioeconomic burdens and health inequalities as well as inequities compared with the wider population (AIHW, 2018; Commonwealth of Australia, 2013). The health outcomes that you will see as a clinician result from a complex interplay between the determinants of historical, social, financial, environmental and cultural factors, among many others. It is not just about determinants of health, but about the factors that have entwined to create impacts and cycles of generations of oppression and poverty. The social determinants of health are widely accepted and understood. As clinicians, it is about listening and developing skills and practices that will enable us to work with Aboriginal and Torres Strait Islander people to achieve better outcomes overall.

The inequality between the health status of and care for Aboriginal and Torres Strait Islander children and non-Aboriginal Australians has been documented extensively. Wise (2013, p. 3) states that:

> one of Australia's greatest challenges is the elimination of the gap between the developmental outcomes of Aboriginal and Torres Strait Islander children to non-Aboriginal children in the early years of life. Not only is eliminating inequality and inequities a fundamental moral responsibility, but child development is also a determinant of health, wellbeing and learning skills across the balance of the life-course and therefore critical for Australia's progress.

Research by Education Services Australia Ltd (2010) shows that early childhood development needs a collaborative and intersectional approach in policies to safeguard all children so they will have equal opportunities to flourish and prosper in order to address 'Closing the Gap' goals (Department of the Prime Minister and Cabinet, 2020). One way to achieve these outcomes is through the evidence-based Family Matters building blocks (see Box 3.3).

BOX 3.3 FAMILY MATTERS BUILDING BLOCKS

1. All families enjoy access to quality, culturally safe, universal and targeted services necessary for Aboriginal and Torres Strait Islander children to thrive.
2. Aboriginal and Torres Strait Islander people and organisations participate in and have control over decisions that affect their children.
3. Law, policy and practice in child and family welfare are culturally safe and responsive.
4. Governments and services are accountable to Aboriginal and Torres Strait Islander people.

Source: Family Matters (2021).

Until this can be acknowledged and addressed, Aboriginal and Torres Strait Islander children will remain over-represented in out-of-home care (SNAICC, 2019). Aboriginal and Torres Strait Islander children continue to be incarcerated at unacceptable rates (Brown, 2020), and continue to have significantly poorer health than other children (Lowitja Institute 2020; SNAICC & NATSILS 2012). Figure 3.1 provides a visual of key data from 2020.

There are serious concerns about the overall mental health and wellbeing of our Aboriginal and Torres Strait Islander children. Suicide was the leading cause of death for Aboriginal and Torres Strait Islander children aged 5–17 years between 2015 and 2019 (ABS, 2019).

Figure 3.2 shows some of the issues and solutions proposed by Aboriginal community-run organisations. It emphasises the importance of youth learning about culture and Elders being able to hand down key cultural knowledge.

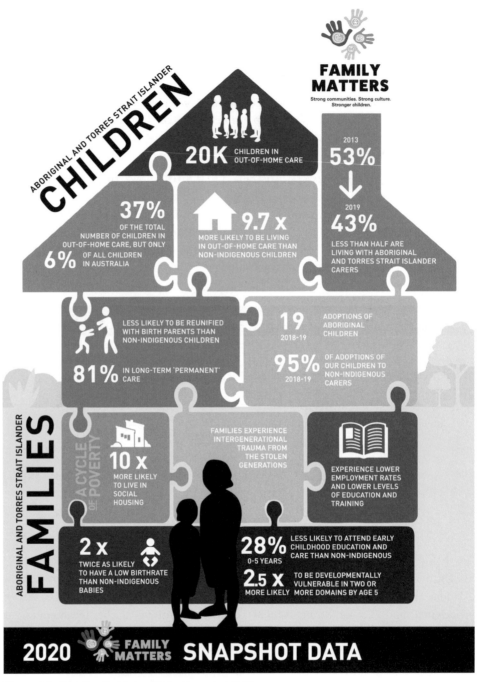

Figure 3.1   The Family Matters Data Snapshot 2020

Source: Reproduced from SNAICC (2020).

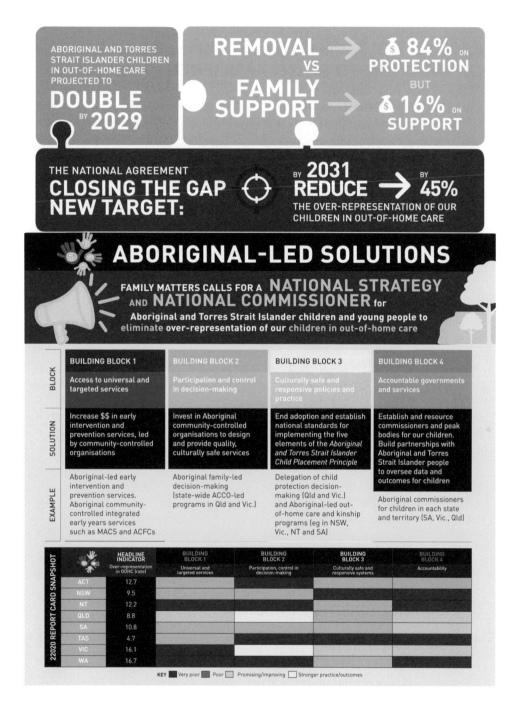

Figure 3.2   2020 Report Card Snapshot: The Solutions, The Family Matters Data Snapshot 2020
Source: Reproduced from SNAICC (2020).

CASE STUDY 3.2 LOTTIE: ESTABLISHING CONNECTION TO BUILD RESILIENCE

Lottie is a 5-year-old who lives in a small remote community. She is the youngest of five children. Her mother, Molly, is an artist and her father works for the local council. Lottie's immunisation is up to date and the community's immunisation is around 98 per cent for young people. This is due to the work of Aboriginal health workers and health professionals (such as nurses and doctors) who visit the school and family members who have had babies. A number of lifestyle factors impact the growth and development of Lottie and her siblings. Some of the issues include:

- poor access to fresh foods in community shop (processed food is five times cheaper)
- running water in her home does not work well (due to plumbing issues and lack of access to a good plumber)
- overcrowding (relatives and extended family often stay and visit)
- education (Lottie's pre-school has a high turnover of teachers).

As a nurse in the community, what other issues (lifestyle factors) can you think of that might affect Lottie and her siblings?

In many Aboriginal and Torres Strait Islander communities, the above issues are outside the control of the families. It is important to look at the big picture and apply a wholistic approach when considering the impacts on Lottie's growth and development. This allows practitioners to create outcomes that meet the needs not just of Lottie and her siblings, but the whole community, as the definition of Aboriginal health reflects.

After reading the case study, what is one way that you, as a nurse working in the community, can advocate on behalf of the family and community?

Cultural determinants of health

The National Aboriginal Health Strategy (NAHS) provides the following definition of health:

> Aboriginal health is not just the physical well-being of an individual but refers to the social, emotional and cultural well-being of the whole community in which each individual is able to achieve their full potential as a human being, thereby bringing about the total well-being of their community. It is a whole-of-life view and includes the cyclical concept of life-death-life. (cited in Gee et al., 2014, p. 56)

Brown (n.d.) explains cultural determinants of health as 'acknowledg[ing] the extensive and well-established knowledge networks that exist within communities, the National Aboriginal Community Controlled Health Organisation (NACCHO) movement, human rights and social justice sectors' and suggests that these are 'consistent with the thematic approach to the Articles of the United Nations Declaration on the Rights of Indigenous Peoples (UNDRIP)'.

Cultural determinants include:

- self-determination
- freedom from discrimination
- individual and collective rights
- freedom from assimilation and destruction of culture
- protection from removal/relocation
- connection to, custodianship, and utilisation of Country and traditional lands
- Reclamation, revitalisation, preservation and promotion of lanuage and cultural practices
- Protection and promotion of traditional knowledge and Aboriginal and Torres Strait Islander intellectual property
- understanding of lore, law and traditional roles and responsibilities. (NACCHO, 2013, cited in Brown, n.d.)

This is seen in programs such as child ear health in Ceduna Koonibba Aboriginal Health Service Aboriginal Corporation, where the organisation identified that it could improve its service by increasing screening and training to have early detection and management of middle ear disease. It included the South Australian Department of Education, a multidisciplinary team from the child health team at the Aboriginal health service, local childcare centres and the local hospital, all working to achieve the best outcome measures for the population of Aboriginal children (NACCHO, 2018, p. 23).

REFLECTION POINTS 3.2

- Aboriginal and Torres Strait Islander children have lower health outcomes than their non-Aboriginal and Torres Strait Islander counterparts.
- Closing the Gap requires engagement with Aboriginal and Torres Strait Islander people, communities and organisations.
- Watch the Close the Gap TEDx talk (Fitzpatrick, 2015) and reflect on the way engagement was used to help Close the Gap. What roles had to alter for the change in outcomes from the community and staff? List the adverse impacts of social and cultural factors. What do you think about their protective effects?

Cultural safety in paediatric nursing practice

Drawing from the many Aboriginal and Torres Strait Islander ways of knowing, being and doing, parents have an understanding of 'what works' to keep our children from harm and nurture them. Most significant is being an active participant in their family and community. There are many obstacles such as racism, cultural disconnection, intergenerational trauma and family disruption. The inequalities and inequities confronted by many Aboriginal and Torres Strait Islander families and communities are now broadly recognised, as is the need for an ongoing commitment to building awareness, learning, education and training that is embedded in cultural safety (Bowes & Grace, 2014; Close the Gap Steering Committee, 2010; Price-Robertson & McDonald, 2011).

Roles of health professionals working with Aboriginal and/or Torres Strait Islander children, their families and the wider community

As healthcare professionals caring for Aboriginal and Torres Strait Islander children, we carry enormous responsibility and the potential to not only improve the health of the children for whom we care, but also to help enable empowerment to make improvements in their health in a more wholistic sense, including their family, their community, their ongoing health into adulthood and that of future generations. It is a privilege as healthcare professionals in this field that we hold and should honour. We may not all have the ability to influence social or political policies, but we can understand the role they play; advocate when we can in our position of power, privilege and influence; and ensure that our interactions are respectful and collaborative. This influence on a child is especially important in the early years of childhood. Enormous work has been done through the National Framework for the Health Services for Aboriginal and Torres Strait Islanders (Department of Health, 2016) that explains the significance of the development from conception to early childhood in providing a strong establishment for lifelong wholistic health and wellbeing.

According to this document, care for Aboriginal and Torres Strait Islander children should be characterised by:

- access to culturally safe and competent services
- health services that are evidence-based, strengths-based and accountable
- collaboration between primary, secondary and tertiary services with Aboriginal and Torres Strait Islander communities and organisations, and with other sectors such as housing, justice and education services.
- development of Aboriginal and Torres Strait Islander healthcare professionals within the broader workforce that supports their cultural safety in the health system.
- trust and rapport that allow effective therapeutic relationships to be built over time (Department of Health, 2016).

The roles of Aboriginal and Torres Strait Islander health workers and health practitioners are invaluable when working with Aboriginal and Torres Strait Islander children and families and it is important to understand and respect their roles as healthcare practitioners. Depending upon the work setting and individual scope of practice, they can provide a range of health services, ranging from clinical services, health promotion, advocacy and language interpretation to health management and education of other health practitioners (Department of Health, 2016).

We need to tap into our Dreaming to respond to the challenges and changes that need to occur around us and within us, our families and communities for positive change to be addressed. We need to approach political leaders to champion change as well as meet the challenges head on. As nurses in the field of paediatric nursing, the challenge is *Ganna* (listening) from Bundjalung, meaning listening with not just your ears but with understanding, and advocating, supporting and networking to develop relationships and a sense of rapport with children, their carer/s and the key people around them who have influence.

Establishment of Aboriginal organisations and services including Aboriginal Community Controlled Organisations for self-determination

In 1971, the first Aboriginal Medical Service (AMS) in Redfern, also known as an **Aboriginal Community Controlled Health Service (ACCHS)**, was established as a reflection of the aspirations of Aboriginal and Torres Strait Islander people for **self-determination**. ACCHSs work on the social and cultural determinants of health, and were a response to the urgent need to provide decent, accessible and culturally safe health services for the expanding and mostly medically uninsured Aboriginal and Torres Strait Islander populations around the country.

Figure 3.3 shows the community-based establishment of Aboriginal and Torres Strait Islander health organisations working together to meet the needs and advocate better outcomes for their communities. A number of the organisations and structure of Aboriginal health organisations historically come from humble beginnings in Redfern. Over time, the national body, NACCHO, has been developed from these. Figure 3.3 shows only some of the structures, such as the Aboriginal Health & Medical Research Council (AH&MRC) of New South Wales, which has four membership regions across New South Wales: Metropolitan, Northern, Southern and Western. This is an example of a state-based service, in contrast to our national body, NACCHO, which has a number of affiliates.

Aboriginal Community Controlled Health Service (ACCHS) – Non-profit incorporated Aboriginal Community Controlled Health Organisations (ACCHOs) that deliver 'holistic and culturally appropriate primary healthcare and Aboriginal health related services to the communities they serve' (AH&MRC, 2019). An ACCHS is managed by an Aboriginal board elected by local Aboriginal and Torres Strait Islander community membership.

Self-determination – The right of Aboriginal and Torres Strait Islander people to control our own lives and develop our own futures for ourselves, as championed in the United Nations Declaration on the Rights of Indigenous Peoples. Evidence shows self-determination is essential to benefit the health of every Aboriginal and Torres Strait Islander person (Queensland Aboriginal and Islander Health Council, 2020, p. 1).

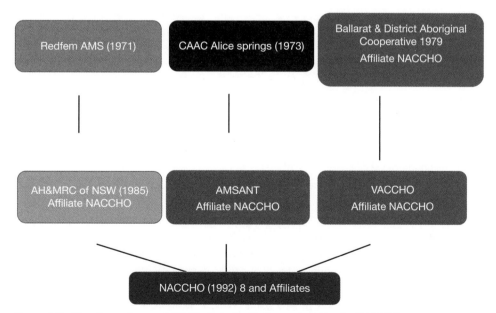

Figure 3.3   Structure of some ACCHOs linked with the national body, NACCHO

SUMMARY

- There are several layers within the New Zealand healthcare system that are designed to drive better outcomes for Māori *tamariki* and *rangatahi*. However, it is clear that change is needed to meet the needs of Māori families. Māori families, or *whānau*, must be central to the health and wellbeing of the Māori child and young person, and must have the resources to meet the determinants of good health for the growing child.

- Although services exist that are aimed at providing culturally safe care to Māori *whānau*, it has become evident through *whānau* stories that Māori needs are not being considered or met when it comes to effective and timely support for mothers and their *tamariki* and *rangatahi*.

- Throughout this chapter, we have emphasised various ways to look through the lens of Aboriginal and Torres Strait Islander children's connections and worldviews to create appropriate ways to look at doing, being and knowing through the interconnection of children and their families, as well as the involvement of community in raising and developing Aboriginal and Torres Strait Islander children.

- There are many obstacles to the health and wellbeing of Aboriginal and Torres Strait Islander children, and it is only by listening and working together with their family members and the wider Aboriginal and Torres Strait Islander communities that change can occur.

- Using the resources of Aboriginal and Torres Strait Islander people, and research and funding from the health sector, in communities and other services can result in better outcomes.

- Paediatric health practitioners must use a culturally safe and sensitive manner to address racism, oppression and the marginalisation of our most vulnerable Aboriginal, Torres Strait Islander and Māori children, their families and communities.

LEARNING ACTIVITIES

3.1 Read through the New Zealand government *Child and Youth Wellbeing Strategy 2019* (Department of the Prime Minister and Cabinet, 2019).
  - What are some key features of the vision that stand out to you?
  - What were two existing relevant models and frameworks considered in developing the current strategy?
  - What were some methods used to ensure that the strategy was culturally safe for Māori people?

3.2 Read through some of the reports from The Longitudinal Study of Indigenous Children (LSIC, also known as *Footprints in Time* – Department of Social Services, 2021). How children connect with those around them is key to their development and growth.
  - Draw a diagram of your connections when you were a child, showing what was significant to your connections about your development – whether it is family, community, sports, and so on. Draw in another colour the disconnections that would be experienced by the experiences if you were from the Stolen Generations.

Write down your feelings and try to explain why you have these feelings. Explain what determinants maybe impacted.

3.3 Consider which key points from this chapter resonate with you and why. Explain this to a fellow student or friend in a few sentences.

3.4 Think about what this chapter has taught you about the historical context of the health systems in New Zealand and Australia. List the similarities and differences in relation to how they assist Māori, and Aboriginal and Torres Strait Islander children and their families.

ACKNOWLEDGEMENTS

The authors would like to thank Marilyn Clarke for her contribution to the early drafts of this chapter.

FURTHER READING

The New Zealand Ministry of Health provides a range of resources developed to support the health and wellbeing of Māori *tamariki* and *rangatahi* and their *whānau*. This site is updated regularly with reports regarding the recent inquiries, which are freely available online:

- Ministry of Health website: Publications: www.health.govt.nz/publications
- Overview of the New Zealand Health and Disability System: www.health.govt.nz/new-zealand-health-system/overview-health-system?mega=NZ%20health%20system &title= Overview

Information and resources related to Te Tiriti o Waitangi and the Treaty of Waitangi can be found via the website: www.health.govt.nz/our-work/populations/maori-health/te-tiriti-o-waitangi

In addition, a range of groups and organisations regularly publish updates and reports about specific conditions or health priorities. To read more information on the Māori inquiry into Oranga Tamariki, see: https://whanauora.nz/wp-content/uploads/2021/06/OT-REVIEW-REPORT.pdf

The Australian Institute of Aboriginal and Torres Strait Islander Studies Map of Indigenous Australia demonstrates the cultural diversity of Aboriginal and Torres Strait Islander peoples, their languages and their regions: https://aiatsis.gov.au/explore/map-indigenous-australia

The Australian Institute of Family Studies has a useful website to learn more about some of the characteristics of traditional Aboriginal and Torres Strait Islander cultural practices that contribute to effective family functioning, and how these practices can have positive effects on children and communities (Lohoar, Butera & Kennedy (2014), see https://aifs.gov.au/cfca/sites/default/files/publication-documents/cfca25.pdf

The AHPRA Statement of Intent is a joint agreement between AHPRA and a number of other organisations relating to its visions and values for Aboriginal and Torres Strait Islander healthcare: www.ahpra.gov.au/About-AHPRA/Aboriginal-and-Torres-Strait-Islander-Health-Strategy/Statement-of-intent.aspx

REFERENCES

Aboriginal Health and Medical Research Council of NSW (AH&MRC) 2019, About, viewed 2 February 2021, www.ahmrc.org.au/about

Australian Bureau of Statistics (ABS) 2019, *Causes of death, Australia: Statistics on the number of deaths, by sex, selected age groups, and cause of death classified to the international Classification of Disease (ICD)*, viewed 2 February 2021, www.abs.gov .au/statistics/health/causes-death/causes-death-australia/latest-release

Australian Health Practitioner Regulation Agency (AHPRA) & National Boards 2020, *Aboriginal and Torres Strait Islander health and cultural safety strategy 2020–2025*, AHPRA, Sydney.

Australian Indigenous Doctors' Association (AIDA) 2018, *Cultural safety factsheet*, AIDA, Canberra.

Australian Institute of Health and Welfare (AIHW) 2018, *Australia's health 2018: In brief*, cat. no. AUS222, AIHW, Canberra.

Barber, J A. 1999, Concerning Our National Honour: Florence Nightingale and the Welfare of Aboriginal Australians, Collegian: Journal of the Royal College of Nursing Australia, 6(1), 36–9.

Bowes, J & Grace, R 2014, *Review of early childhood parenting, education and health intervention programs for Indigenous children and families in Australia*, Closing the Gap Clearinghouse, Canberra.

Brown, L 2020, In my blood it runs: Challenges the inevitability of Indigenous youth incarceration, *The Conversation*, 2 July, viewed 2 February 2021, https:// theconversation.com/in-my-blood-it-runs-challenges-the-inevitability-of-indigenous-youth-incarceration-140624

Brown, N n.d., Promoting a social and cultural determinants approach to Aboriginal and Torres Strait Islander affairs, *Checkup,* viewed 2 February 2021, www.checkup.org .au/icms_docs/183362_Prof_Ngiare_Brown.pdf

Close the Gap Steering Committee for Indigenous Health Equality 2010, *Shadow report: On the Australian Government's progress towards closing the gap in life expectancy between Indigenous and non-Indigenous Australians*: Oxfam Australia, Sydney.

Common Ground 2021, First Nations, Aboriginal and Torres Strait Islander, or Indigenous?, Common Ground, 28 January, viewed 2 February 2021, www.commonground.org .au/learn/aboriginal-or-indigenous

Commonwealth of Australia 2013, *National Aboriginal and Torres Strait Islander Health Plan 2013–2023: Closing the Gap*, Commonwealth of Australia, Canberra.

Department of Health 2016, *National Framework for Health Services for Aboriginal and Torres Strait Islander Children and Families*, Australian Government, Canberra, viewed 2 February 2021, www.coaghealthcouncil.gov.au/Portals/0/National% 20Framework%20for%20Health%20Services%20for%20Aboriginal%20and% 20Torres%20Strait%20Islander%20Children%20and%20Families.pdf

Department of the Prime Minister and Cabinet 2019, *Child and youth wellbeing strategy,* Australian Government, Canberra, viewed 2 February 2021, https:// childyouthwellbeing.govt.nz/sites/default/files/2019-08/child-youth-wellbeing-strategy-2019.pdf

—— 2020. *Closing the Gap Report 2020*, Australian Government, Canberra, viewed 2 February 2021, https://ctgreport.niaa.gov.au/sites/default/files/pdf/closing-the-gap-report-2020.pdf

Department of Social Services, 2021, *Footprints in Time - The Longitudinal Study of Indigenous Children (LSIC),* Australian Government, Canberra, viewed 2 February 2021, www.dss.gov.au/about-the-department/publications-articles/research-publications/longitudinal-data-initiatives/footprints-in-time-the-longitudinal-study-of-indigenous-children-lsic

Education Services Australia for the Ministerial Council for Education, Early Childhood Development and Youth Affairs (MCEECDYA) 2010, *Engaging families in the early childhood development story*, Early Childhood Service, Department of Education and Children's Services, Adelaide.

Family Matters 2021, Our vision, viewed 2 February 2021, www.familymatters.org.au/our-vision

Fitzpatrick, J, 2015, *Close the Gap*, TEDxPerth, viewed 2 February 2021, www.youtube.com/watch?v=EEJbB-Ke2tc

Gee, G, Dudgeon, P, Schultz, C, Hart, A & Kelly, K 2014, Aboriginal and Torres Strait Islander social and emotional wellbeing, in P Dudgeon, H Milroy & R Walker (eds), *Working together: Aboriginal and Torres Strait Islander mental health and wellbeing principles and practices*, Commonwealth of Australia, Canberra, pp. 55–68.

Gilmore, M 1934, *Old days, old ways: A book of recollections*, Angus & Robertson, Sydney.

Hauora Report 2019, *Report on stage one of the Health Services and Outcomes Kaupapa Inquiry*, Waitangi Tribunal, Lower Hutt, viewed 2 February 2021, https://forms.justice.govt.nz/search/Documents/WT/wt_DOC_152801817/Hauora%20W.pdf

Jones, JN 2012, Birthing: Aboriginal women, *Journal of Indigenous Policy*, 13, pp. 103–9.

Lohoar, S, Butera, N & Kennedy, E 2014, *Strengths of Australian Aboriginal cultural practices in family life and child rearing*, Australian Institute of Family Studies, Canberra.

Lowitja Institute 2020, *We nurture our culture for the future, and our culture nurtures us, Close the Gap Steering Committee*, Lowitja Institute, Melbourne, viewed 2 February 2021, https://humanrights.gov.au/our-work/aboriginal-and-torres-strait-islander-social-justice/publications/close-gap-2020

Magick Dennis, F & Keedle, H 2019, Birthing as Country, *Women and birth*, 32, pp. 383–90.

Ministry of Health 2015, Well child Tamariki Ora visits, viewed 2 February 2021, www.health.govt.nz/your-health/pregnancy-and-kids/first-year/6-weeks-6-months/well-child-tamariki-ora-visits.

—— 2017a, Immunise your child, viewed 2 February 2021, www.health.govt.nz/your-health/pregnancy-and-kids/services-and-support-you-and-your-child/immunise-your-child

—— 2017b, Overview of the health system, viewed 2 February 2021, www.health.govt.nz/new-zealand-health-system/overview-health-system

—— 2020a, *Indicator of potentially avoidable hospitalisations for the Child and Youth Wellbeing Strategy: A brief report on methodology*, Ministry of Health, Wellington, viewed 2 February 2021, www.health.govt.nz/publication/indicator-potentially-avoidable-hospitalisations-child-and-youth-wellbeing-strategy-brief-report

—— 2020b, *Wai 2575 Health Services and Outcomes Kaupapa Inquiry*, viewed 2 February 2021, www.health.govt.nz/our-work/populations/maori-health/wai-2575-health-services-and-outcomes-kaupapa-inquiry

—— 2020c, *Ministry of Health Annual Report for the year ended 30 June 2020*, viewed 2 February 2021, www.health.govt.nz/system/files/documents/publications/ministry-of-health-annual-report_2020.pdf

Moeke-Maxwell, T, Mason, K, Toohey, F & Dudley, J 2019, Pou Aroha: An Indigenous Perspective of Māori Palliative Care, Aotearoa New Zealand. In RD. MacLeod & L Van den Block (eds), *Textbook of Palliative Care*, Cham: Springer, pp. 1247–63.

National Aboriginal Community Controlled Health Organisation (NACCHO) 2013, *Official Records of the General Assembly, Sixty-first Session, Supplement No. 53 (A/61/53), part one, chap. II, sect. A. NACCHO Intervention on Indigenous Health Equality to the 12th Session of the UNPFII, New York,* viewed 2 February 2021, www.checkup.org.au/icms_docs/183362_Prof_Ngiare_Brown.pdf

—— 2018, *National Framework for Quality improvement in Primary Health Care for Aboriginal and Torres Strait Islander People 2018–2023*, NACCHO, Canberra.

NZ Digital Government 2018, SmartStart a new type of service, viewed 2 February 2021, www.digital.govt.nz/showcase/smartstart-a-new-type-of-service

Papps, E & Ramsden, I 1996, Cultural safety in nursing: The New Zealand experience, *International Journal for Quality in Health Care,* 8(5), pp. 491–7.

Plunket 2021, Our vision and our mission, viewed 2 February 2021, www.plunket.org.nz/plunket/about-plunket/who-we-are/our-vision-and-mission

Price-Robertson, R & McDonald, M 2011, *Working with Indigenous children, families and communities: Lessons from practice*, Communities and Families Clearinghouse, Canberra.

Queensland Aboriginal and Islander Health Council 2020, Submission DR173, viewed 2 February 2021, www.pc.gov.au/__data/assets/pdf_file/0008/255608/subdr173-indigenous-evaluation.pdf

Simpson, J et al. 2017, *Te Ohonga Ake: The health status of Māori children and young people in New Zealand.* New Zealand Child and Youth Epidemiology Service, Wellington, viewed 2 February 2021, http://hdl.handle.net/10523/7390

Secretariat of National Aboriginal and Islander Child (SNAICC) 2020, *The Family Matters data snapshot 2020*, viewed 2 February 2021, www.familymatters.org.au/wp-content/uploads/2020/11/FamilyMatters2020SnapshotData.pdf

SNAICC – National Voice for our Children 2019, *The Family Matters report, 2019*, viewed 2 February 2021, www.familymatters.org.au/the-family-matters-report-2019

SNAICC & NATSILS [National Aboriginal and Torres Strait Islander Legal Services] 2012, *Aboriginal and Torres Strait Islander Child Rights Report Card*, viewed 2 February 2021, www.snaicc.org.au/wp-content/uploads/2015/12/02918.pdf

Te Puni Kōkiri 2016, *The Whānau Ora outcomes framework: Empowering whānau into the future*, viewed 2 February 2021, www.tpk.govt.nz/docs/tpk-wo-outcomesframework-aug2016.pdf

—— 2020, Whānau Ora, viewed 2 February 2021, www.tpk.govt.nz/en/whakamahia/whanau-ora

—— n.d., Publications about Whānau Ora, viewed 2 February 2021, www.tpk.govt.nz/en/a-matou-mohiotanga/whanau-ora

UNICEF 2018, *Annual Report 2017*, viewed 2 February 2021, www.unicef.org/media/47861/file/UNICEF_Annual_Report_2017-ENG.pdf

Whānau Ora 2019, *Whānau story: Orange Tamariki – Porirua*, viewed 2 February 2021, https://whanauora.nz/successstories/whanau-story-oranga-tamariki-2

Wise, S 2013, *Improving the early life outcomes of Indigenous children: Implementing early childhood development at the local level*, Closing the Gap Clearinghouse, Canberra.

Legislation cited

Aborigines Protection Act 1909 (Aust)

Māori Development Act 1991 (NZ)

New Zealand Public Health and Disability Act 2000 (NZ)

State Owned Enterprises Act 1986 (NZ)

4

Research with children and youth

Donna Waters

LEARNING OBJECTIVES

In this chapter you will:

- Review the definitions of research, evidence and evidence-based practice and discuss how these interact with person- and family-centred approaches to care
- Explore the core principles of human research ethics and research governance in relation to researching with children and young people
- Develop your knowledge of safe and meaningful research co-design with children and youth, and reflect on how you can use this knowledge to support your own research development and evidence-based practice improvements in care

Introduction

To understand how we can more fully engage with children and young people to discover which research and services are important to them, we first need to understand our own use of language relating to research and evidence. As health professionals, there are two main pathways by which findings from research can be shared with children and young people, and then collectively implemented in practice. First, new knowledge from research is continuously added to the health professionals' bank of clinical understanding and expertise, influencing their individual approach to care. At other times, this new knowledge may be so compelling as to demand a change to practice. It is through this constant exchange of gaining and applying knowledge in partnership with children, young people and their families that research and evidence are intimately linked, thus becoming prioritised and contextualised as 'best practice'.

In this chapter, we will broadly distinguish research as a process for deriving new knowledge, and evidence as the knowledge that is produced and used within a specific context. Evidence from other sources (not research) is also used to inform health and treatment decisions. These often subtle differences can be confusing to those entering the world of evidence-based practice as the word 'evidence' can be used broadly to encompass all forms of evidence, or specifically to refer only to evidence that derives from quality research. When navigating the healthcare setting, it is sometimes difficult to understand which context is being used.

We will also introduce audit and benchmarking as important tools for measuring healthcare quality and safety, and discuss their relevance to the generation of clinical research questions. Within the construct of research co-design and evidence-based decision-making, this chapter will also discuss special considerations for conducting ethical research with children and young people. Acknowledging that there may be age or developmental challenges, we will explore ways in which children and young people can be supported to become more involved in setting their own research priorities and designing and 'doing' research.

Research and evidence

What is research?

Research is a systematic and rigorous process used for the generation of new knowledge. A simple way to decide whether or not something is research is to critically appraise the research method to determine whether it is sufficiently systematic and rigorous to produce a valid result. Only then is it possible to ask what these results contribute that was not known before (generation of new knowledge). This is why the very successful *User's Guides to the Medical Literature* series (see the JAMA Network online) has consistently recommended assessing the quality of research studies by first asking 'Are the results of the study valid?' before moving to 'What are the results?' and 'Can they be applied in my practice?' Clearly, if the research methods are not valid, there will always be uncertainty about the knowledge generated, with potential negative impacts on practice, inefficiency and possibly even harm.

Research – A systematic and rigorous process for the generation of new knowledge.

Generating new knowledge through research

Methodology – Analysis of the approach, practices, activities, sampling and other working methods used to engage in the steps of the research process for the formation of new knowledge (research) – for example, phenomenology uses the method of in-depth interview.

Method – Application of a common process, tool or technique to collect research data – for example, a questionnaire.

Research question – A clearly articulated and focused question that is framed to maximise the efficiency and effectiveness of searching literature and choosing an appropriate research design to answer the question. A research question must be able to be answered – that is, be *answerable*.

Researchers choose from a range of **methodological** approaches and select **methods** to find the answer to a focused and answerable **research question**. A popular approach to asking an answerable question is to build the question using the PICO acronym by defining the **p**opulation, **p**erson or **p**roblem; an **i**ntervention, **i**ssue or **e**xposure; and a **c**omparison group (if used). The question will also have clearly defined **o**utcomes. It is also common to see the **t**imeframe or **t**ype of study included in research questions, written as either PICOT or PECOT (see Boluyt et al., 2012; Jarrett et al., 2015).

While the process of research proceeds systematically through a series of steps (see below), the theoretical and methodological approach chosen by the researcher will determine exactly what each step looks like. Theories guide decisions about assumptions underlying the research method, and what is accepted as valid and reliable evidence of these assumptions. Theories therefore act as a scaffold to inform the context of the investigation (the methodology) and the way evidence or data is gathered (the method). In their simplest form, the main steps of the research process are:

1. Define the problem.
2. Pose an answerable research question.
3. Search the literature to see what is already known and/or review methods used for similar questions.
   - Develop a research design and choose an appropriate method.
   - Secure funding (if required).
   - Gain ethical and site approvals.
   - Collect data to conduct the study.
   - Analyse the data to answer the question.
   - Disseminate (and publish) the results.

Research design – A detailed plan of how the research will proceed from the research question through to the dissemination of results.

The steps of the research process are presented within a framework known as the **research design**. Essentially, the design is a plan that determines boundaries for the research project and is an important reference for the research team. The co-design of research occurs when end-users (people, patients, children, families and communities) are engaged in any or all stages of the research process, such as defining the problem and question, selecting the study site and sample, ethics, analysis, funding and timelines.

Clinical audit and benchmarking

Clinical audit – The routine and consistent measurement of clinical indicators for the purpose of monitoring health outcomes across groups and organisations.

The process of routinely and consistently measuring health outcome data is called a **clinical audit**. Used mostly as a tool for measuring safety and quality in healthcare, audits and benchmarking are also important for the generation of research questions.

Outcomes measurement offers health services an *indication* of the quality of healthcare delivered across groups of people as well as across institutions. Consequently, health outcomes measures are often called clinical *indicators*. Audits compare and contrast clinical indicators between peer facilities or against aspirational targets set by a health service or national/global best-practice standards – a process known as **benchmarking**. Benchmarking within and between services is undertaken primarily for the purpose of making improvements, but organisations are also alerted to possible system or process compromises when upward or downward trends occur.

The monitoring, collation and benchmarking of clinical indictors are critically important for driving internal quality and other improvement activities, but they do not constitute research. For example, we expect clinical indicator measurement to be standardised and consistent, but clinical audit is not rigorous in the same way as a scientific research method must be. Similarly, benchmarking is a process rather than an outcome. The results of clinical audit are not intended to be generalisable (applied to others) and are not generally submitted to peer review or publication outside the organisation (except perhaps for accreditation purposes) in the same way as research findings.

Audits and benchmarking are therefore specific techniques for capturing, comparing and contrasting systems data within the context of safety and quality in healthcare. However, a natural response when looking at trends in benchmarking data may be to ask *why* one place is performing better than another on a particular measure. Health professionals may then decide to formulate a research question to discover new knowledge about why such trends are occurring.

Translating knowledge from research

Disciplinary and geographical conventions reveal a range of terms for translating knowledge from research into practice. For example, the term **knowledge translation** is used to describe the process of moving what we have learned from research through to application in health policy and practice settings. But this process is also variously referred to as 'knowledge transfer', 'research/knowledge diffusion' and 'dissemination'. The term 'evidence implementation' is also often used, as well as 'research utilisation' and 'evidence transfer'. With so many terms for the same process, it is little wonder that we become confused by the language of research and evidence.

Possibilities for translating knowledge from research are not only impacted by the quality of the research itself, but by personal, environmental and contextual factors. Kitson et al. (2008) modelled the translation of research evidence using the now well-known Promoting Action on Research Implementation in Health Services (PARIHS) framework. This framework recognises variation in research evidence and context, while adding a critical component that is often missing from other models: the need for active facilitation. While some research is ground-breaking and triggers immediate and significant impacts, the reality is that most research will not be translated into practice without active facilitation over time.

One way to think about drivers of research translation is from a supply and demand perspective. Figure 4.1 illustrates that the success of using research evidence in practice relies not only on the research supply side but also on appropriateness and demand for evidence. For example, there may be no (or limited) research, or no access to research (as sometimes occurs in resource-poor settings). Alternatively, good-quality research may exist but the healthcare environment may be unable or unwilling to act on it. This may be due to lack of finance, workforce or equipment to implement change (lack of supply), or barriers in political and policy settings. Equally, a child, young person or their family

Benchmarking – The process of assessing and comparing performance measures.

Knowledge translation – The pathway or period during which findings from either basic or applied research are disseminated, implemented as evidence and have a measurable impact on patients, policy or practice.

may choose not to accept an evidence-based treatment or service and/or clinicians and other stakeholders may not be supportive of practice change (lack of demand).

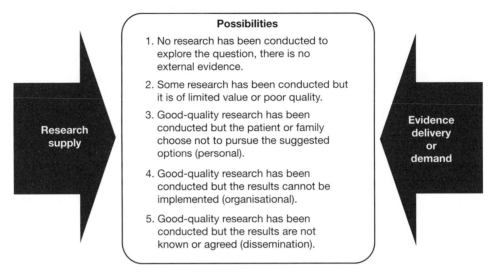

Figure 4.1   Possibilities for generating and using research evidence

We will return to this discussion of factors related to the research and evidence interaction after we define the meanings of evidence.

CASE STUDY 4.1 THE MEANING OF EVIDENCE

In order to understand what nurses and midwives understand as evidence, the chapter author (Waters et al., 2009) interviewed professional opinion leaders from metropolitan and rural areas of New South Wales, Australia. The 23 participants were in senior academic or health leadership positions and 21 had completed a doctorate.

The results of the study showed that nursing and midwifery opinion leaders used very different approaches to understand relationships between research and evidence. Views on the meaning of evidence were related to personal and professional experiences, and participants varied regarding where they thought research was positioned in relation to evidence – for example, local or global, internal or external. The results imply that opinion leaders ascribe meaning to evidence-based practice in very different ways because of their personal understanding of *evidence*.

A lack of a common meaning around basic terms such as 'research' and 'evidence' among nursing and midwifery opinion leaders reveals a somewhat confusing landscape for the wider clinical, professional, educational and cultural context of evidence-based practice.

What is evidence?

We have broadly distinguished research as a process for deriving new knowledge, and now define evidence as the knowledge that is produced and used within a specific context. Other ways to categorise evidence are to describe sources of knowledge as *external* (from research) or *internal* (relating to the child, young person, family, clinician or setting). External evidence from good-quality, contextually relevant research (also termed 'research evidence') offers proven treatment options and introduces new ways to design and deliver care. But *internal* evidence arising from intrinsic cultural and ethical values and preferences plays an equally significant role in the success of service and treatment decisions, and the implementation of research into practice.

The context of evidence is therefore broad and ever-changing. At every encounter, the experience of the clinician or carer, the healthcare environment and the specific values and priorities of the young person, their family and community are likely to be different. This fluid interrelationship ultimately shapes decisions about what constitutes the quality of evidence and how evidence is used within different contexts (evidence-based practice).

Evidence-based practice

We have identified that evidence can come from both external and internal sources. Rather than ignoring internal evidence, synthesis of this knowledge with external evidence from research is what permits us to deliver personalised, high-quality and safe care to children and young people in a culturally safe and contextually appropriate way. When care is delivered in this way, we are performing 'best practice'.

Thirty years after the introduction of what was originally called evidence-based *medicine* (EBM), it is perhaps unsurprising that a large part of the success (or otherwise) of implementing research into practice is found to be dependent on 'human' factors – the way clinicians and others use research evidence to make decisions about the care of individual patients and what individual people care about and value (Accad & Francis, 2018). **Evidence-based practice (EBP)** offers a framework to translate knowledge from research into health professional practice while taking the quality of research and personal, environmental and contextual factors into account.

Evidence-based practice (EBP) – Application of the best available research evidence in health decisions that are appropriate to the context and aligned to the values and priorities of children, young people and their families.

While there are many critics of EBM, Djulbegovic and Guyatt (2017, p. 416) argue that the movement was never intended to offer a new scientific theory, but rather a 'coherent heuristic structure' for optimising practice using credible and trustworthy evidence. EBP extends the 'coherent structure' of EBM to all health disciplines, recognising the many different ways that multidisciplinary teams partner with people in health decisions while using quality research evidence that is appropriate to the context of care. This partnering is also at the basis of person/patient or family-centred care.

The EBP framework refers to a series of steps to support the implementation of evidence (Table 4.1). The researcher follows steps consistent with the research process; however, note that when we are *using* evidence (as a practitioner), a major deviation occurs in the research process after we have found out what the literature tells us. Evidence-based practitioners have many tools and resources at their disposal to judge the quality of research and the *strength* of the evidence for practice – for example, see GRADE (Grading of Recommendations, Assessment, Development and Evaluations) at BMJ Best Practice online.

Table 4.1 Contrasting the research process and evidence-based practice

A researcher	An evidence-based practitioner
• Asks a research question • Conducts a review of literature • Develops a research design • Determines the best method to use • Secures funding (if required) • Gains ethical and site approval • Conducts the research study • Analyses the results • Answers the question • Disseminates (publishes) the results	• Asks a practice question • Conducts a review of literature • Determines the quality of evidence from the literature • Summarises the results • Answers the question • Applies results or implements practice changes • Evaluates the impact or effectiveness of change

The evidence-based practitioner derives questions directly from their practice. How often have you had a thought such as, 'This child keeps pulling their bandages off – I wonder whether there is another dressing I could use to keep the wound covered?' Using the EBP framework, you can ask a practice question (*ask*), conduct a search of the research literature (*access*), determine the quality and appropriateness of the literature you find (*appraise*), answer your question and *apply* your new knowledge to your practice, then *assess* (using audit or research) to evaluate whether the change has made a difference. Sometimes you see the five 'As' of evidence-based practice written as **a**ssess the problem or patient, **a**sk the question, **a**cquire the evidence, **a**ppraise it, then **a**pply it to practice.

Evidence implementation

Healthcare is not delivered in a vacuum, and it is usually in the implementation of EBP (applying evidence to practice) that contextualised knowledge from internal and other sources most significantly impacts the process. Despite the seemingly large amount of published research, there are still many areas for which good-quality evidence does not yet exist. Alternately, the available evidence may be of good quality, but cannot be applied within the setting or context. Further, every healthcare encounter will be different because every child and family is different – as are individual competing factors, barriers and environmental influences. Similarly, a young person might exercise their choice to disregard your advice, regardless of how strong the evidence might be for a particular recommendation. The complex interplay of research evidence with clinician contribution (or lack of contribution) and patient and family preference take place within many different environments – all of which are moderated by economic, environmental, social and political contexts. In essence, the evidence alone is not enough.

While nurses generally accept EBP as a positive strategy, basing practice on evidence is definitely not easy. In a systematic review designed to understand how long it takes before findings from health research are converted to patient benefit (the process of research translation), Morris, Wooding and Grant (2011) concluded that while a number of studies had coincidentally landed on the answer of 17 years, the use of different approaches and outcome measures in the 23 studies included in their review made it difficult to arrive at a definitive answer. However, the range of this estimate has not substantially changed in the 20 years since the US Agency for Healthcare Research and Quality (AHRQ) proposed that 'it may take as long as one or two decades for original research to be put into routine clinical practice' (AHRQ, 2001, p. 1).

Considering the many internal and external factors influencing the implementation of evidence, we clearly have a lot of work to do in speeding up this translation pathway. It is encouraging that recent efforts have focused on testing ways to construct more effective, inclusive and collaborative ways to actively facilitate evidence transfer. The more rapid translation of research evidence is not only of benefit to children, young people and their families, but is necessary to ensure efficient and effective outcomes from ever-dwindling research funding and resources.

Implementation science is the study of approaches and methods used for evidence transfer or knowledge translation. Implementation science has already resulted in the creation of a vast array of frameworks and models for what essentially remains a simple (albeit not easy) process of getting research into practice (Curran, 2020). The goal of implementation science is not to establish impact or outcome, but rather to identify those factors that affect the uptake of evidence-based interventions that, if successful, will ultimately impact on quality improvement and effectiveness (Bauer & Kirchner, 2020).

> **Implementation science** – The study of approaches and methods to improve the translation of research evidence into policy and practice.

Researching with children and young people

As health professionals, we are privileged to have the opportunity to conduct research *with* children, youth, families, carers and communities. No researcher, however esteemed, has the right to assume ownership of the human rights or health choices of another adult or a child, nor to use the language of research to assume power. Children, young people and those who care for them have the same access to research as we do! We rely on the judgement of parents and carers of children and young people to use their own internal and external sources of evidence for decisions they are making on behalf of, or with, those in their care.

Similarly, the people for whom we care should be able to assume that health professional education is based on the best available evidence from research, and that this evidence underpins knowledge and skills for the delivery of care. In addition to professional conduct and ethics, the tenet of using the best available evidence for decision-making is so fundamental to healthcare that expectations relating to quality, safety, research and evidence-based practice can be found in the professional registration standards of all health disciplines.

Research ethics are similarly based on the principle of respect and the rights of all people. At a time when we know that children and young people around the world are being denied basic human rights, it is important to remember that the principles of research and research governance, founded in the 1947 Nuremburg Code (discussed further in the section on research ethics below) are intended to be applied fully and globally.

REFLECTION POINTS 4.1

- *Research* and *evidence* are terms that are often used interchangeably, but in fact their meanings are different. Do you think the careless use of these words has had any impact on how nurses working in neonatal and paediatric settings feel about research? Do you understand what is expected of you as an evidence-based practitioner?
- Evidence can be derived from research (external evidence) or from other sources (internal evidence). What impact do you think your geographical location, health-care environment and patient population have on your ability to use evidence in your practice?
- Evidence-based practice is usually presented as a series of five steps, consisting of asking a question, accessing evidence, appraising the quality of the evidence, applying results in practice, and assessing or evaluating the effect of the change. Which of these five steps do you think would be the most challenging in your nursing practice and why?

Human research and ethics

Human research includes any research that is 'conducted with or about people, or their data or tissue' (NHMRC, 2018d, p. 3). Human research therefore includes everything from primary and secondary personal data, observations, questionnaires, images, interviews and surveys; body fluids and tissues (including exhaled breath); through to psychological, physiological and medical interventions and tests. There are specific ethical considerations related to research with potentially vulnerable human participants such as the following: women or girls who are pregnant and the human foetus; people in dependent or unequal relationships; people highly dependent on medical care who may be unable to give consent; people involved in illegal activity; people with cognitive or intellectual disabilities or mental illness; Māori, Pacific Islander, Aboriginal and Torres Strait Islander people; and, of course, children and young people – who may also fit into many of the previous categories (NEAC, 2019; NHMRC, 2018d).

The paediatric and adolescent health setting presents some specific challenges related to the ethical conduct of human research. Children and young people have a range of developmental capacities for understanding their involvement in healthcare and research decisions. Research with children and young people often raises questions about maturity for the consent process and the possibility of conflicting values when parents or carers are giving consent for participation on behalf of children and young people in their care. The issue of whether it is acceptable to pay money or offer incentives for the recruitment of children, young people or their families may also carry the risk of exploitation (Resnik, 2015).

The future will present even greater challenges for human research ethics as personal data are collected, shared and stored in international data registries and biobanks, social media and cloud networks. For example, access to specimens stored in human biobanks will continue to raise important ethical questions into the future. At the same time, such technologies also permit residual blood or tissue obtained from clinical procedures to be stored for long periods, offering enormous potential for future research, genomics and personalised medicine.

History and human research ethics

The principles of human research ethics arose from the Nuremberg Trials of 1945–46, an investigation into crimes committed during World War II (1939–45). This was a pivotal moment in history, prompting development of a universal written code of medical ethics known as the Nuremberg Code of 1947. Of the 10 principles in the Code, the first relates to the giving of voluntary consent by the human subject. While we now refer to this as the principle of **autonomy** (discussed later in the chapter), at the time the Code technically precluded children or any other person unable to give direct *voluntary* consent for participation in research (Davidson & O'Brien, 2009). The 1964 Declaration of Helsinki later attempted to reflect the major principles of the Nuremberg Code within the specific context of biomedical research. Revised several times over the intervening 50 years, the most recent Declaration is available online.

Autonomy – Respect for human beings to make their own decisions about participation in research.

Another pivotal point in the history of human research ethics was a report commissioned by the US Congress, published as the Belmont Report in 1979 (see Brothers et al., 2019). This report identified three core ethical principles (respect for persons, beneficence and justice), and offered important guidance for research involving humans. The three principles are applied as actions for gaining informed consent, assessing benefit against risk and the appropriate selection of research participants. In an attempt to further clarify and articulate principles from the Nuremberg Code and Declaration of Helsinki, the report also defined what we now call *basic* research (laboratory or bench-top experimentation with biological specimens or animal models) and *clinical or applied* research conducted directly with people. With US Federal Agencies agreeing to adopt a uniform set of rules for the protection of human subjects in 1991, the principles of the Belmont Report are now often referred to as the *Common Rule*.

Subsequently, a range of international organisations have developed and published guidelines for the ethical conduct of health and biomedical research, including the International Ethical Guidelines for Health-related Research Involving Humans, a collaboration between the World Health Organization (WHO) and the Council for International Organizations of Medical Sciences (CIOMS). Under the auspices of the National Health and Medical Research Council (NHMRC), the Australian Health Ethics Committee has developed the *National Statement on Ethical Conduct in Human Research* in collaboration with the Australian Research Council (ARC) and Universities Australia (NHMRC, 2018d). In New Zealand, the National Ethics Advisory Council (NEAC) produces the National Ethical Standards for Health and Disability Research and Quality Improvement (NEAC, 2019) – hereafter collectively referred to as the National Statements. All guidelines are easily searchable, updated regularly and freely available online. Further, every guideline developed since the Nuremberg Code specifically contains sections relating to research with vulnerable groups, including children and young people.

Principles of human research ethics

The principles of human research ethics broadly attest that any risks from research will be outweighed by the contribution of the research to improving health and healthcare, and that the dignity, privacy and wellbeing of the research participant will be protected at all times.

The National Statements of Australia and New Zealand (NEAC, 2019; NHMRC, 2018d) organise the discussion of ethical values in research around the central principles of the original Belmont Report (respect for people, beneficence and justice), with additional guidance for research merit and integrity. Brothers et al. (2019) have recently questioned the interpretation of original Belmont principles in relation to twenty-first century technologies such as bio-specimen storage, genomics, stem-cell and animal-to-human transplants; however, there will always be ethical challenges in research. Many national and international guides are available to support shared discussion and decisions between human research ethics committees, researchers and participants about values and priorities for mutual benefit. You will find some of these guides in the Further reading list at the end of this chapter. Contemporary research design demands consideration of altruism, power relationships, societal and community benefit, respect for culture and all forms of diversity, inclusion of LGBTQI+ people, cultural safety and alignment with nationally specific priorities and values – all within the context of constantly challenged healthcare environments.

Research merit and integrity

The principles of respect for persons, beneficence and justice exist under the assumption that any research of poor scientific quality will be unethical. Any child, young person or adult has a right to expect that before their participation in a study is considered, the proposed research has a clear and answerable aim or question, is informed by current research literature, uses an appropriate design and method, is practically possible to complete and results are disseminated (remember the steps of the research process). Further, it is expected that the study will be conducted or supervised by researchers with appropriate training and experience, and within a safe and adequately resourced environment.

Research governance – The processes by which institutions establish and oversee the legal, ethical and safe conduct of human research. This includes establishing and operating institutional or geographically based human ethics committees and monitoring (or receiving recommendations from specialist committees) regarding individual researcher accountabilities for the ethical design, conduct, scientific rigour and personal and cultural safety of their studies.

The role of Human Research Ethics Committees (HRECs) in Australia, or Health and Disability Ethics Committees (HDECs) in New Zealand, is discussed later, but for now we can say that it is also expected that any research involving humans will have undergone prior ethical review by a HREC or HDEC from the institution or area within which the study will be conducted. While human ethics committees have an important oversight role in monitoring **research governance** processes, the increasing complexity of research designs, and requirements for meaningful consultation with research participants and their communities, have seen the establishment of locally specific committees to review and make recommendations. For example, institutional scientific committees may conduct a prior peer review of the scientific validity and merit of a study or clinical trial, thus enabling the HREC and HDEC to concentrate on *ethical* standards.

With specific consideration of children and young people, research governance principles focus on whether the research design and methods are appropriate for the age and developmental maturity of the intended participants, and whether the researchers have the appropriate education and experience to work with children and young people within the context of their research question. The research must be in the best interests of the child, young person or family, and should only be conducted where the question relates directly to children and young people, and comparable research with adults could not answer the research question. These considerations must also be viewed under the broader provisions of the United Nations Convention on the Rights of the Child (UNOHCHR, 1990), specifically Article 24, and the World Medical Assembly (WMA) Declaration of Ottawa on Child Health, adopted in 1998 and amended in 2009 (WMA, 2017).

Respect for children and young people is fundamental to recognising their intrinsic value as human beings and their capacity to make autonomous decisions about participation in research. The project and all risks should be explained in developmentally appropriate language, including rights to privacy and confidentiality, and with consideration of what is important and valued by the child and their family. It is therefore important that any research design will describe the following: how children and young people will be approached for participation (recruited to the study); whether the facility or environment in which the study is to be conducted is appropriate to their needs; any potential impact on the child's family or community, such as may occur in school-based research; and a clear description of how researchers will judge the capacity of potential participants and their families to understand the project and its risks, and give both assent (agreement) and consent (permission) to participate.

Autonomy and respect for persons

As one of the three fundamental ethical principles of research contained in the Belmont Report, respect for persons refers to valuing the privacy, confidentiality, customs, perceptions and cultural freedoms of research participants, and recognises the value and intrinsic right of individuals and collectives (groups and communities) to make autonomous decisions about their participation in research – a principle we earlier referred to as *autonomy*. In its broadest meaning, autonomy also encompasses relational concepts such as interdependence. In New Zealand, for example, the principles of partnership and sharing implicit in the Treaty of Waitangi are expected to be respected by all, and in all health research proposals. Signed in 1840, this Treaty frames the rights of New Zealand Māori to determine and protect their culture, lands and other possessions in relationships with the New Zealand government.

Recognising that individuals have intrinsic human value, it is expected that all researchers and research designs will inherently respect the interactions human beings have with each other through common beliefs, customs, perceptions and culture, as well as individual rights to privacy and confidentiality of information and other data. For children and young people, these interactions extend to relationships with parents and carers, and include the responsibilities of parents and carers to protect and support children and young people with diminished developmental capacity to make autonomous decisions.

In addition, the National Statements of Australia and New Zealand (NEAC, 2019; NHMRC, 2018d) specify participants who are considered vulnerable within the context of research and for whom studies requiring participation must be reviewed by a human research ethics committee. These vulnerable groups were identified above, where we also noted that in addition to being named as a vulnerable group in their own right, children and young people may be represented in any or all of the other vulnerable groups.

The differing developmental capabilities of children and young people are respected in the National Statements in two ways: first, while guidance is given, the exact circumstances in which autonomous consent may or may not be appropriate are not specifically dictated; and second, the guidelines are flexible about decisions regarding a child's level of maturity and subsequent capacity to understand the complexities of the proposed research. Apart from suggesting responsiveness to a child's developmental capacity to understand their involvement, the Australian statement proposes that 'even young children ... should be engaged *at their level* in discussion about the research and its likely outcomes' (NHMRC, 2018d, p. 65). Similarly, the New Zealand statement confirms that 'age alone has been shown to be an inaccurate marker of the level of children's competence' (NEAC, 2019, p. 67).

Assent and consent in research with children and young people

It is the recognition of the many internal and external factors that impact the capacity of a child or young person to make decisions about their participation in research that precludes a simple answer to questions about the age of consent for research. It is important to distinguish that while the capacity of a child or young person to consent to medical procedures is prescribed by specific legislation, consent for participation in research is not. In New Zealand, the age of consent for medical procedures is 16 years, and this age also guides decisions around consent for research. However, the National Statements of both Australia and New Zealand (NEAC, 2019; NHMRC, 2018d) are not directive regarding the capacity of a minor (defined variously as 16 or 18 years) to consent to research participation. Therefore, while a non-verbal infant clearly cannot participate in research discussions, a young child is often capable of understanding aspects of the research design sufficient to ask relevant and important questions – for example, 'Will it hurt?' – and, particularly in later childhood, may be deemed sufficiently mature to give fully informed and free consent. As children and young people with communication difficulties use various technologies to navigate daily life, solutions can also be found to facilitate their 'voice' and engagement in research (UNOHCHR, 1990).

You may see the word 'assent' used in discussions about the participation of children and young people in research. Assent relates to a child agreeing to participate in research without the giving of free and informed consent (for the reasons discussed above). Assenting is much more than passive acceptance or non-refusal. It relates to the giving of explicit and active agreement that, like the giving of consent, should be reviewed as the child or young person matures (Dockett & Perry, 2011). In general, both parental and child assent are required for participation in research – except, of course, where a child is not mature enough to give assent (such as an infant), or where possibilities of therapeutic benefit from the research are such that the parent chooses to overrule their child's assent – for example, a trial of an experimental treatment where no medically acceptable alternative currently exists. This is discussed below under the ethical principle of beneficence. Where a child or young person is deemed mature and competent to exercise their right not to assent (or dissent), it is inappropriate to proceed.

Free and informed consent implies a dynamic and voluntary decision. Consent is *free* when it is not influenced by coercion, pressure or inducement from family, peers or others, and is *informed* when sufficient information is given to permit adequate understanding of the benefits and risks of participation (Davidson & O'Brien, 2009). When a child is unable to give free and informed consent to participate in research, parents or guardians are asked to make a judgement based on their interpretation of the child's best interests and the level of risk to be endured for the sake of others. Parents and children are also both at risk of the sometimes subtle coercion that may exist when a favourite nurse or doctor asks them to join a research project. Table 4.2 suggests a number of ways to support the giving of free and informed consent by children and young people.

Table 4.2   Facilitating free and informed consent

Consent is free	Consent is informed
• Research protocol clearly identifies age-appropriate and developmentally appropriate process for gaining assent and consent • Process minimises risk of coercion by parents, peers, healthcare team or others • Any financial reimbursement or inducement is proportionate to inconvenience • Any participant deemed mature and competent must assent to participation • Any participant deemed mature and competent must provide their own informed consent • A child or young person gaining capacity for assent and/or consent during the study is given the opportunity to do so	• Information appropriate to age, developmental stage and level of literacy • Use of visual and digital aids, such as charts, illustrations, videos, apps • Sufficient time is given to digest and understand the information • Engaged in discussion: early and appropriate to age, cognitive and communication ability • Questions encouraged and answers appropriate to level of maturity • Participant able to demonstrate understanding of potential consequences and risks • Special provisions made for privacy around collection of sensitive information

Source: Adapted from Davidson & O'Brien (2009); Isles (2013).

As the National Statements suggest, it is inappropriate to define individual maturity by age, or to assume that the complexity of the research is beyond the understanding of a child of a particular age. Factors such as experience of illness, personality, independence, ethnicity, culture and life circumstances all have potential to influence capacity for individual decision-making. However, it is clear that infants are unable to give free and informed consent because they cannot take part in discussion about the research. Consent for the participation of infants and very young children must be given by at least one parent or legal guardian – keeping in mind that for any child, the legal guardian may sometimes be an organisation and sometimes the legal guardian may change.

Further guidance for gaining consent for participation in research from children and young people assumes assent and can be considered within three broad categories:

1. For a child or young person able to understand some relevant information about the research but remaining vulnerable to undue influence due to developmental immaturity, consent must be obtained from at least one parent or the legal guardian.

2. A young person of developing maturity may give consent when they have capacity to understand information about the research. However, due to potential developmental vulnerabilities, their consent alone is not sufficient and additional consent must be given by at least one parent or the legal guardian. In the context of the New Zealand National Statement (NEAC, 2019, p. 66), guidance for the giving of shared consent with a parent or guardian broadly refers to young people under the age of 16 years.

3. A young person may give sole consent for research participation when a research ethics committee is satisfied of the following: the young person is mature enough to understand all relevant information; the research involves no more than a low risk; the research will be of benefit to the group of young people to which the participant belongs; the young person is estranged or separated from their parents or guardian; or it would be contrary to the best interests of the young person to seek parental consent (NHMRC, 2018d, p. 66). In the context of the New Zealand National Statement (NEAC, 2019, p. 68), legally effective consent for participation in health research is aligned to capacity to consent for medical treatment; sole consent is therefore possible from the age of 16 years unless the young person is deemed incapable due to unconsciousness, cognitive disability or mental illness, for example.

Exceptions to these general rules occur when conditions are contrary to state or territory legislation (for example, see report from Rallis Legal in the Further Reading section). Similarly, where vulnerabilities exist in aspects of the life of a young person that are unrelated to their understanding of consent, an ethics review board may decide that the nature of the research requires the consent of both parents. For example, this might include developmental aspects of accepting risk and burden for moral or altruistic reasons, social immaturity or homelessness.

As children and young people continue to grow and mature over time, researchers must take the evolving capacity of each individual child or young person into consideration during the period of study. Assent and consent are reviewed regularly, in tandem with dynamic developmental, physical and environmental changes occurring for each child or young person (see Case study 4.2). As an example of one of the many guides available to support ethical research with children and young people, the Australian Paediatric Research Ethics and Governance Network (APREGN) offers a companion interpretation of the Australian National Standards within the specific context of consent for participation in clinical trials (APREGN, 2017).

Opting-in, opting-out and refusal to participate

A large amount of personal information is now stored in data registries with residual biological and genetic material from routine care and treatment residing in large biobanks. An *opt-in* procedure requires a participant to actively consent for the future use and storage of their data or residual samples for research occurring into the indefinite future. Increasingly, persons who participate in research studies are enrolled using opt-out strategies – that is, their data and/or samples will continue to be included in future research until they issue an express request to exclude them (opting out). It is also often not appreciated that for some minimal and low-risk projects, researchers may have been given permission to waive the need to obtain assent and consent under an opt-out strategy (sometimes called *passive consent*). In other words, if you haven't said no, then this means yes! This may also occur when project deliverables cannot be achieved without a waiver of this kind.

There remains a great deal of speculation about appropriate opt-in and opt-out procedures with children and young people, and parents are often unaware of their rights and responsibilities around consenting or opting out (Giesbertz, Bredenoord & Delden, 2012). Research consent forms and participant information sheets will outline specific information about the privacy and confidentiality of research data and samples, and detail exactly how and when these will be disposed of. Participants are also informed that they have a right to actively refuse to continue their participation in a study at any time and/or refuse permission for their data or biological samples to be stored beyond the life of the study.

This is another reason for building flexibility into research design around consent procedures. The right of a child or young person to refuse or discontinue participation in a research study is generally judged commensurate to their capacity to give consent. For example, where a child is unable to demonstrate capacity and maturity to fully participate in decisions about the current study, the judgement of parents or guardians will take precedence, as long as these remain in the best interests of the child. Alternatively, young people who have reached an age or stage at which they can give autonomous consent may have different views from their parents regarding how or whether their personal genetic material (such as neonatal screening cards) may be stored for future research.

Standing parental consent

The Australian National Statement has provision for parents to give **standing parental consent** to certain types of research conducted within educational settings (NHMRC, 2018d, p. 67). Schools may, for example, seek standing parental consent at the beginning of a school year for their child's involvement in research, provided that the research is deemed to be of benefit to children of a similar age and does not compromise learning or involve disclosure of sensitive personal or family relationships and/or potentially identifiable information.

Beneficence

In general, **beneficence** implies improving or offering some benefit to people or communities. The ethical principle of beneficence in research relates to balancing

Standing parental consent – Enables parents to give consent to their child's involvement in one or more research projects about which they have been informed on the understanding that they may withdraw consent for their child's participation for any individual project or withdraw standing consent at any time.

Beneficence – The act of benefiting others or contributing to the greater good. In research ethics, beneficence relates to actions taken to remove or reduce any risk or harms associated with the research.

benefit with risk of harm. For many studies, there will be minimal or no direct benefits to current research participants – with potentially beneficial outcomes from the research occurring only in the future. Researchers are responsible for ensuring the rigour and validity of their research design and methods, and to do whatever they can to minimise any actual or potential risk to participants (NEAC, 2019; NHMRC, 2018d). The researcher must demonstrate to the ethics committee how the emotional, physical, cultural and psychological safety of the child or young person is maintained throughout the research, and that risk of participation remains lower than would be ethically acceptable when there are likely benefits.

Beneficence is also demonstrated by some research participants who estimate their own personal level of risk to be less than the risk of *not* contributing to future benefits that may arise from the research. But it is important to remember that what counts as risk and benefit can be very different between people.

Non-maleficence (or doing no **harm**) is another term used in the discussion of risk versus benefit in research. Harm can be *perceived* or *real*. The idea of potential harm to a research participant is balanced by the notion that any perceived or real harm will be outweighed by the benefit accrued by the individual on behalf of the greater good. In the context of research ethics, a risk is anything with the potential for harm, discomfort or inconvenience.

Discomfort is a less serious form of risk, which can also be physical or psychological – perceived or real. For example, a young person might become psychologically distressed or feel uncomfortable about discussing their personal experience of a recent diagnosis of epilepsy with a research interviewer, but they are unlikely to suffer long-term harm as a result of sharing this information. In this case, it is appropriate for the researcher to consider where and how the interviews can be made more comfortable, for example, by giving the young person choice of interview location and time, or options for in-person or virtual communication.

There will always be some level of inconvenience associated with participation in research. This is especially relevant for parents or carers of children and young people, who may incur financial or emotional costs connected with their child's participation in research such as taking time off work, travelling, meeting with researchers, and completing consent and testing procedures. In general, modest compensation (e.g. parking, accommodation or food vouchers) is regarded as acceptable. Similarly, while offering payments and rewards directly to children and young people is associated with an increased likelihood of their participation in research, the level of reward must be balanced with the risk of undue influence (Taplin et al., 2019). For example, iTunes® vouchers are not likely to cause parents or participants to ignore risks associated with participation in the research, whereas upfront cash payments may prompt a different reaction.

Harm – May be physical (such as pain or injury) or psychological (such as feeling guilty, upset or humiliated). Social harm may damage relationships within social networks, while economic or legal harm relates to the imposition of costs or exposure to legal risk as a result of participation in research.

Best interests

The concept of maintaining the best interests of the child or young person is related to ensuring our research design provides the best possible approach to protecting the emotional, psychological and physical safety of participants. *Best interests* relate to many of the principles we have already discussed, such as respecting the right to refuse to participate, supporting the capacity of the child or young person to understand the research and give consent, and provision for refusal to be overridden by the parent's judgement if this is deemed to be in the best interests of the child or young person. An example demonstrating the failure of researchers to maintain the best interests of children comes from a now famous study published in *The Lancet* in 1998, proposing a causative relationship between measles, mumps and rubella (MMR) vaccination, autism and bowel disease. More than 20 subsequent studies and reviews have proven this study to be fraudulent, but not before significant harm was caused in the form of vaccine avoidance (Godlee, Smith & Marcovitch, 2011).

CASE STUDY 4.2 BALANCING BENEFIT AND HARM

Arianna has just turned 5 and attends the cystic fibrosis outpatient clinic each month. Her father, Christos, tells you that he has been approached by a researcher who is conducting a study to look at vitamin E and peripheral nerve function in children with cystic fibrosis. He shows you the patient information sheet and consent form, which state that participants will be required to undergo nerve conduction studies and electromyography on two occasions over the next 12 months as part of a randomised controlled trial of high-dose vitamin E supplementation. Christos asks, 'Do you think this study would be of any benefit to my Arianna?'

Below are some points you might like to discuss with Christos and Arianna. The related principal of research ethics is in brackets.

- Is the researcher part of Arianna's current healthcare team? (coercion)
- Does Christos understand that in a randomised controlled trial, Arianna may be allocated to a treatment or control group and may or may not receive additional vitamin E? (beneficence and autonomy)
- Is Arianna willing to undergo additional testing and take additional medication? (assent)
- Nerve conduction studies can be painful. (risk of harm)
- Is the family willing and able to undertake two additional healthcare visits and give time to attend testing and medication management? (inconvenience and cost)
- Children with chronic illnesses are often approached to join research studies. Is this the first study in which Arianna has participated? How does she feel about it? (justice)

Level of risk

Risk is the potential for harm, discomfort or inconvenience to occur. It is generally accepted that the level of risk to which children and young people are exposed through participation in research should be lower than that for adult research participants. However, the assessment of risk is different for everyone, and it is important to remember that like harm, risk can be actual or perceived. The assessment of risk is also about weighing the relative probabilities associated with the likelihood of risk

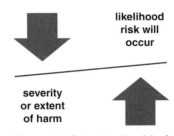

likelihood
risk will
occur

severity
or extent
of harm

Figure 4.2   Balancing the risk of
harm in research participation

occurring, and the severity or extent of harm that may result if the risk occurs (see Figure 4.2). Knowing the probability and severity of risk is one of the ways in which children, young people and their parents or guardians can judge the extent to which they are at risk from participating in research, and researchers and ethics committees can determine how these risks might be mitigated or managed.

Human research ethics committees will generally allocate research to a category of risk to determine the level of ethical review required. Research of *low or negligible risk* refers to types of research in which the actual or perceived risk is gauged to be no greater than discomfort (low) or inconvenience (negligible). In some countries, the term *minimal risk* is used to denote risk that is no greater than what a child might expect to encounter in everyday life – for example, a child might expect to fall off a bike. However, as Davidson and O'Brien (2009) suggest, a single blood test on a calm infant performed by an experienced venipuncturist using a topical anaesthetic can present an entirely different level of risk to performing the same procedure on a distressed and wriggling infant.

Justice

Justice is an integral part of all ethical research because this principle is concerned with fairness and equity. The consideration of justice starts with the experience of researchers within a paediatric and adolescent setting, and their ability to focus the research question and design the study to be consistent with how children and young people feel comfortable in the world. For example, has the research been designed to maximise the chances of participation? Is the process of recruitment fair? Will all children and young people benefit equally from the results?

We often see examples of research inequity in the Australian and New Zealand contexts. There are also many sub-populations of children and young people we know to be excluded from both participation and translation of benefits of research and new discoveries. For example, opportunities for participation in research may be translated to innovative care and treatment in large city teaching hospitals, whereas rural and remote health services may miss out. Similarly, there are families in both New Zealand and Australia with limited access to health services, poor health literacy, difficulties with language, homelessness or poverty.

Fairness also relates to the burden of the research. When discussing the ethical principle of beneficence, we asked whether the inconvenience caused to children, young people and their parents through participation in research could be judged *reasonable* when compared with the actual benefit that the individual child or young person might gain. Another fundamental question is whether the participation of children and young people is essential to the research, or could the research question be answered by the recruitment of adult participants only? Have the researchers considered every possible alternative to an invasive procedure – could a stored human biospecimen be used instead? Within the context of autonomy and beneficence, the principle of justice is deeply embedded in decisions around whether it is justifiable to involve children and young people in research when they may not benefit directly. This is particularly relevant to the consideration of maturity and capacity of minors to give assent, and free and informed consent, and the role of human research ethics committees.

Human research ethics committees

Human research ethics committees undertake the ethical review of research relative to levels of risk. As noted earlier, ethics committees consider the scientific merit (validity, quality and safety) of a study in order to make decisions about actual or potential risk to participants, and weigh these risks against the stated aims and benefits of the research (research ethics). The Health Research Council (HRC) of New Zealand HRC Research Ethics Guidelines (HRC, 2017) and Australian Code for the Responsible Conduct of Research (NHMRC, 2018a) advise that any research that is perceived to have anything more than a low level of risk must be reviewed by an appropriately constituted human research ethics committee. As discussed above, low risk is defined as actual or perceived risk being no greater than a level of discomfort, and negligible risk is described as that which has 'no foreseeable risk of harm or discomfort' (NHMRC, 2018d, p. 15). Many institutions have provisions for the approval or exemption of low and negligible-risk research, often through a 'low-risk' sub-committee. Quality projects may also be referred to low-risk sub-committees if any doubt exists over safety or risk to the public, or where there is intention to publish findings.

There is an expectation that research proposals submitted to ethics committees have integrity and demonstrate the research to be sufficiently feasible (able to be completed) and scoped (able to produce a reliable result) to make a meaningful new contribution to knowledge (the definition of research). No research that is judged to present any risk to participants may commence until approval is received, and often full funding of the research is withheld until evidence of approval has been presented. Research participants must be provided with direct contact information for an independent ethics committee representative if they wish to complain, and annual declarations verifying the continued safe and ethical conduct of the research are required.

The New Zealand Guidelines (HRC, 2017) and Australian Code (NHMRC, 2018a) explain the specific role of institutions and researchers in promoting research integrity, and offer guidance on managing departures from best practice, such as research misconduct. Further, the National Statements of Australia and New Zealand (NEAC, 2019; NHMRC, 2018d) provide guidance on all processes associated with research governance and ethical review, including recommendations for the operation, resourcing and membership of research ethics committees. Human research ethics committees must include laypersons in their membership (at least one man and one woman) who are independent of the organisations or institutions represented by the committee, and not currently engaged in work related to health and medical research.

Collectively, these national documents dictate processes that enable ethics committees to undertake the standardised ethical review of all types of research, including clinical trials, research with Indigenous and Pacific Islander peoples, migrant and non-English speaking populations, people living with disability, people living in other countries and research with human tissue, genetic and other sensitive personal data, and of course research involving children and young people (HRC & Peart, 2007; NHMRC, 2018d, p. 65). For example, research conducted with Aboriginal and Torres Strait Islander people in Australia requires review by an Aboriginal Human Research Ethics Committee, the membership of which is predominantly Aboriginal and Torres Strait Islander people (NHMRC, 2018b). A companion document, *Keeping Research on Track II* (NHMRC, 2018c), offers further support for respectful and culturally safe research co-design and conduct.

In New Zealand, questions relating to cultural safety, sensitivity and consultation with Māori people are reviewed in consultation with representative members of geographically (rather than institutionally) based human ethics committees. *Te Ara Tika: Guidelines for Māori Research Ethics* (HRC, 2010a, 2010b) offers a framework for researchers and members of HDECs to discuss ethical issues that may arise for Māori participants. The New Zealand Health Research Council (HRC) document *Māori Research Ethics: An Overview* has been prepared as a background resource to assist researchers with the implementation of Te Ara Tika (NEAC, 2012).

Human research ethics committees are integral to maintaining the safety of children and young people participating in research. Their role in interpreting recommendations from the National Statements supports researchers, reviewers and funders of research to identify their responsibilities and accountabilities for ethical research. They monitor specific criteria for managing conflicts of interest and the handling of complaints, and protect the interests of vulnerable and marginalised groups within our populations. Ethics committees have an equally important role to play in supporting and suggesting appropriate consultation with potential participants and the monitoring of research studies to their conclusion.

REFLECTION POINTS 4.2

- Autonomy and respect in human research ethics value the intrinsic rights of a human being to hold individual and collective beliefs, perceptions, customs and cultural norms. These principles also imply that the design and scope of research with children and young people will respect their individual capacity and developmental maturity to make their own decisions. What steps can you take to ensure that competing values and power relationships between health professionals, parents, children and young people are not unduly influencing their decisions about participation in research?
- Research data that expose the human genome may have significant longer-term consequences for the child, their family and other blood relatives. There is also the possibility of increasing stress around reproductive choices or paternity. What other potential risks of genetic research can you identify for the child or young person and their family?
- In research ethics, the principle of justice requires that any potential benefits or burdens from the research are equally and fairly distributed across population sub-groups (e.g. age, gender, social, economic, cultural and ethnic groups). Think about research in which you have been involved, or with which you are familiar, and consider whether this research was 'just'.

Meaningful research participation

In this final section, we discuss how to encourage and facilitate participation and partnership in research with children and young people. Finally, we will close the research 'loop' by suggesting ways in which shared knowledge about research, evidence and research ethics can be used to support a truly participatory approach to evidence-based practice.

Partners in research

Meaningful participation in research can be defined as that which refers to an 'explicitly described, defined and auditable role or task necessary to the planning and/or conduct of health research' (Slattery, Saeri & Bragge, 2020, p. 3). However, the academic literature continues to reveal only moderate success in establishing meaningful research partnerships with children and young people. Imbalances of power and a lack of control over the funding and design of research programs are commonly cited. Historically, academic institutions and health services are hierarchically structured, and are difficult enough to navigate for adults, let alone children and young people. Minority communities can experience institutional racism, along with privilege and power challenges, in their relationships with academic organisations (Andrews et al., 2012). Gaining the trust of family and community stakeholders is another frequently identified roadblock, as is securing commitment to the extra time, money and effort required for effective communication between health professionals, researchers, academic institutions and end-users to truly partner in research (Allen et al., 2010; Bailey et al., 2014).

However, for those with access, online and social media platforms have rapidly increased opportunities for children and young people to lead and engage with environmental, social, political and economic agendas – for example, in climate change – and to be more actively involved with the research process. Further opportunity comes with increasing expectations from government and research funding bodies for the demonstration of safe and meaningful research engagement with those for whom the research is most relevant, and articulation of ethical research practices in the online environment.

Supporting participation

In a scoping review of research studies using online recruiting and tracing of families and children for research follow-up, Hokke et al. (2018) found that while at least 10 relevant guidelines for online participation in research were found, these were rarely referenced. Problems concerning the researchers' ability to judge capacity for consent, engage parents, assess vulnerability and maintain online privacy and confidentially were raised but rarely discussed.

Frameworks and models for engaging children, young people, their families and their communities in participatory decision-making in education, community and government are continuously emerging (Donnelly & Kilkelly, 2011; Ohlin et al., 2010). Successful examples should not be excluded just because they fall outside the perceived context of 'health'. However, it may be that institutional and national systems are yet to reconcile the broad individual characteristics of children and young people with increasingly complex ethical and safety issues, particularly those related to health research conducted in the online environment.

The National Health and Medical Research Council (NHMRC) of Australia and Consumers Health Forum of Australia Inc (CHF) issued a joint Statement on Consumer and Community Involvement in Health and Medical Research (the Statement) in 2016. While silent on the specific involvement of children and young people, the Statement is broad in its definition of consumers and communities (NHMRC, 2016). A range of resources have since been developed to support the Statement (NHMRC, 2020). The New Zealand Ministry of Youth Development (NZMYD, n.d.), and Youth Councils in most states and territories of Australia similarly offer online resources and toolkits to support youth participation in many aspects of personal and community development, including research.

Research co-design – A defined, auditable contribution by research end-users to the planning, conduct and/or monitoring of research.

Research co-design occurs when end-users are engaged in any or all stages of the research process (Slattery, Saeri & Bragge, 2020). Participatory research methods (sometimes called participatory action research) are one example where research engagement is planned within the actual context in which healthcare and treatment is to be delivered (Haijes & van Thiel, 2016). Co-design can be facilitated through face-to-face activities such as focus groups and interviews, through online surveys and Delphi methods, phone apps and other digital feedback processes. Approaches can range from low-effort/low-risk through to complex co-production and co-publication designs (Slattery, Saeri & Bragge, 2020).

Other key factors for the successful engagement of children, young people and their families as partners and co-designers of health research include:

- early participation in prioritising and planning the research, including assessment of needs, clarifying values, vision, roles and responsibilities, and scoping the program and extent of involvement (Slattery, Saeri & Bragge, 2020)
- support for the formation of partnerships (Allen et al., 2010), with attention paid to communication mechanisms, well-structured physical or virtual interactions and training of stakeholders and consumers (Andrews et al., 2012; Bailey et al., 2014)
- clear processes for deciding stakeholder capacity for collaboration, managing conflict and expectations, establishing norms for decision-making (Allen et al., 2010) and planning for ending the engagement when the research is complete
- agreeing the desired rewards or outcomes for all members and organisations involved, including predetermined arrangements for shared reporting, publication and dissemination of findings (Slattery, Saeri & Bragge, 2020).

Representation is not the same as meaningful participation; however, children and young people can be supported towards engagement in research through peer-activities such as Child and Youth Advisory Committees, and conferences and camps associated with support groups and charities – for example, Children with Disability Australia, Camp Quality NZ, Canteen or the Starlight Foundation.

Finally, it is important for researchers and others to remain aware of the potential to *over-research* specific groups. Children and young people who spend a large part of their lives engaging with hospitals, clinics and other health services – for example, those with genetic or chronic childhood illnesses or disabilities – form a highly accessible research population. Reiterating the three fundamental principles of research ethics above, the research design must offer an explicit and easy way for children and young people to say *no* if they do not wish to participate, or if they wish to withdraw from the study (see Case Study 4.3).

CASE STUDY 4.3 REFUSAL TO PARTICIPATE

Jackson was diagnosed with Spinal Muscular Atrophy (SMA) Type 3 when he was 2 years old. SMA is a rare genetic disorder that affects nervous system control of muscle movement. Jackson and his family have managed his medical, pharmacological and physiotherapy treatment largely as an outpatient.

Now a teen, Jackson knows members of his treating team well. He has been eager to participate in hospital quality and research activities and sits on the hospital Youth Advisory Council. Jackson's mother, Lila, gave consent for him to participate in a longitudinal cohort study about quality of life for children with SMA when he started school.

As Jackson approaches his thirteenth birthday, he can no longer walk unassisted and is losing interest in his physio and other activities. He requests to leave the Youth Advisory Council and wants to opt out of his six-monthly visits with the research team.

Lila seeks your advice. She is distraught, as she sees her son's participation in research as being of potential benefit to his overall health and of significant value to other children and young people with SMA. What might you discuss with Lila regarding Jackson's right to refuse participation in research? What might you discuss with Jackson?

Partners in evidence implementation

Evidence implementation and evaluation are practice initiatives for improving the quality, safety and appropriateness of care for all children and young people. This chapter has encouraged you to reflect on how you can use your knowledge of research and evidence to focus on issues and questions that are of primary concern to children, young people and their families, to support evidence-based practice, and to encourage the meaningful partnership of children and young people in research that is ethical and of value to them and their future.

With much already achieved to support the searching and appraisal of quality research evidence in health, this chapter has also emphasised the complex environment and myriad contexts in which evidence implementation occurs. Implementation science is continuously developing methods to improve our ability to identify those factors that affect the uptake of evidence-based interventions (Bauer & Kirchner, 2020); regardless, evidence-implementation models always propose the initial development of an implementation plan.

A large number of implementation frameworks have been developed and tested across health and other contexts (Nilsen, 2015), the common indicator of success

being that these models must be multi-faceted and must include stakeholder participation. We have already referred to the PARIHS Model (Kitson et al., 2008; Rycroft-
Malone et al., 2013). Another popular model is the Knowledge to Action (KTA)
framework (Graham et al., 2006).

In the clinical research context, children and young people involved in the research
co-design and conduct phases are in the best position to contribute excellent ideas for
the implementation of findings. However, any child or young person who is interested
can be involved in the implementation of research that will inform their own future
care and that of others:

- Children and young people can be asked to identify what they think might be
  potential barriers to implementing research evidence into practice change.
- Children and young people who will be affected by the change in treatment or
  healthcare can become evidence champions to lead and promote the acceptance,
  implementation and maintenance of change.
- Children and young people will become researchers of the future.

REFLECTION POINTS 4.3

- Research fatigue can be experienced by anyone, but it is a specific risk to children,
  young people and families who are frequent users of health services, and
  therefore more accessible for research recruitment. What effects might over-
  researching have on the quality and outcomes of research? How do Australian
  human research ethics committees support researchers to respect the needs and
  interests of children and young people as research participants?
- Children and young people can be involved in the prioritisation, co-design and
  implementation of research that will inform their care by being part of the research
  or evidence implementation team. What kind of digital solutions can you think of to
  support their participation?
- The successful and timely translation of research into practice remains challenging, but can be accelerated through the identification of practice gaps. Have you
  seen quality and safety reports from your own workplace? Have you asked 'why'
  questions about the data you have seen – and have you then thought about
  translating your 'why' question into an answerable research question?

SUMMARY

- Research and evidence are intimately linked in nursing and healthcare, but each
  makes a slightly different contribution. We can broadly distinguish research as a
  rigorous and systematic process for deriving new knowledge, and evidence as
  the knowledge that is produced and used. However, evidence from other sources
  is also used to inform health and treatment decisions. The experience of the
  clinician, the context of the healthcare environment and information about the

specific values and priorities of the child or young person receiving care ultimately shape decisions about how evidence is used and determine how successfully it is implemented.

- The ethics of human research are based on the fundamental principles of research integrity, autonomy and respect, beneficence and justice. These principles collectively attest that any risks from the research will be outweighed by the contribution of the research to improving health and healthcare, and that the dignity, privacy and wellbeing of the research participant will be protected at all times.

- Obtaining consent for participation in research is central to respect for persons. While Australia and New Zealand have specific legislation concerning the age at which minors are deemed to have capacity to consent to medical treatment, this may not apply to participation in research. The age of consent for participation in research is defined by individual maturity. Younger children may have the capacity to understand the nature of the research and may give their consent in addition to their parent doing so. Mature children and young people capable of understanding the risks and benefits of their participation in research may give sole consent, with parental consent being waived in some circumstances.

- In the context of research ethics, a risk is anything that has the potential for harm, discomfort or inconvenience. Harm can be perceived or real, physical or psychological. Discomfort is a less serious form of risk.

- The inconvenience associated with participation in research may seem minimal to the researcher, but is especially relevant to the parents or carers of children and young people who may need to take time away from work or family and may incur financial or emotional costs as a result of their child's participation in research.

- Practical ways of involving children and young people in the co-design, conduct and monitoring of research are still developing. Active training for representation and meaningful participation is already undertaken by a number of community-based organisations and charities representing adults. These organisations have begun to extend this training to young people. There are a range of models and methods used outside the health context that present possibilities for application to increasing children and young persons' engagement in health research and expanding their role in implementing evidence-based healthcare.

LEARNING ACTIVITIES

4.1 There is often debate about whether a systematic review of literature can be defined as 'research'. What features would need to be present in a systematic review for it to be classified as research?

4.2 Imagine that you are following the steps of the research process to design a research project about effective post-operative pain management in infants (the population). For each step of the research process, think about how this question would be applied to both an infant *and* adult post-operative setting. Make a table to show differences for each population.

Consider, for example:
- differences between children and adults in the common types of surgery
- the post-operative management of these different surgical procedures

- the medications that are used for post-operative pain in adults and children (the intervention)
- how pain is measured (the outcome) in infants and adults
- procedures for gaining participant consent and project ethics approval
- project budget and timeline.

4.3 You are part of a research team that will be conducting in-depth qualitative interviews with children and young people who have had epilepsy for at least two years. Your research study is called 'Young People's Experience of Living with Epilepsy'. A member of the team has come to you with concerns about the study. He asks you what options have been built into the research design to maximise choice and minimise inconvenience, discomfort and potential harm to the participants.

What might you discuss with him? The following headings might help:

- Human research ethics committees – roles and responsibilities
- Research team – roles and responsibilities for the ethical conduct of research
- Participant rights to assent, consent and withdrawal
- Strategies to engage and encourage participant involvement in research process and implementation of findings.

FURTHER READING

Evidence-based practice

Ioannidis, JPA 2016, Evidence-based medicine has been hijacked: A report to David Sackett, *Journal of Clinical Epidemiology*, 73, pp. 82–6.

Ethical conduct of research involving children and young people

Field MJ & Berman RE (eds) 2004, *The ethical conduct of clinical research involving children,* National Academic Press, Washington, DC, viewed 16 August 2020, www.nap.edu/catalog/10958/ethical-conduct-of-clinical-research-involving-children

Powell, MA, Fitzgerald, R, Taylor, NJ & Graham, A 2012, *International literature review: Ethical issues in undertaking research with children and young people*, Southern Cross University, Centre for Children and Young People, Lismore and University of Otago, Centre for Research on Children and Families, Dunedin, viewed 8 August 2016, http://childethics.com/wp-content/uploads/2013/09/Powell-et-al-2012.pdf

Rallis Legal 2016, *Laws relating to the giving of consent for persons with impaired capacity to provide informed consent to participate in research in each Australian State and Territory*, NHMRC, Canberra.

Spriggs, M 2010, *Understanding consent in research involving children: The ethical issues. A handbook for human research ethics committees and researchers*, Royal Children's Hospital, Melbourne, viewed 16 August 2020, https://childethics.com/wp-content/uploads/2013/01/ERIC-Spriggs-2010.pdf

REFERENCES

Accad, M & Francis, D 2018, Does evidence based medicine adversely affect clinical judgement? *BMJ*, 362, p. k2799, viewed 16 August 2020, https://doi.org/10.1136/bmj.k2799

Agency for Healthcare Research and Quality (AHRQ) 2001, *Translating research into practice (TRIP) II,* US Department of Health and Human Services, Rockville, MD, viewed 7 August 2020, http://archive.ahrq.gov/research/findings/factsheets/translating/tripfac/trip2fac.pdf

Australian Paediatric Research Ethics and Governance Network (APREGN) 2017, *Clinical trials, the child participant and consent: A practical guide for investigators and sponsors*, Royal Children's Hospital, Melbourne, viewed 9 August 2020, www.rch.org.au/uploadedFiles/Main/Content/ethics/APREG%20Guide%20to%20child%20consent%20in%20CT%20revised%2019%20May%202017_FINAL%20VERSION.pdf

Allen, ML, Culhane-Pera, KA, Pergament, SL & Call, KT 2010, Facilitating research faculty participation in CBPR: Development of a model based on key informant interviews, *Clinical and Translational Science*, 3(5), pp. 233–8.

Andrews, JO, Newman, SD, Meadows, O, Cox, MJ & Bunting, S. 2012, Partnership readiness for community-based participatory research, *Health Education Research*, 27(4), pp. 555–71.

Bailey, S, Boddy, K, Briscoe, S & Morris, C 2014, Involving disabled children and young people as partners in research: A systematic review, *Child: Care, Health and Development*, 41(4), pp. 505–14.

Bauer, M & Kirchner, J 2020, Implementation science: What is it and why should I care? *Psychiatry Research*, 283: 112376.

Boluyt, N, Rottier, BL, de Jongste, JC, Riemsma, R, Elianne, JLE, Vrijlandt, EJLE & Brand, PLP 2012, Assessment of controversial pediatric asthma management options using GRADE, *Pediatrics*, 130(3), pp. E658–68.

Brothers, KB, Rivera, SM, Cadigan, J, Sharp, RR & Goldenberg, AJ 2019, A Belmont reboot: Building a normative foundation for human research in the 21st century, *Journal of Law, Medicine & Ethics*, 47(1), pp. 165–72.

Curran, G 2020, Implementation science made too simple: A teaching tool, *Implementation Science Communications*, 1, p. 27.

Davidson, A & O'Brien, M 2009, Ethics and medical research in children, *Pediatric Anesthesia*, 19, pp. 994–1004.

Djulbegovic, B & Guyatt, GH 2017, Progress in evidence-based medicine: A quarter century on, *The Lancet*, 390, pp. 415–23.

Dockett, S & Perry, B 2011, Researching with young children: Seeking assent. *Child Indicators Research*, 4, pp. 231–47.

Donnelly, M & Kilkelly, U 2011, Child-friendly healthcare: Delivering on the right to be heard, *Medical Law Review*, 19, pp. 27–54.

Giesbertz, N, Bredenoord, A & Delden, JV 2012, Inclusion of residual tissue in biobanks: Opt in or opt out? *PLoS Biology*, 10(8), viewed 16 August 2020, www.plosbiology.org/article/fetchObject.action?uri=info%3Adoi%2F10.1371%2Fjournal.pbio.1001373&representation=PDF

Godlee, F, Smith, J & Marcovitch, H 2011, Wakefield's article linking MMR vaccine and autism was fraudulent (editorial), *BMJ*, 342, doi:10.1136/bmj.c7452

Graham, I, Logan, J, Harrison, M, Straus, S, Tetroe, J, Caswell, W & Robinson, N 2006, Lost in knowledge translation: Time for a map? *Journal of Continuing Education in the Health Professions*, 26(1), pp. 13–24.

Haijes, HA & van Thiel, GJMW 2016, Participatory methods in pediatric participatory research: A systematic review. *Pediatric Research*, 79(5), pp. 676–83.

Health Research Council (HRC) of New Zealand (on behalf of the Pūtaiora Writing Group) 2010a, *Te Ara Tika: Guidelines for Māori research ethics: A framework for researchers and ethics committee members Me whakatika te matatika ki roto i te tikanga kia tika ai*, NZ Ministry of Health, Wellington, viewed 13 August 2020, www.hrc.govt.nz/resources/te-ara-tika-guidelines-maori-research-ethics-0

—— 2010b, *Guidelines for researchers on health research involving Māori, version 2*, NZ Ministry of Health, Wellington, viewed 13 August 2020, https://hrc.govt.nz/resources/guidelines-researchers-health-research-involving-maori

—— 2017, *HRC research ethics guidelines 2017*, NZ Ministry of Health, Wellington, viewed 9 August 2020, https://hrc.govt.nz/resources/hrc-research-ethics-guidelines-december-2017

Health Research Council (HRC) of New Zealand & Peart, N. 2007, *Research involving children*, NZ Ministry of Health, Wellington, viewed 13 August 2020, https://hrc.govt.nz/resources/research-involving-children

Hokke, S et al. 2018, Ethical issues in using the internet to engage participants in family and child research: A scoping review. *PLoS ONE*, 13(9), doi:10.1371/journal.pone.0204572

Isles, AF 2013, Understood consent versus informed consent: A new paradigm for obtaining consent for pediatric research studies. *Frontiers in Pediatrics*, 1, Article 38, viewed 16 August 2020, www.ncbi.nlm.nih.gov/pmc/articles/PMC3864257/pdf/fped-01-00038.pdf

Jarrett, I, Wilson, R, O'Leary, M, Eckersberger, E & Larson, HJ 2015, Strategies for addressing vaccine hesitancy: A systematic review, *Vaccine*, 33, pp. 4180–90.

Kitson, AL, Rycroft-Malone, J, Harvey, G, McCormack, B, Seers, K & Titchen, A 2008, Evaluating the successful implementation of evidence into practice using the PARIHS framework: Theoretical and practical challenges. *Implementation Science*; 3(1), doi:10.1186/1748-5908-3-1

Morris, Z, Wooding, S & Grant, J 2011, The answer is 17 years, what is the question? Understanding time lags in translational research, *Journal of the Royal Society of Medicine*, 104, pp. 510–20.

National Ethics Advisory Committee (NEAC) – Kāhui Matatika o te Motu 2012, *Āhuatanga ū ki te tika me te pono mō te Rangahau Māori: Māori Research Ethics: An overview*, NZ Ministry of Health, Wellington, viewed 15 August 2020, https://neac.health.govt.nz/publications-and-resources/neac-publications/m%C4%81ori-research-ethics-overview

National Ethics Advisory Committee (NEAC) 2019, *National ethical standards for health and disability research and quality improvement*, NZ Ministry of Health, Wellington, viewed 7 August 2020, https://neac.health.govt.nz/publications-and-resources/neac-publications/national-ethical-standards-health-and-disability

National Health and Medical Research Council (NHMRC) 2016, *Statement on consumer and community participation in health and medical research*, Commonwealth of Australia, Canberra, viewed 9 August 2020, www.nhmrc.gov.au/about-us/publications/statement-consumer-and-community-involvement-health-and-medical-research

—— 2018a, *Australian Code for the Responsible Conduct of Research 2018*, National Health and Medical Research Council, Australian Research Council and Universities Australia, Canberra, viewed 9 August 2020, www.nhmrc.gov.au/about-us/publications/australian-code-responsible-conduct-research-2018

—— 2018b, *Ethical conduct in research with Aboriginal and Torres Strait Islander peoples and communities: Guidelines for researchers and stakeholders,* Commonwealth of Australia, Canberra, viewed 9 August 2020, www.nhmrc.gov.au/about-us/resources/ethical-conduct-research-aboriginal-and-torres-strait-islander-peoples-and-communities

—— 2018c, *Keeping research on track II: A companion document to ethical conduct in research with Aboriginal and Torres Strait Islander peoples and communities: Guidelines for researchers and stakeholders,* Commonwealth of Australia, Canberra, viewed 9 August 2020, www.nhmrc.gov.au/about-us/resources/keeping-research-track-ii

—— 2018d, *National statement on ethical conduct in human research 2007 (Updated 2018),* National Health and Medical Research Council, Australian Research Council and Universities Australia, Canberra, viewed 7 August 2020, www.nhmrc.gov.au/about-us/publications/national-statement-ethical-conduct-human-research-2007-updated-2018

—— 2020, *Toolkit for consumer and community involvement in health and medical research*, Commonwealth of Australia, Canberra, viewed 16 August 2020, www.nhmrc.gov.au/about-us/consumer-and-community-engagement

New Zealand Ministry of Youth Development (NZMYD) – Te Manatū Whakahiato Taiohi n.d. *Working with young people,* Ministry of Social Development, Wellington, viewed 16 August 2020, www.myd.govt.nz/working-with-young-people

Nilsen, P 2015, Making sense of implementation theories, models and frameworks, *Implementation Science*, 10, p. 53, doi:10.1186/s13012–015-0242-0

Ohlin, J, Heller, A, Bryne, S & Keevy, N. 2010, *How young people participate in civic activities using internet and mobile technologies*, report to the National Youth Affairs Scheme (NYAS), Commonwealth of Australia, Canberra, viewed 16 August 2020, https://docs.education.gov.au/system/files/doc/other/how_young_people_participate_in_civic_activities_using_internet_and_mobile_technologies.pdf

Resnik, DB 2015, Bioethical issues in providing financial incentives to research participants, *Medicolegal and Bioethics*, 5, pp. 35–41.

Rycroft-Malone, J, Seers, K, Chandler, J, Hawkes, CA, Crichton, N, Allen, C, Bullock, I & Strunin, L 2013, The role of evidence, context, and facilitation in an implementation trial: Implications for the development of the PARIHS framework, *Implementation Science*, 8, p. 28.

Slattery, P, Saeri, AK & Bragge, P 2020, Research co-design in health: A rapid overview of reviews, *BMC Health Research Policy and Systems*, 18, p. 17.

Taplin, S, Chalmers, J, Hobin, B, McArthur, M, Moore, T & Graham, A 2019, Children in social research: Do higher payments encourage participation in riskier studies? *Journal of Empirical Research on Human Research Ethics*, 14(2), pp. 126–40.

United Nations Office of the High Commissioner of Human Rights (UNOHCHR) 1990, *UN convention on the rights of the child (UNCRC)*, UNOHCHR, Geneva, viewed 16 June 2020, www.ohchr.org/en/professionalinterest/pages/crc.aspx

Waters, DL, Rychetnik, L, Crisp, J & Barrett, A 2009, Views on evidence from nursing and midwifery opinion leaders, *Nurse Education Today*, 17(4), pp. 829–34.

World Medical Assembly (WMA) 2017, *WMA declaration of Ottawa on child health 2009*, viewed 10 August 2020, www.wma.net/policies-post/wma-declaration-of-ottawa-on-child-health

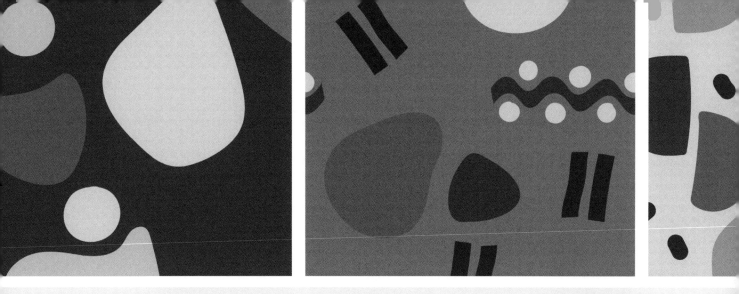

PART B

Nursing infants, young children and their families

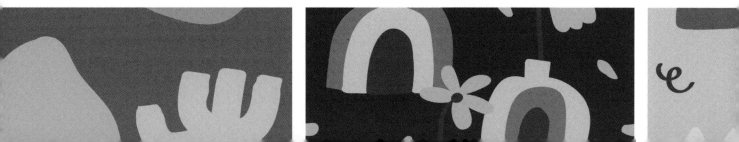

Working with new families throughout the transition to parenthood

5

Nicola Brown

LEARNING OBJECTIVES

In this chapter you will:

- Discuss preconceptual health and wellbeing as an emerging focus for care of women and families
- Outline current approaches to the nursing care of women and their babies during the antenatal and postnatal periods

Introduction

In paediatric nursing, families are central to the care of children – in fact, the patient is considered to be both the child and their whole family. In this chapter, you will begin to explore current approaches to the care of the woman and family during pregnancy, birth and parenting.

Becoming a parent is a life-changing transition for women and their partners, resulting in a range of changes during pregnancy and after birth that can present challenges to parents and impact their babies. In addition to the profound physical changes that take place during pregnancy, women and their partners experience changes in their roles and relationships with themselves and others in their social networks. In this chapter, preconception health, and antenatal and postnatal care will be discussed, including considering the factors influencing maternal and infant health and wellbeing.

Preconception and antenatal care

Our understanding of the importance of maternal health and its impact on maternal and child health outcomes over the lifespan has influenced approaches to perinatal healthcare services. An emerging area of focus for healthcare is improving the health and wellbeing of women and their partners before conception (**preconception care**).

Preconception care – Aims to identify the health risks that may exist for a woman and/or her partner prior to conception and intervene to ensure the best possible health outcomes for the mother and baby throughout their lifespan (WHO, 2013).

Fertility – The ability of an individual or couple to reproduce.

Some examples of preconception care strategies include efforts to improve nutrition; reduce adverse lifestyle factors such as maternal obesity, tobacco, drug and alcohol consumption; and reduce the risk of foetal abnormalities such as neural tube defects through supplementation with folic acid. Care extends to ensuring access to effective contraception and planning of reproduction prior to pregnancy (Dorney & Black, 2018).

Fertility is an important consideration in Australia. The average age of first-time parents in Australia has been increasing for several decades, as women and their partners delay parenting for economic and social reasons (AIHW, 2020). For example, the percentage of Australian women birthing their first child after the age of 30 years rose from 23 per cent in 1991 to 48 per cent in 2016 (AIFS, 2021).

There can be medical consequences to delaying childbearing, including difficulties conceiving due to ageing factors. Female fertility declines from approximately 30 years of age, and this decline accelerates from 35 years. The risk of miscarriage, obstetric and neonatal complications also increases. Male fertility also declines after the age of 40 years, including diminished sperm quality. Older fathers are associated with higher risk of schizophrenia and autism in their biological children.

The health of the infant across the lifespan is influenced by their intrauterine environment – otherwise 'known as the developmental origins of health and disease' (Dorney & Black, 2018). For example, maternal nutritional status and weight both before and during pregnancy can influence foetal growth and birth outcomes, and can impact the child's health and wellbeing in the long term. Infants born to mothers who were obese at the time of conception may have a higher risk of being overweight during their lifespan and may endure the cardiovascular risk factors associated with obesity (Hanson et al., 2017). Maternal malnutrition is associated with greater risk of poor foetal development and low birth weight (WHO, 2013).

The Australian government has developed and published recommendations for **antenatal** care (Department of Health, 2020). These evidence-based guidelines developed at a national level provide a consensus statement for the care of healthy pregnant women who do not have pre-existing conditions and are not at risk of pregnancy complications. The main recommendations include:

- promoting health and wellbeing in the antenatal period, including nutrition and exercise recommendations
- health information on preparing for pregnancy, birth and parenting
- promoting and preparing for breastfeeding
- monitoring of foetal wellbeing during pregnancy
- monitoring the health of the woman, including for any risk arising for premature birth or pre-eclampsia, gestational diabetes, anaemia, STIs or mental health
- managing the symptoms of pregnancy (reflux, nausea, haemorrhoids)
- discussing the option of testing for chromosomal abnormalities.

> **Antenatal care** – The routine care of pregnant women during pregnancy. This can include physical assessment and monitoring of maternal health and wellbeing, lifestyle counselling and monitoring of the developing foetus.

Preconceptual and antenatal health and wellbeing

Most of the recommendations for optimal health prior to pregnancy also apply to women who are pregnant and their families. Good health before, during and after pregnancy, which includes physical and psychosocial wellbeing, is an important area of focus for health promotion in women and their partners as they plan for pregnancy and birth, and raise families (Dorney & Black, 2018; RACGP, 2019).

Women should be encouraged to continue a healthy diet during preconception and pregnancy, in accordance with adult dietary guidelines (NHMRC, 2013), including drinking plenty of water. Women who are overweight or obese can be encouraged to lose weight prior to pregnancy (RACGP, 2019). Women who are underweight during pregnancy may need to consume more food for adequate weight gain. Women who are overweight or obese may benefit from avoiding large portions of energy-dense foods; however, diets are not generally recommended during pregnancy. Low- to moderate-intensity physical exercise is associated with health benefits during pregnancy. Weight changes, diet and physical activity should be discussed regularly during antenatal visits, in a respectful, positive and supportive manner.

Screening tools can help the healthcare provider to identify women who have risk factors, including the use of addictive substances. Avoidance of tobacco, alcohol and other addictive substances is an important aspect of preconceptual and antenatal care. There is no safe amount of smoking or alcohol consumption during pregnancy, and the growing foetus can be adversely affected by these substances. For example, smoking is associated with lower birth weight and premature birth (Lawder et al., 2019), while alcohol is associated with foetal alcohol spectrum disorder (Forray, 2016). Parents may be motivated to improve health and wellbeing, and therefore be open to interventions for the cessation of smoking and the use of alcohol and other drugs.

Use of medications during the preconceptual and antenatal periods needs careful consideration. While consumption of some medications may negatively impact fertility or foetal development, in turn medication cessation may negatively impact maternal wellbeing. Few medications have been assessed as categorically safe during pregnancy, including herbal preparations. Use of medications needs to be considered in discussion with the woman by her healthcare providers, taking into account her unique health circumstances and considering the relative risk versus benefit of the medication for its purpose.

Some nutritional supplements are recommended during preconception and the antenatal period, due to their potential to reduce risk of disability in infants. As a result of recommendations regarding the use of folic acid during preconception and early pregnancy, the rate of neural tube defects such as anencephaly and spina bifida have decreased significantly. Women who are planning pregnancy should be encouraged to take folic acid supplementation from at least 12 weeks before conception and throughout the first trimester. Iodine supplementation is recommended in pregnancy. Maternal thyroid dysfunction due to iodine deficiency can have an adverse impact on foetal brain and central nervous system development, leading to infant mortality and disability. Many foods are fortified with iodine in Australia; however, consumption of iodine-fortified foods may not be consistent in women of childbearing age. Iron supplements may be warranted for women at risk of iron deficiency only. Other supplements are not routinely recommended.

Some women may experience more dental issues and poorer oral health during pregnancy. For example, vomiting can increase exposure of the oral mucosa and teeth to acid, and women are more likely to experience gingivitis (inflammation of the gums) during pregnancy, possibly due to greater vascular permeability and changes in the microbiome of the gut, influenced by the hormones changes in pregnancy (Morelli et al., 2018). Poorer periodontal health has been associated with an increased risk of preterm birth or low birth weight (Iheozor-Ejiofor et al., 2017). Current Australian pregnancy guidelines (Department of Health, 2020) recommend that all healthcare professionals caring for women during pregnancy promote oral health practices such as regular brushing with a fluoride toothpaste, flossing and regular dental checks and descaling, and oral care after vomiting.

Preparation for parenting

Planning to have a baby is a significant step in the lives of family members, and the confirmation of pregnancy is a time for great excitement and celebration. However, depending on the individual circumstances, the woman and her partner may face challenges for a variety of reasons that may include physical and psychological health and wellbeing, and social factors such as employment and social support. Furthermore, the addition of a new family member in the form of a newborn infant will require adjustments to the relationship of the parents between themselves and with extended family members and friends.

Antenatal education

In Australia and New Zealand, as part of antenatal care, expectant parents can attend classes designed to help them prepare for birth and parenting. Antenatal classes are most commonly offered by maternity services. Course content may include the physiologic and emotional changes experienced during pregnancy, the process of birth, plans and options for birth, pain management during labour, postnatal care of the infant, and preparation for breastfeeding. The effectiveness of such education classes to influence the outcomes or experience of birth has not been established, and concerns have been expressed that the course content tends to focus on preparation for birth, rather than parenting (Entsieh & Hallström, 2016).

Birthing choices

Women who are experiencing a normal, healthy pregnancy can give birth at home or in a birthing centre within a hospital. Women with risk factors for their pregnancy or birth, or adverse health outcomes for either themselves or their infant, may only be able to give birth in a hospital setting. In Australia and New Zealand, most babies are born in a hospital setting, although increasing numbers of woman are choosing to birth at home.

There are concerns that the place of birth can increase the chance for women receiving medical interventions. For example, women who give birth in a private hospital setting are more likely to have a caesarian section, and women with low-risk pregnancies who give birth in labour ward in a hospital setting are more likely to have medical interventions than women who deliver in a birth centre or their home (AIHW, 2018). In Australia, there is a growing push for continuity of care models, as there is evidence that such models may reduce the rates of medical intervention and thus improve outcomes for women and their babies (Sandall et al., 2016).

REFLECTION POINTS 5.1

Our own experiences or those of friends and family can influence perceptions of healthcare. What are your own experiences of pregnancy, birth and early parenthood? How might these experiences influence your views of different care models during pregnancy?

Monitoring of maternal health in the antenatal period

Monitoring and promoting maternal health during pregnancy are important for both maternal and child wellbeing. It is recommended that women attend an appointment with their healthcare provider in the first trimester, and regularly for monitoring during the pregnancy. Depending on their preference and circumstances, women may be cared for during pregnancy by a midwifery team, general practitioner and/or obstetrician. As the pregnancy progresses, the visits become more frequent (Department of Health,

2020). A range of clinical assessments are offered during the antenatal period to promote and enhance physical and emotional wellbeing.

During the first antenatal visit, maternal height and weight are assessed, and body mass index (BMI) is calculated to help estimate predicted weight gain during pregnancy. Maternal blood pressure is screened at the first visit to identify women with hypertension and establish their individual baseline. Up to 15 per cent of women may experience hypertension (Wu et al., 2020) and oedema during pregnancy. Tests are routinely undertaken to identify women who may be developing signs of **pre-eclampsia**, a serious disorder in pregnancy that is not well understood.

Pre-eclampsia – Hypertension occurring after 20 weeks' gestation, detected during two or more assessments and including the involvement of one or more systems (e.g. renal, hepatic, respiratory, haematological, neurological).

Approximately 3 per cent of Australian women develop mild to severe pre-eclampsia during pregnancy (Department of Health, 2020), usually during the last few months of pregnancy. Pre-eclampsia usually resolves within a few days of the birth of the baby (Duhig, Vandermolen & Shennan, 2018). The level of hypertension is used as the primary measure of severity, in addition to the presence of proteinurea and the extent of oedema. Women may also experience neurological effects including dizziness, headache or visual disturbances, nausea and vomiting. If severe pre-eclampsia develops, women may be at risk of seizures, renal or liver failure, thromboembolism or death. Risk factors include women with pre-existing hypertension, those who are overweight and obese, or those with a family history of pre-eclampsia (Department of Health, 2020). Women with severe pre-eclampsia may require bed rest and monitoring, with consideration of the need for anti-hypertensive and anti-convulsant medications. Calcium supplementation and aspirin may be indicated as preventative treatments in women who are at high risk of pre-eclampsia. An important part of antenatal care is to assess the relative risk of pre-eclampsia and provide education to women on signs that indicate they may need to seek help, including headache, visual disturbances, vomiting, epigastric pain and/or rapid swelling (face, hands and feet).

Infectious diseases during pregnancy can have an adverse effect on the developing foetus. Women who are planning to become pregnant, or who are currently pregnant, are offered screening for a range of infectious diseases including human immunodeficiency virus (HIV), and hepatitis B and C. Women may also be offered screening for syphilis and other sexually transmitted diseases, including chlamydia. Testing for cytomegalovirus may be offered to women who work in childcare settings. A rubella infection in the mother during pregnancy can result in serious congenital disabilities in the infant (e.g. hearing loss, global developmental delay, cardiac defects, cleft lip and palate), miscarriage, stillbirth and foetal growth delay. Rubella immunisation is recommended prior to pregnancy, and women with a previous immunisation history are offered a test to check their immunity as part of antenatal care (Department of Health, 2020).

Group B streptococcus is a common bacterium colonising the gastrointestinal tract, urethra and vagina, which can be transferred to the baby during labour and delivery (Department of Health, 2020). Women are generally unaware that they carry the bacterium unless they are screened in the antenatal period (around 35–38 weeks). A positive Group B streptococcus test indicates a higher risk for preterm labour or infection in the newborn, such as pneumonia, meningitis or sepsis. Women who are screened and receive a positive result are offered intravenous antibiotics during labour to reduce the risk of infection in the newborn.

Monitoring of foetal growth and development

Foetal growth and development are monitored during pregnancy in several ways including physical assessment of the mother, ultrasound and monitoring of foetal movements and heart rate. During the first antenatal visit, the due date for the birth is estimated, based on the first day of the woman's last menstrual period (LMP) plus 280 days. If women are uncertain about the date of conception, an ultrasound may be offered to assess the gestational age of the foetus.

From approximately 12 weeks, the foetal heart rate can be detected and monitored by Doppler. An ultrasound is offered between 18 and 20 weeks to assess foetal well-being and development. Some congenital abnormalities may be able to be detected at this point, including neurological and cardiac abnormalities. This can provide time for parents and their healthcare team to consider a plan/treatment options, depending on the nature of the condition detected.

At around 20 weeks, most women will start to sense early signs of foetal movement, and these will become more obvious as the pregnancy progresses. Women should be provided with information about normal foetal movement, including the changing patterns that can occur during sleep and waking periods and advised to seek help promptly if they have concerns about decreased or notable changes in foetal movements.

CASE STUDY 5.1 GINA: ANTENATAL CARE

Gina (30 years) is 20 weeks pregnant. This is Gina's second pregnancy – she had a miscarriage approximately two years ago at 12 weeks' gestation. After the miscarriage, Gina and her partner Sean had decided to wait for some time before attempting to become pregnant again, while they grieved for their lost baby.

Gina has elected to have her antenatal care provided by the midwifery team at the local hospital. Gina experienced considerable nausea and some vomiting, fatigue and anxiety during the first trimester. She is now feeling well and beginning to feel very light sensations of her baby moving. Yesterday she had her 18–20 week ultrasound and found out that the baby was a girl.

Gina and Sean are hoping that Gina will be able to have a normal vaginal birth in the birth centre of their local hospital. They are planning to attend antenatal classes, and Gina also wants to attend a breastfeeding preparation class.

Discomforts of pregnancy

Women can experience a range of pregnancy symptoms, some of which can impact wellbeing and quality of life. The most common include nausea and vomiting, fatigue, constipation and haemorrhoids, urinary frequency, physical pain and ankle swelling.

Nausea, retching and vomiting, often called 'morning sickness', is a well-known and commonly experienced symptom and discomfort of early pregnancy, experienced by most women to varying degrees of severity during the first trimester. In severe cases, nausea is accompanied by severe and unremitting vomiting, a condition known as hyperemesis gravidarum. Women experiencing severe vomiting can become dehydrated and may require medical intervention, including hospital admission for medical management and intravenous rehydration. In extreme cases, hyperemesis may continue throughout pregnancy. Although nausea and vomiting are not associated with any negative impact on the pregnancy, these are unpleasant symptoms to experience. A systematic review of interventions to manage nausea and vomiting in early pregnancy (Matthews et al., 2015) was unable to identify compelling evidence for any particular intervention. Table 5.1 outlines the current evidence for commonly used interventions as recommended by the Australian Department of Health (2020).

Table 5.1 Interventions to manage nausea and vomiting in pregnancy

Intervention	Evidence
Ginger products	Limited and inconsistent evidence of the effectiveness of ginger products Dosages of up to 250 mg four times per day appear to be safe
Acupressure, acustimulation, acupuncture	Some evidence supports the use of P6* acupressure and appears to be safe in pregnancy Evidence of effectiveness of acupressure, acustimulation and acupuncture is inconsistent and limited No significant benefit of acupuncture demonstrated
Pyridoxine (vitamin B6)	Limited evidence to support use of pyroxidine Concerns about potential risk of toxicity – seek advice on recommended dosages in pregnancy from a medical practitioner
Antihistamine	May have some benefit in the management of nausea Seek advice on type and dosage from a medical practitioner
Other pharmacological treatments	Antiemetics may be indicated in severe nausea and vomiting Seek advice on type and dosage from a medical practitioner

* P6: pressure point located on the centre of the inner wrist
Source: Adapted from Department of Health (2020).

The growing foetus can cause pressure on organs in the abdominal cavity that contribute to urinary frequency, constipation and haemorrhoids. Avoiding fluids due to nausea can further contribute to constipation. Women are encouraged to drink plenty of water and maintain a high-fibre diet. Urinary frequency should be monitored, as it may be an indication of urinary tract infection and may require treatment.

Women can experience pain in several ways during pregnancy. As the growing foetus gains weight and size, women adjust their posture and gait to accommodate the change in centre of gravity and maintain balance. These changes in posture can lead to back and neck ache. These discomforts may be relieved by rest and by the application of heat to the local area.

In late pregnancy, most women will begin to report that their ankles swell as the day goes on. The swelling is often relieved by resting with the legs elevated. Lower limb oedema is also one of the potential signs of pre-eclampsia, and thus any oedema should be considered in relation to other signs of pre-eclampsia such as proteinurea and hypertension.

Mental health and wellbeing during pregnancy

It is common for women to experience mental health issues in pregnancy and the first years after birth. If maternal mental health issues are not recognised or treated, it may have an adverse impact on infant wellbeing (Hazell Raine et al., 2020). As many as one in five women reports depression, anxiety or stress during the perinatal period (AIHW, 2012). Maternal mental health and wellbeing may impact on foetal and child development. There is some evidence that maternal and/or paternal mental health problems are associated with preterm birth, and child emotional and behavioural difficulties (Stein et al., 2014).

Some women and their partners will have a history of mental health disorders prior to pregnancy, which may re-emerge during pregnancy and during the postnatal period. This is a particular challenge for pregnant women who need to cease the medications used to manage their condition due to the risk of side-effects from the medication for the developing foetus. For other women and men, mental health difficulties can arise for the first time during the transition to parenting. Anxiety may arise in response to fears about aspects of the pregnancy – including the risks associated with pregnancy and the changing role of becoming a parent. Higher levels of anxiety in pregnancy are associated with a higher risk of post-natal depression.

As there is the potential for mental health issues to arise, screening for perinatal mental health conditions is recommended during pregnancy and during the perinatal period. The Edinburgh Postnatal Depression Scale (EPDS) is a commonly used, validated screening tool for early detection of signs of depression and anxiety, used with women during antenatal and postnatal periods. It has also been validated for use in men (Matthey et al., 2001). It is widely used internationally and is available in a range of languages. The tool consists of 10 items, which ask the woman to report on symptoms of emotional distress during the previous seven-day period. One of the items (item 10) asks the women to disclose any thoughts of self-harm. In administering the EPDS, clinicians are required to calculate an overall score, and also to note the response to item 10 in determining the level of risk indicated by the screening tool. The higher the overall score, the more likely the woman is to be experiencing more severe symptoms of depression or anxiety. It is important to note that the EPDS is a screening tool only – referral is required for further clinical assessment, diagnosis and intervention. Healthcare professionals require training in appropriate and sensitive administration and scoring of the EPDS. Training should include use of the tool when screening for women from different cultural backgrounds, and on local policies and guidelines for responding when risk of self-harm or suicidal ideation is identified from the screening.

Family and domestic violence are serious risk factors for the health and wellbeing of the pregnant women and the foetus. In addition to the physical risks of injury, miscarriage, haemorrhage, trauma and death, women who experience violence during pregnancy are more likely to develop depression in the postnatal period (Department of Health, 2020). Domestic and family violence, and violence against women, represent an international problem. Almost 17 per cent of Australian women report experiencing partner physical or sexual violence (ABS, 2020). For some families, becoming pregnant or the birth of children can increase the risk of domestic violence at the same time that families are more likely to be accessing healthcare services. As a result, contact with healthcare professionals in maternity and child and family health services provides an opportunity to screen and refer women at risk or experiencing domestic violence to services for assistance. Opportunistic screening has been integrated into services that cater to women with higher risk. For example, in New South Wales, women are routinely screened when attending antenatal, child and family health, mental health, and drug and alcohol services (NSW Ministry of Health, 2019). Even though healthcare professionals have opportunities to screen, there is some evidence that indicates women are not routinely screened when engaging with services, such as general practice services (O'Reilly & Peters, 2018).

There is some variation in approaches to screening, such as the use of different screening tools across different states and territories. Irrespective of the tool used, clinicians are advised to undertake additional training in the administration of the tool. For example, one of the key elements of screening requires that clinicians ask screening questions without the woman's partner present.

Postnatal care

Postnatal care focuses on responding to the infant's and mother's needs after birth. There is an initial period of assessment and observation of the mother and baby to ensure that they have both recovered from the birth process and that there are no complications. Depending on the model of maternity care that is chosen, a woman and her new baby may stay in hospital for up to 24 hours after birth. If complications have arisen during birth for the mother or baby, or a caesarean section was performed, a longer stay in hospital may be required. In most instances, the family will be visited in the home in the days following the birth by midwives to monitor the mother's and infant's wellbeing and recovery.

Once the baby is born, the midwife's role extends to assessing and optimising the newborn's wellbeing. If the newborn requires additional monitoring, assessment or treatment, they may be admitted to a neonatal unit or paediatric services following discharge.

Postnatal care of the mother

After the placenta has been birthed, women will experience a bloody discharge (lochia) for several weeks. In the first few days, the lochia is bright red, heavy and contains clots. Over time, the discharge becomes lighter and is less intensely red. In addition to the discharge, women may experience mild contractions, especially during breastfeeding.

Women who have had a vaginal birth requiring episiotomy or stitches for a tear will have perineal discomfort for several days from the swelling and stiches. Regular bathing is encouraged to help keep any wounds clean and mild analgesics can be used for pain. To avoid further discomfort that may be caused by constipation, women can be encouraged to consume fibre-rich foods and maintain a good fluid intake.

Postnatal care of the newborn infant

Assessment of newborn transition

In the first minutes after the baby is born, the focus is on newborn wellbeing and the infant's transition to extrauterine life. As a baby takes its first breath after birth, a range of physiological changes begin to take place as the baby adapts to the new, external environment.

The baby will start to appear progressively more red or pink than grey/purple, will have greater muscle tone and may cry. All these are positive signs of changes occurring in newborn physiology, including the initiation and maintenance of regular respirations, conversion from to air filled lungs and the redirection of blood flow toward the newborn's lungs and normal circulation. If this does not occur, the baby may need stimulation to encourage the first breath or may need respiratory resuscitation.

From approximately 35 weeks' gestation, maturation of the adrenal glands leads to an increase in cortisol production, which increases further during and immediately after birth. The increased cortisol influences the maturation of the respiratory system and metabolism, and is important to the transition to external life (Graves & Mumford Haley, 2013).

Respiratory changes

A range of factors contribute to the stimulation and initiation of respiration in the moments after birth. These include a decline in pH and increased carbon dioxide, drop in environmental temperature, exposure to light and noise, position and movement, and the recoil of the newborn's chest after delivery (Davidson, 2020).

Fluid production in the lungs decreases before labour and birth, and surfactant production increases. The compression of the baby's torso during birthing and the initiation of respiration help to expel fluid from the lungs. Surfactant production helps to maintain inflation of the alveoli (Graves & Mumford Haley, 2013).

Taking the first breaths helps to clear the airway of any fluids in the mouth or airway – sometimes babies may require suctioning to help clear these.

Circulatory changes

Initial respirations influence the transition to normal circulation. With the first breaths, the infant's oxygen level increases, leading to an increased dilation of the pulmonary arteries and increased pulmonary circulation. The increase in pulmonary blood flow decreases pressure in the right atrium and ventricle, with increasing flow to the left atrium and ventricle (Davidson, 2020; Graves & Mumford Haley, 2013). Vasoconstriction of the umbilical arteries reduces blood flow from infant to placenta, while blood continues to transfuse from the placenta to the newborn for approximately five minutes, facilitated by contractions of the uterus (Graves & Mumford

Haley, 2013). Structures that formed part of foetal circulation including the ductus arteriosus, ductus venosus and foramen ovale begin to close as the pressures change (Davidson, 2020).

Thermoregulation

Prior to birth, foetal thermoregulation is maintained in the consistent intrauterine environment of warm amniotic fluid, through heat generated by the placenta and foetal metabolism. After birth, the external environment is less constant, and the infant can rapidly lose heat. Infants who experience a decrease in temperature will respond by increasing physical activity and thermogenesis, increasing oxygen and glucose consumption, as well as increasing the risk of hypoglycaemia and hypoxia (Graves & Mumford Haley, 2013). Keeping the newborn in skin-to-skin contact with the mother's chest after birth helps to maintain newborn thermoregulation and reduces the risk of hypoglycamia and hypoxia (Moore et al., 2016).

At birth, an assessment of the infant's wellbeing is undertaken with the first few minutes, using an **Apgar score**. The score consists of five criteria, including colour, respiratory effort, reflexes, muscle tone and heart rate. A score of 0, 1 or 2 is assigned to each of the criteria. A higher overall score (7–10) indicates little difficulty in adjusting to extrauterine life, while low scores indicate need for further intervention that may include resuscitation. Tables showing the Apgar score criteria are readily available online.

Promoting skin-to-skin care as soon as possible after birth, and continuing for as long as possible, has a range of benefits for the infant and mother, including stabilisation of physiological parameters such as heart rate and initiation of breastfeeding (Moore et al., 2016). In some instances, infants may need further support to maintain their body temperature. Newborn infants lack a mature thermoregulation system, and may need support to maintain body temperature including warmed blankets, or an incubator if hypothermic.

After birth, the parents will usually spend time with their baby, with healthcare professionals supporting and promoting time together.

After the initial, brief physical assessment of the infant at birth, a more extensive assessment is undertaken to assess infant wellbeing. This systematic, head-to-toe assessment seeks to identify any indicators of congenital disorders, neonatal conditions or developmental concerns that may require further investigation and referral (RACP, 2009). It also establishes birth weight and length, important indicators of intrauterine growth (Villar et al., 2017).

The average infant birthweight is Australia is 3.3 kilograms (AIHW, 2020) and average length is 50 centimetres. Most infants will lose about 10 per cent of their body weight in the first few days following birth, mainly via insensible fluid loss through the urinary system and bowel, and due to low fluid intake. Birthweight is generally regained by the second week.

Newborn infants may have some transient physical characteristics, including head moulding and body hair. Infants may have an elongated head shape due to moulding that takes place during birth. The bones of the skull shift during birth, and in the days following the head shape gradually returns to a more rounded shape. The

Apgar score – A brief assessment undertaken at one minute and five minutes after birth. It provides an initial assessment of the newborn infant's clinical status (American Academy of Pediatrics, 2015).

spaces between skull bones, including fontanelles and suture lines, can be palpated during examination of the head. There are specific newborn reflexes that are normally present at birth (see Table 5.2). Some of these reflexes help the baby to begin feeding.

Table 5.2 Newborn reflexes

Reflex	Description
Rooting	When touched on cheek or lip, infant turns head toward the touch and opens mouth.
Sucking	Stimulation of the mouth cavity causes infant to suckle.
Swallow	When mouth cavity is filled with liquid, infant swallows.
Gag	Stimulation of the posterior third of the tongue and mouth causes infant to gag.
Extrusion	Stimulation of the tongue causes infant to thrust tongue forward.
Moro 'startle'	Sudden jarring, noise or 'startle' causes infant to extend limbs, arch back and head, then flex limbs back inwards.
Tonic neck	Turning of the infant's head to one side, causes opposing arm to bend and arm on head side to extend.
Grasp	Stimulation of the palm of the infant's hand causes fingers to close in a grasp.
Babinski	Stoking the outside edge of the sole of the foot causes the toes to extend with big toe flexing upwards.
Crawl	Placing infant on their abdomen causes them to make crawling movements with arms and legs.
Stepping	When held upright with infant's feet touching a surface, the infant begins to 'walk' their feet and legs.

The administration of vitamin K is recommended at birth (NHMRC, 2010) to reduce the risk of bleeding in neonates, including vitamin K deficiency bleeding. Newborns are considered to be at risk of low vitamin K at birth, as maternal vitamin K does not transfer via the placenta and there is limited vitamin K present in breastmilk. A single injection of vitamin K, or oral formulation of vitamin K, is administered at birth and a further two doses in the early weeks (NHMRC, 2010). These methods provide vitamin K coverage while the infant's gut microbiome develops in the first few weeks; they are then able to produce vitamin K. Injection is the preferred method of administration; however, some parents may be hesitant or resistant to the administration of vitamin K, due to a study several years ago that indicated a possible association between injected vitamin K and childhood leukaemia. However, the cause has not been substantiated, and thus vitamin K is still recommended and encouraged. Parents should have received written information during pregnancy, and prior to the administration of vitamin K, regarding the rationale and importance of vitamin K and methods of administration (NHMRC, 2010).

REFLECTION POINTS 5.2

- Why might parents be concerned about health initiatives such as vitamin K and immunisation?
- What skills and strategies can be used to help support parents who are reluctant or hesitant to accept these interventions?

CASE STUDY 5.2 GINA: POSTNATAL CARE

Gina gives birth to her baby girl, Anna, in the birth centre with Sean present as her support person. Gina has a small perineal tear that did not require sutures. Baby Anna is placed skin to skin at birth with Gina, and then the cord is cut and clamped by Sean, with help from the midwife. Over the next few hours, Gina and Sean hold Anna in turn, initially skin to skin, while staying warm under a blanket. Anna has her first breastfeed from Gina, with support from the midwife.

After the birth, Gina and her baby daughter are cared for in the postnatal ward for 24 hours, and are now ready to go home. Anna wakes and feeds every one to three hours, and mostly sleeps between feeds. Gina asks the midwives to help her with breastfeeding each time, as she is still not sure that Anna is latching properly.

The midwife records Anna's feeds and nappy changes on a chart, noting that Anna is having wet nappies at each feed. Gina asks about the first bowel motion, a soft, sticky, green stool. The midwife explains that this is a normal meconium stool, the first bowel motion passed by babies after birth.

Prior to discharge, the paediatric registrar asks Gina whether she may examine Anna. The registrar explains that she is performing a head-to-toe assessment to check Anna's general health prior to discharge. Gina consents, and undresses Anna.

Anna is awake, alert and active, with good muscle tone for all limbs. Her skin is generally pink and intact, with no signs of central cyanosis or jaundice, and no bruising or rashes. Anna's temperature is 36.7°C per axilla, and she has a respiratory rate of 38 per minute and a heart rate of 135 per minute. Anna's head is visually and tactically examined by the registrar. Her head is slightly elongated due to moulding during the vaginal birth. The registrar explains that Anna's head shape will change as the moulding resolves over the next few days. The fontanelles are level. Anna's eyes are clear with no discharge. The registrar examines Anna's mouth and notes there is a normal palate and sucking reflex. Her chest, back and limbs are symmetrical and all normal reflexes are present. Her abdomen is soft and not distended. The umbilical clamp and cord are still in situ and clean.

Following discharge from the postnatal ward, Gina and Anna will be visited at home in the next week by a midwife and will then visit child and family health nursing services for Anna's next check. Gina will see her GP at approximately six weeks to check her postnatal recovery.

Each family in Australia is provided with a personal health record for their newborn infant during their postnatal stay. This record documents the infant's birth details and is used as an ongoing record of their growth and development through childhood, immunisation status, hospital and other healthcare visits. It also contains useful health information for the parents. The record is in a book format and varies between states and territories with regard to colour of the book and some differences in the information provided within. There are plans to create an electronic or application-based record.

Fostering attachment and bonding in the early postnatal period

In the case study, baby Anna is placed directly on her mother's skin immediately after birth and then kept close to her parents in the hours that follow. These actions help to foster the development of **attachment** between the infant and her mother, and **bonding** of the parents to Anna. Infant to primary caregiver attachment is developed throughout the first year, based on repeated positive and responsive interactions during the care of the infant. In the weeks and months to come, Gina and Sean will begin to recognise Anna's cues and behaviours, which indicate her need for help with hunger, tiredness and other emotions. The consistent, responsive, loving behaviours of the mother towards the infant help to develop secure infant attachment to the mother. These responsive maternal behaviours, supported by a caring partner and extended family, help to foster infant mental health and wellbeing, and impact mental health throughout childhood and adulthood (Galbally et al., 2020).

Attachment – Refers to the development of an enduring relationship between the infant and their primary caregiver – usually their mother – during infancy (Bowlby, 1958).

Bonding – The emotional tie from the parent to the infant (Bicking Kinsey & Hupcey, 2012).

Infant care: Focus on feeding

The early days and weeks of infant care are focused on responding to the baby's need for food and sleep. Infant sleep and settling are addressed in Chapter 6. In this section, we will explore infant feeding.

In Australia and New Zealand, the World Health Organization (WHO) recommendations for exclusive breastfeeding of infants until 6 months of age are widely supported by child and family health clinicians and organisations. Research has consistently demonstrated that breastmilk is ideal and the only food required by infants in the first six months of life (NHMRC, 2012; WHO, 2013). Breastfeeding should be encouraged and supported for as long as the baby and the mother wish (NHMRC, 2012). In our work as healthcare professionals, it is important to promote breastfeeding and the use of breastmilk as the best and safest first food for newborns and infants.

In some circumstances, parent may need to feed their baby with a bottle. This may be due to parent choice to feed their baby breastmilk with a bottle or to use infant formula. As a result, healthcare professionals working with children and families promote and support breastfeeding while also respecting the woman's right to choose to breastfeed or not; they must therefore be able to support parents who need to feed their baby with a bottle. In this section, we will discuss the importance of supporting breastfeeding in the newborn and early period of infancy. Feeding of infants via a bottle will also be explored. At birth and for the first few days and weeks afterwards, the caregiver and infant are getting to know each other and both can find feeding takes a bit of effort to adjust to. The support of healthcare professionals, family and friends during this time is important to the establishment of infant feeding.

Breastfeeding

Breastfeeding is associated with short- and long-term advantages for the infant, including improved general health, physical and cognitive growth and development, and protection against a number of diseases during childhood and through the life-course (NHMRC, 2012). Initiation of breastfeeding is high in most but not all Australian population groups. Unfortunately, the early cessation of breastfeeding in the early months after birth is also high (COAG Health Council, 2019). Our role as healthcare professionals is to support the breastfeeding mother, her infant and family, and promote and advocate for the initiation and maintenance of breastfeeding.

As the benefits of breastfeeding are so well established (see Table 5.3), national and international organisations promote breastfeeding widely. The WHO and UNICEF promote the Baby-Friendly Health Initiative (BFHI) to encourage acute and community health services to promote breastfeeding. The BFHI requires organisations to demonstrate specific criteria to identify themselves as 'baby friendly' via an audit process (Box 5.1).

Table 5.3   Potential beneficial effects of breastfeeding

Mothers	Infants
Decreased association with risk for: • Breast cancer • Ovarian cancer • Diabetes • Postpartum haemorrhage • Cardiovascular disease (including hypertension and hyperlipidaemia) • Maternal depression • Postpartum weight retention **Menstruation is postponed** when feeding frequently – may confer some contraceptive effect and reduce iron loss via menstruation **No direct household cost** for breastfeeding	**Nutritional benefit** – best source of nutrition for infant and confers immunological benefits that are not available via alternative food sources, including for infant microbiome **Reduced risk/severity for a range of health conditions** in infancy and childhood (e.g. infections, SID, pyloric stenosis, gastroesophageal reflux, leukaemia) and life course (e.g. diabetes, obesity, cardiovascular disease, asthma)

Source: Adapted from NHMRC (2012); COAG Health Council (2019).

BOX 5.1 TEN STEPS TO BABY-FRIENDLY HEALTH INITIATIVE

Critical management procedures

1a. Comply fully with the International Code of Marketing of Breastmilk Substitutes and relevant World Health Assembly resolutions.

1b. Have a written infant feeding policy that is routinely communicated to staff and parents.

1c. Establish ongoing monitoring and data-management systems.

2. Ensure that staff have sufficient knowledge, competence and skills to support breastfeeding.

Key clinical practices

3. Discuss the importance and management of breastfeeding with pregnant women and their families.

4. Facilitate immediate and uninterrupted skin-to-skin contact and support mothers to initiate breastfeeding as soon as possible after birth.

5. Support mothers to initiate and maintain breastfeeding and manage common difficulties.

6. Do not provide breastfed newborns any food or fluids other than breastmilk, unless medically indicated.

7. Enable mothers and their infants to remain together and to practise rooming-in 24 hours a day.

8. Support mothers to recognise and respond to their infants' cues for feeding.

9. Counsel mothers on the use and risks of feeding bottles, teats and pacifiers.

10. Coordinate discharge so that parents and their infants have timely access to ongoing support and care.

Source: Reproduced from WHO (2015).

Supporting breastfeeding

Women may experience initial difficulties with the transition to breastfeeding. Good support from healthcare professionals can make a significant difference, and help women to establish and continue breastfeeding. Sore nipples, pain, mastitis, engorgement and low supply are a few of the challenges faced by some breastfeeding mothers. Sometimes these challenges result in the cessation of breastfeeding. It is important for the health professional to have a working knowledge of the signs, symptoms and management of common breastfeeding problems. For further discussion about supporting breastfeeding, refer to Forster and Roache (2018) in the Further reading section.

Feeding infants with a bottle

Infants may be fed using a bottle for many different reasons, ideally with expressed breastmilk. These reasons may include the need for the breastfeeding mother to return to work, a mother's personal choice not to breastfeed, or to enable the infant to take formula required for medical reasons. When the informed decision not to breastfeed has been made, the only safe alternative for feeding infants to meet their primary nutritional needs is infant formula.

Parents who feed their infant with a bottle require just as much information and support as a breastfeeding mother. It is important that healthcare professionals remain supportive and non-judgemental, regardless of the method of infant feeding. Many parents worry that bottle feeding will adversely affect their relationship with their infant; however, infants can still form healthy attachments with their caregivers while bottle feeding. As healthcare professionals, we play an important part in reminding parents and caregivers that it is positive interactions with their baby that build the relationship, regardless of whether the baby is bottle-fed or breastfed.

Irrespective of the method, feeding is an essential social and emotional interaction between the infant and the parent or caregiver. When feeding a baby with a bottle, the caregiver should hold the baby close with their face visible to the baby so that the caregiver and baby can observe each other. Infants should not be prop-fed or placed in their cot or pram with the bottle.

In general, bottle feeding should only be used to provide infants with expressed breastmilk or infant formula. There may be some circumstances where cooled boiled water is offered when the infant has additional fluid requirements. Fluids such as juice, cordials, soft drinks, and teas are not appropriate fluids for infants (NHMRC, 2012).

BOX 5.2 PRINCIPLES FOR PREPARATION OF INFANT FEEDING BY BOTTLE

- Wash hands and prepare bottle feed (expressed breastmilk or infant formula) in a clean area.
- Wash bottles, teats, caps and other equipment used to prepare feed and sterilise.
- If using infant formula:
  - Prepare only one bottle at a time, just prior to feeding.
  - Read and follow manufacturer's instructions for preparation.
  - Use water that has previously been boiled and cooled to reconstitute formula.
  - Only use the infant formula pack scoop to measure the powder.
  - Do not use any more or less formula than recommended on the infant formula pack.
  - Store infant formula in accordance with manufacturer's instructions.
- Check the temperature of the feed – it should feel just warm to touch when a few droplets of feed are dropped on your wrist.
- Any feed left in the bottle should be discarded at the end of the feed.

Source: Adapted from NHMRC (2012, p. 76).

Some parents initially find storing expressed breastmilk, preparing infant formula and cleaning feeding equipment confusing. Ideally, parents will be using expressed breastmilk for their baby. If that is not possible, then parents will need to prepare an appropriate infant formula according to the manufacturer's directions so that the infant's nutritional requirements are adequately met.

Infant formula available in Australia is prepared to a high level of quality and in accordance with national standards (see Box 5.2). However, while produced as closely as possible to similar nutritional components as human milk, infant formula lacks a number of biological and immunological factors (NHMRC, 2012).

As with preparing and storing expressed breastmilk, high standards of hygiene should be used for the preparation and storage of infant formula. Bottles, teats and other feeding equipment need to be cleaned and washed after use, prior to boiling, chemical or steam sterilisation.

Expressing of breastmilk and storage of expressed breastmilk is covered in Forster and Roache (2018) (see Further reading section).

SUMMARY

- Planning for parenthood can be a time to intervene to help improve and enhance the health and wellbeing of parents. There is growing evidence that the preconceptual health of parents can impact on the health of their offspring throughout the life-course.
- The focus of antenatal and postnatal care is on monitoring the health and wellbeing of the mother and developing foetus/baby, and assisting parents in their adjustment to parenting, recognising and responding to the needs of their infant.
- There are a range of care models for women during pregnancy, birth and the postnatal period. Best outcomes may be achieved with a continuity of care model.

LEARNING ACTIVITIES

5.1 Learning about breastfeeding is an important area of knowledge for all healthcare professionals, including paediatric nurses. If you have never watched a woman breast-feed closely before, it can be daunting to do it in person for the first time with a parent of a patient for whom you are caring. We recommend that you begin to observe breastfeeding by watching recorded feedings. The website of the Australian Breastfeeding Association has a range of excellent resources for parents and professionals, and is a good place to begin observing women breastfeed.

5.2 Pregnancy and parenthood can be triggers for experiencing psychosocial and mental health difficulties and concerns. Locate and review your state/territory Health Department guidelines on the screening for women during pregnancy and the postnatal period.

5.3 The Stillbirth Centre of Research Excellence has developed an e-learning module (the 'Safer Baby Bundle') to provide healthcare professionals with current and evidence-based guidelines on strategies to reduce the risk of preventable stillbirths. These modules are freely available by registering at the Centre's website: hwww.stillbirthcre.org.au/safer-baby-bundle/elearning

FURTHER READING

Forster, E & Roache, B 2018, Supporting breastfeeding, in E Forster & J Fraser (eds), *Paediatric Nursing Skills for Australian Nurses*, Cambridge University Press, Melbourne, pp. 233–52.

Infant health record, viewed 21 February 2021, www.pregnancybirthbaby.org.au/infant-health-record

National Health and Medical Research Council (NHMRC) 2012, *Infant feeding guidelines: A summary*, National Health and Medical Research Council, Canberra, viewed 21 February 2021 www.eatforhealth.gov.au/sites/default/files/content/The%20Guidelines/170131_n56_infant_feeding_guidelines_summary.pdf

Silbert-Flagg, J & Pillitteri, A 2017, *Maternal and child health nursing*, 8th ed., Philadelphia, PA: Lippincott Williams & Wilkins.

REFERENCES

American Academy of Pediatrics Committee on Fetus and Newborn, American College of Obstetricians and Gynecologists Committee on Obstetric Practice 2015, The Apgar score, *Pediatrics*, 136(4), pp. 819–22.

Australian Bureau of Statistics (ABS) 2020, *Partner violence – in focus: Crime and justice statistics*, viewed 22 January 2021, www.abs.gov.au/statistics/people/crime-and-justice/focus-crime-and-justice-statistics/latest-release

Australian Institute of Family Studies (AIFS) 2021, *Births in Australia*, viewed 22 January 2021, www.aifs.gov.au/facts-and-figures/births-in-australia#:~:text=Nowadays%2C%20the%20late%2020s%20and,2011%20and%2048%25%20in%202016

Australian Institute of Health and Welfare (AIHW) 2012, *Experience of perinatal depression: Data from the 2010 Australian National Infant Feeding Survey*, cat. no. PHE 161, AIHW, Canberra.

—— 2018, *Australia's health in brief*, cat. no. AUS 222, AIHW, Canberra, viewed 5 July 2020, www.aihw.gov.au/reports/australias-health/australias-health-2018-in-brief/contents/births-in-australia

—— 2020, *Australia's mothers and babies 2018 – in brief*, AIHW, Canberra.

Bicking Kinsey, C & Hupcey, JE 2012, State of the science of maternal–infant bonding: A principle-based concept analysis, *Midwifery*, 29(12), pp. 1314–20.

Bowlby, J 1958, The nature of the child's tie to his mother, *International Journal of Psychiatry in Medicine*, 39, 350–73.

COAG Health Council 2019, *Australian national breastfeeding strategy 2019 and beyond*, COAG Health Council, Canberra, viewed 12 November 2020, www.coaghealthcouncil.gov.au/Portals/0/Australian%20National%20Breastfeeding%20Strategy%20-%20Final.pdf

Davidson, M 2020, *Fast facts for the neonatal nurse: Care essentials for normal and high-risk neonates*, Springer, Dordrecht.

Department of Health 2020, *Clinical practice guidelines: Pregnancy care*, Australian Government Department of Health, Canberra.

Dorney, E & Black, KI 2018, Preconception care, *Australian Journal of General Practice*, 47(7), pp. 424–9.

Duhig, K, Vandermolen, B & Shennan, A 2018, Recent advances in the diagnosis and management of pre-eclampsia, *F1000Research*, 7, p. 242.

Entsieh, AA & Hallström, IK 2016, First-time parents' prenatal needs for early parenthood preparation: A systematic review and meta-synthesis of qualitative literature. *Midwifery*, 39, pp. 1–11.

Forray A 2016, Substance use during pregnancy, *F1000Research*, 5, p. F1000 Faculty Rev-887.

Forster, E & Roache, B 2018, Supporting breastfeeding, in E Forster & J Fraser (eds), *Paediatric Nursing Skills for Australian Nurses*, Cambridge University Press, Melbourne, pp. 233–52.

Galbally, M, Stein, A, Hoegfeldt, CA & van Ijzendoorn, M 2020, From attachment to mental health and back, *The Lancet Psychiatry*, 7(10), pp. 832–4.

Graves, B & Mumford Haley, M 2013, Newborn transition, *Journal of Midwifery & Women's Health*, vol. 58, pp. 662-70.

Hanson M et al. 2017, Interventions to prevent maternal obesity before conception, during pregnancy, and post partum, *The Lancet Diabetes & Endocrinology*, 5(1), pp. 65–76.

Hazell Raine, K, Nath, S, Howard, LM, Cockshaw, W, Boyce, P, Sawyer, E & Thorpe, K 2020, Associations between prenatal maternal mental health indices and mother–infant relationship quality 6 to 18 months postpartum: A systematic review, *Infant Mental Health Journal*, 41(1), pp. 24–39.

Iheozor-Ejiofor, Z, Middleton, P, Esposito, M & Glenny, A 2017, Treating periodontal disease for preventing adverse birth outcomes in pregnant women, *Cochrane Database of Systematic Reviews*, 6(6), CD005297.

Lawder, R, Whyte, B, Wood, R, Fischbacher, C & Tappin, DM 2019, Impact of maternal smoking on early childhood health: A retrospective cohort linked dataset analysis of 697 003 children born in Scotland 1997–2009, *BMJ Open*, 9(3), p. e023213.

Matthews, A, Haas, DM, O'Mathúna, DP & Doswell, T 2015, Interventions for nausea and vomiting in early pregnancy, *The Cochrane Database of Systematic Reviews*, 2015(9), CD007575-CD.

Matthey, S, Barnett, B, Kavanagh, DJ & Howie, P 2001, Validation of the Edinburgh Postnatal Depression Scale for men, and comparison of item endorsement with their partners, *Journal of Affective Disorders*, 64(2–3), pp. 175–84.

Moore, ER, Bergman, N, Anderson, GC & Medley, N 2016, Early skin-to-skin contact for mothers and their healthy newborn infants, *Cochrane Database of Systematic Reviews*, 11(11), CD00351.

Morelli, ER et al. 2018, Pregnancy, parity and periodontal disease, *Australian Dental Journal*, 63, 270–8.

National Health and Medical Research Council (NHMRC) 2010, Joint statement and recommendations on vitamin K administration to newborn infants to prevent vitamin K deficiency bleeding in infancy – October 2010, viewed 14 November 2020, www.nhmrc.gov.au/about-us/publications/vitamin-k-administration-newborns-joint-statement

—— 2012, *Infant feeding guidelines*, National Health and Medical Research Council, Canberra.

—— 2013, *Australian dietary guidelines*, NHMRC, Canberra.

NSW Ministry of Health 2019, *Domestic violence routine screening program,* viewed 14 November 2020, www.health.nsw.gov.au/parvan/DV/Pages/dvrs.aspx

O'Reilly, R & Peters, K 2018, Opportunistic domestic violence screening for pregnant and post-partum women by community based healthcare providers, *BMC Women's Health*, 18(1), 128.

Royal Australasian College of Physicians (RACP) 2009, *Examination of the newborn*, RACP, Sydney.

Royal Australian College of General Practitioners (RACGP) 2019, Preventive activities prior to pregnancy, in *Guidelines for preventive activities in general practice: The red book*, viewed 12 November 2020, www.racgp.org.au/clinical-resources/clinical-guidelines/key-racgp-guidelines/view-all-racgp-guidelines/red-book/preventive-activities-prior-to-pregnancy

Sandall, J et al. 2016, Midwife-led continuity models versus other models of care for childbearing women, *Cochrane Database of Systematic Reviews*, 4, CD004667.

Stein, A et al. 2014, Effects of perinatal mental disorders on the fetus and child. *The Lancet*, 384(9956), pp. 1800–19.

Villar, J et al. 2017, Body composition at birth and its relationship with neonatal anthropometric ratios: The newborn body composition study of the INTERGROWTH-21st project, *Pediatric Research*, 82, 305–16.

World Health Organization 2013, *Preconception care: Maximising the gains for maternal and child health*, viewed 5 July 2020, www.who.int/maternal_child_adolescent/documents/preconception_care_policy_brief.pdf

—— 2015, *Ten steps to support breastfeeding*, viewed 12 November 2020, www.who.int/activities/promoting-baby-friendly-hospitals/ten-steps-to-successful-breastfeeding

Wu, R et al. 2020, Hypertensive disorders of pregnancy and risk of cardiovascular disease-related morbidity and mortality: A systematic review and meta-analysis, *Cardiology*, 145(10), 633–47.

Supporting families to manage child behaviour and sleep patterns, and promote optimal child development

Amy E Mitchell

LEARNING OBJECTIVES

In this chapter you will:

- Be introduced to current challenges in child health and development in Australia and New Zealand
- Take a social ecological approach to examining the influence of physical and psychosocial factors on children's development
- Explore approaches to supporting families to optimise child development from policy and clinical practice perspectives
- Consider evidence-based principles for supporting child development through managing behaviour, sleep, nutrition, physical activity and screen use

Introduction

This chapter focuses on supporting families to promote optimal child development. It takes a systems-based approach to examining factors that influence child development, explores some of the most common problems and concerns encountered by nurses who care for children and young people on a regular basis, and draws on the latest research evidence to outline foundational principles for improving health and developmental outcomes.

This chapter is grounded in an understanding that the family environment has a tremendous influence on children's health and development, and that a strong working partnership with parents and caregivers is essential. It begins with a brief overview of current challenges faced by children in Australia and New Zealand before examining important social and environmental determinants of children's development. The remainder of the chapter comprises a series of case studies illustrating common child development concerns and outlines current best-practice, evidence-based strategies to support families with child behaviour, sleep, nutrition, physical activity and technology use.

Current issues in child health and development

There have been enormous advances in recent decades in terms of improving children's health and development in many countries around the world, including Australia and New Zealand. Global and national policy and initiatives aiming to improve health across the lifespan now focus on the long-term benefits of supporting healthy development from the earliest years of life. The Australian Medical Association (2010, p. 1) states that:

> Developmental health and wellbeing ... is concerned with individuals achieving their maximal competencies intellectually, physically and emotionally as a result of interactions within a positive social environment and avoidance of poor health, educational, behavioural and criminal outcomes and the resulting huge social and economic cost to society.

Despite advances in knowledge and practice, factors that impact children's development still pose problems at the population level. Likewise, at the community level, many families present with concerns about their child's development that may be long-standing or complicated by socioeconomic, cultural or other factors that require prompt and thorough assessment and intervention to improve short- and long-term outcomes.

Children's health and development: A snapshot

Recent reports from the *Australia's Health* series (AIHW, 2020b, 2020c) and *New Zealand Health Survey* (Ministry of Health, 2018, 2019) reveal changing patterns in health indices relevant to children's development. Some improvements are evident –

for example, the proportion of Australian households where children are exposed to tobacco smoke has fallen from 19.7 per cent in 2001 to just 2.1 per cent in 2019. Likewise, rates of smoking among young people (14–17 years) fell from 18 per cent to just 3 per cent over the same period, mirroring drops in alcohol consumption (68 per cent in 2001 to 27 per cent in 2019).

Yet children's health has failed to improve or worsened across other areas, and data reveal ongoing and emerging challenges. Approximately one in four children in Australia and New Zealand is now overweight, and one in 10 is obese. More than 90 per cent of children do not eat the recommended daily serves of vegetables, around a quarter of children do not eat the recommended serves of fruit and almost half regularly consume sugar-sweetened or artificially sweetened drinks. Most children do not engage in enough physical activity and most exceed recommended screen use limits. Mental health and behavioural problems remain common in Australia, affecting boys (13.7 per cent) more often than girls (8.2 per cent) aged 14 years or younger; 9.5 per cent of boys and 6.6 per cent of girls in New Zealand (aged 3 to 14 years) likewise experience social, emotional or behavioural difficulties.

Data collected from other population-level surveys provide further context to these figures. The first RCH National Child Health Poll (Rhodes, 2015) identified the top child health concerns of Australian parents (see Table 6.1), suggesting that community perception of child health challenges roughly align with national data trends. Importantly, many of the issues identified as major concerns for Australian children are risk factors for the development of physical and psychosocial health problems that extend well beyond childhood.

Table 6.1 Top five parent-rated child health concerns by child age

5 years and younger	6 to 12 years	13 years and older
1. Sun safety	1. Excessive screen time	1. Excessive screen time
2. Excessive screen time	2. Not enough physical activity	2. Stress and/or anxiety
3. Not enough physical activity	3. Internet safety	3. Not enough physical activity
4. Poisoning	4. Bullying	4. Internet safety
5. Infectious diseases	5. Stress and/or anxiety	5. Unhealthy diet

Source: Adapted from Rhodes (2015).

Determinants of children's health and development

The environment into which a child is born and where they are raised can have lifelong effects via influences on physical and psychological developmental processes. Although this chapter focuses primarily on optimising children's physical growth and development, it is important to recognise that physical and psychological developmental processes are inextricably linked. Determinants of children's mental health are examined in Chapter 8, and effects of illness on psychosocial development is described in Chapter 9. This chapter will therefore focus primarily on the impact of children's biological and psychosocial environment on physical health and development.

Child development: A social ecological model

Myriad biological, social, and environmental factors combine to determine a child's developmental trajectory. While some are relatively fixed – for example, family history, culture, genetics – others are modifiable and may be targeted by intervention approaches that recognise the strong pathways of influence that exist between a child's environment and developmental processes.

Bronfenbrenner's (1979, 1992) social ecological model provides an overarching framework that explains the ways different aspects of a child's environment influence development (see Figure 6.1). An understanding of the numerous and often complex relationships that exist between a child and their environment is important, and the entire ecological system within which a child is situated should be considered when developing, testing and implementing strategies to improve health and developmental outcomes.

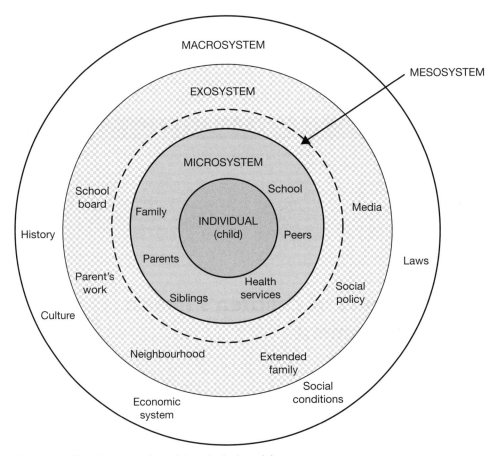

Figure 6.1 Bronfenbrenner's social ecological model
Source: Reproduced from Morawska and Mitchell (2018).

The model comprises five broad ecological systems. The *microsystem* represents the most proximal layer of influence on the child, and includes the family environment and close interpersonal relationships with family members and caregivers. The *mesosystem* represents connections or relationships between two or more settings – in essence, a system of microsystems. The *exosystem* represents processes that are further removed but still influence the child's immediate environment. The most distal layer, the *macrosystem*, includes social and cultural norms and beliefs. Finally, an all-encompassing *chronosystem* describes the ways in which the child and their environment change over time. Taking this ecological perspective, it is evident that almost anything in a child's immediate or more distal environment can affect their health and development.

Child health research, policy and practice are grounded in the understanding that every level of the social ecological model is important and should be considered when developing and testing different approaches to supporting health and development across the lifespan. Recent discoveries in the area of **epigenetics** are building on this established knowledge by shedding light on biological mechanisms by which opportunities or stressors in a child's physical and social environment influence development via direct effects on gene expression (National Scientific Council on the Developing Child, 2010). These exciting discoveries further serve to underline the importance of the first thousand days for children's development and provide impetus to prioritise policy and practice development in this area. Thus, although higher-order layers of the model certainly have a tremendous influence, it is at the microsystem level – with the child and their family – that relatively simple changes in behaviour can exert powerful and enduring effects on children's development, and it is also here that most day-to-day clinical nursing assessment and intervention take place.

Epigenetics – The study of how environmental influences affect gene expression and human development.

The family environment

Early childhood experiences and the family environment arguably have the greatest and most enduring effect on children's development. Parents are our first health educators, health promoters and role models, and experiences in childhood shape the development of skills, behaviours, beliefs and motivations that will underpin health and developmental trajectories across the lifespan. Thus, the way in which families navigate the demands of childrearing and caregiving in an increasingly complex social environment is important, since their choices, values, beliefs and behaviours will support or undermine children's current and future development.

Human babies are born entirely dependent on their parents, and a strong, affectionate bond or attachment relationship with a primary caregiver provides the foundation for physical, emotional, social and cognitive development. From the earliest months of life and throughout childhood, variations in **parenting practices** and **parenting styles** predict variations in children's health and development. For example, parenting practices that provide an infant with an environment that is safe, predictable and engaging, with appropriate levels of stimulation and plenty of opportunities to learn and experience the world around them, will help the infant to flourish. Alongside this, a parenting style that is high in responsiveness, where the primary caregiver is able to read the infant's cues and respond appropriately, strongly supports the infant's

Parenting practices – Specific, observable parenting behaviours that parents use to socialise their children, such as ensuring opportunities for experimentation and play to develop motor or social skills or encouraging healthy lifestyle behaviours.

Parenting styles – Characteristics of the parent that remain relatively stable over time and constitute the general emotional context within which parenting practices are situated.

development. Combining responsiveness with high levels of demandingness, which provides the infant with supportive guidance on boundaries and limits, lays the foundation for the development of self-regulation and supports healthy development.

Parenting styles (see Figure 6.2) are typically characterised by two key dimensions: *responsiveness*, or the parents' capacity to respond to their child in a warm, supportive way; and *demandingness*, or the degree to which the parent enforces expectations of the child through supervision, structure, limit-setting and discipline. The combination of these two dimensions yields the most common typology of parenting styles: *authoritative* parenting, balancing high demandingness with high responsiveness; *authoritarian* parenting, combining high demandingness but low responsiveness; *permissive* parenting, combining low demandingness with high responsiveness; and *neglectful* parenting, low in both demandingness and responsiveness (Maccoby & Martin, 1983).

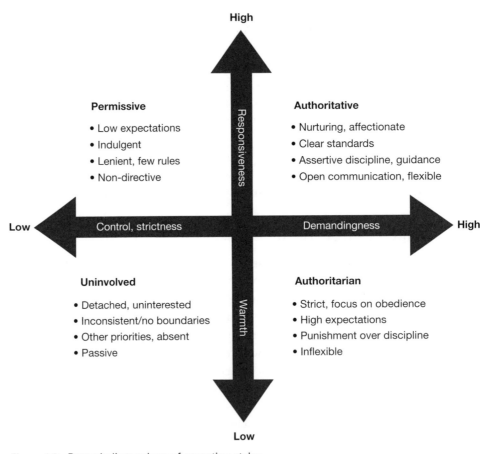

Figure 6.2 Baumrind's typology of parenting styles
Source: Adapted from Baumrind (1967); Maccoby & Martin (1983).

Of these, *authoritative* parenting is typically associated with better child health and developmental outcomes. While acknowledging that parenting style and norms around childrearing vary across and within cultures, encouraging parents to maintain a style of interaction with their child that flexibly balances high levels of both responsive and demanding parenting tends to yield better outcomes for children and families across the boundaries of ethnicity, culture, and sociodemographic status (Steinberg, 2001).

In terms of the impact of childhood adversity on development, parenting has been described as 'the great equaliser'. Responsive parenting and supportive parent–child relationships can improve diverse health outcomes, ameliorating or attenuating the impact of physical and psychosocial risk factors and adversity (Slopen et al., 2016) with benefits extending into adulthood (Chen et al., 2011). Conversely, poorer parent–child relationships, harsh child–parent interactions, poor parental monitoring and supervision, and maltreatment are associated with worse health and developmental outcomes such as increased inflammatory activity (Cicchetti, Handley & Rogosch, 2015), slower brain maturation (Whittle et al., 2016), weakened immune responses to vaccination (O'Connor et al., 2015) and childhood obesity (Woo Baidal et al., 2016).

Optimising child development

Approaches to optimising child development recognise the importance of policies and practices that support families, and ensure that parents have the knowledge, skills, confidence and resources to provide high-quality care to children that will support their development. Supporting children to achieve their full developmental potential is now seen as a basic human right that health professionals have a responsibility to protect (WHO, 2020). Concerns about children's development are a leading reason for attendance at pediatric health services, and nurses and other health professionals are well placed to identify developmental concerns and to engage in assessment, intervention and referral to resolve problems early.

The World Health Organization's first guideline specifically focused on improving early childhood development (WHO, 2020) provides four key recommendations to promote optimal child development:

1. **Responsive caregiving**
   All infants and children should receive responsive care during the first 3 years of life; parents and other caregivers should be supported to provide responsive care.

'Responsive caregiving' describes care that is prompt, consistent, contingent, and appropriate to the child's cues, signals, behaviours or needs. Caregivers are attuned to the child's needs and support them to explore and experiment in their environment. Interventions that target responsive caregiving aim to strengthen the parent-child relationship and show positive effects on growth, motor development, parent-child interactions.

2. **Promote early learning**
   All infants and children should have early learning activities with their parents and caregivers during the first three years of life; parents and other caregivers should be supported to engage in early learning with their children.

A child's earliest learning experiences occur within the family environment, and home environments that provide plenty of opportunities for early learning strongly support children's development. Interventions often focus on improving parents' knowledge, attitudes, behaviours and engagement in early learning activities – for example, shared book reading, play and direct or incidental teaching about nutrition, physical activity, social skills or healthy sleep – and show positive effects on cognition and motor development, and on secure parent–child attachment.

3. Integrate caregiving and nutrition interventions
Support for responsive care and early learning should be included as part of interventions for optimal nutrition of infants and young children.

This recommendation recognises that approaches incorporating parenting support (e.g. responsive caregiving, supporting early learning, supporting children's emotional and behavioural development) into nutrition interventions have better effects on cognitive, language and motor development compared with nutrition interventions alone.

4. Support maternal mental health
Psychosocial interventions to support maternal mental health should be integrated into early childhood health and development services.

Maternal mental health has a strong effect on children's development. Most family-based child development interventions pay some attention to the importance of addressing parental mental health – not only to improve parents' own health and wellbeing, but to buffer the impact of parental mental health difficulties on children's development.

Partnering with families to support child development

Partnering with families to address child development concerns is important to ensure accurate assessment, development of a management plan that is feasible and able to be implemented successfully by the family, appropriate follow-up to track progress, and onwards referral if required. Chapter 5 provides a detailed description of family-centred care and family assessment, which are important in the developmental care context.

Parents presenting with developmental concerns may experience frustration, guilt and a lack of confidence in their parenting role. Frustration may arise when a child's behaviour or development does not align with parental expectations – for example, the infant who will only settle in their parents' arms or the toddler struggling with toilet training. Parents may experience guilt if early signs of a developmental problem were not recognised, help-seeking was unintentionally or intentionally delayed, or they perceive that they contributed to the development or maintenance of the problem. For some, frustration or anger can provide an obstacle to implementation of the child's management plan, and some parents may require psychosocial support prior to and during the management phase.

Some developmental concerns can directly impact parents' own wellbeing, such as sleep problems, which can leave parents sleep-deprived, irritable and exhausted. Whatever the situation, it is important to remember that most parents try to do their best for their child and want to see them flourish. Taking a systematic approach to assessing family strengths, stressors and needs, and normalising difficult feelings and emotions are important to encourage parents to be open and honest about what they perceive as contributors to the problem and their own reaction to the situation.

It is important to be up-front about the likely course of resolution of the problem and the family's role in management. Many common developmental problems require calm, consistent effort from parents to resolve. Helping parents to develop the skills and competencies they need to successfully address the problem, such as coping and self-care strategies alongside strategies to support their child, may be necessary before a management plan is initiated.

Finally, acknowledging that parents are the experts on their own child can help parents to feel heard and validated. Aside from valuable insight into the child's history and current presentation, all families come with a pre-existing history of successes and defeats, beliefs and values, goals and preferences. Adopting a collaborative, respectful approach to assessment and intervention planning increases the chance of commitment from the family and resolution of the problem.

REFLECTION POINT 6.1

- Parents of children with long-standing health or developmental problems are themselves at increased risk of depression, anxiety and stress. Most approaches to addressing children's health and developmental needs rely on parental support engagement to be successful. What implications might this have for assessment and care planning?

Managing behaviour

Behavioural difficulties are common in childhood, may arise at any age or stage of development, and can have broad and far-reaching impacts on the lives of children and families. Around one in four parents reports feeling stressed about their child's behaviour on a daily basis and experiencing difficulty with managing difficult behaviours (Rhodes, 2018).

CASE STUDY 6.1 EVIE

In your role as a community child health nurse you meet 7-year-old Evie. Evie's mother, Eleanor, is concerned about recent changes in her behaviour. Previously a happy, easygoing child, Evie has started refusing to go to school and becomes extremely distressed when it is time to leave the house in the morning. She has also become clingy with Eleanor and stopped cooperating with basic requests – for example, to brush her teeth or tidy up. Evie's father has recently started a fly-in, fly-out job which has him away from home for six weeks at a time. Eleanor is finding parenting alone stressful and exhausting, and has been 'giving in' to Evie's behaviours to avoid more conflict. She is looking for strategies to help support Evie with recent changes and to help reduce her own stress levels.

Behavioural development in childhood

Learning to manage one's own emotions and behaviours is an important developmental task of childhood. Many common behavioural challenges – such as tantruming during toddlerhood – are developmentally normative. However, managing difficult child behaviours, even those that are within the normal range for a child's age and stage of development, can be challenging for parents.

Behaviour difficulties are broadly categorised as *internalising* problems, encompassing emotional difficulties such as anxiety and depression, or *externalising* problems, which comprise disruptive behaviours such as 'acting out', aggression and oppositional behaviour. Child behaviour difficulties lie along a continuum in terms of intensity, frequency and duration, and whether a behaviour is considered a 'problem' or a 'disorder' will largely depend on whether it falls within the normal range for the child's age and stage of development. For example, while low-intensity non-compliant, aggressive or impulsive behaviour is normal in preschool children, frequent, prolonged or destructive tantrums (above the expected norm for intensity) or the same behaviours in a 10-year-old (above the expected norm for age) may suggest a behaviour disorder. More serious behavioural and mental health disorders are examined in Chapter 8. This chapter will focus primarily on supporting healthy behavioural development with typically developing children.

Risk factors and consequences of behavioural problems

Numerous factors combine to explain variation in children's behavioural development. At the individual (child) level, a child's temperament may affect behavioural development via complex mechanisms that are still being uncovered. Sex may also influence behaviour, with higher prevalence of externalising and internalising problems for boys and girls respectively, although whether this is due to genetic influences or socialisation experiences remains unclear. Children with chronic health conditions, intellectual disabilities and developmental delays are also at increased risk of behaviour difficulties, and child behaviour management can be one of the most stressful aspects of parenting for their families.

Overall, however, environmental factors generally have the greatest influence on behavioural development. Adverse events during the perinatal period, including maternal use of alcohol, nicotine and other drugs, preterm birth and low birth weight are all associated with increased risk of behavioural problems in childhood. Chronic stressors within the child's immediate environment, such as disrupted parent–child relationships, inconsistent, harsh or neglectful parenting, domestic violence, parental substance abuse and socioeconomic disadvantage, increase the risk of behavioural problems via numerous pathways, including direct effects on neurological development and functioning. Of course, other more transient factors may also trigger changes in children's behaviour. Major changes or transitions such as starting daycare or school, moving house, a new baby, caregiver illness or incapacitation, the death of a family member, or peer conflict or bullying, and even relatively minor changes such as graduating from a cot to a bed or toilet training, can disrupt children's behaviour.

While most developmentally normative behaviour difficulties can resolve quickly with consistent and supportive parenting, the presence of child-, parent-, or family-level risk factors, as described earlier, can contribute to the onset, maintenance and exacerbation of problem behaviours, which may become a more serious long-term issue (Tremblay et al., 2004). More serious emotional and behavioural difficulties in childhood are associated with adverse short- and longer-term outcomes, including the development of learning difficulties, poorer academic performance, problems with family and peer relationships, and development of more severe conduct and mental health disorders in later life (Tremblay et al., 1992). Difficult child behaviour, parent–child conflict and family stress also contribute to poorer physical health in childhood, including increased risk of accidental injury (Bijur, Stewart-Brown & Butler, 1986), poorer engagement in preventative health behaviours (Berzinski et al., 2019) and less effective management of chronic health conditions (Morawska, Calam & Fraser, 2015).

Approaches to behaviour management

Australia's National Framework for Universal Child and Family Health Services (Department of Health and Ageing, 2011) highlights the role of health professionals in supporting healthy behavioural development by providing anticipatory guidance and general support to parents by normalising child behaviour, promoting parental knowledge of psychosocial development in childhood and supporting parents to develop the skills and competencies they require to prevent and manage challenging behaviours. Most current approaches to child behaviour management take a family-focused approach, recognising the important contribution of parents and parenting to child behaviour and behaviour change. Contemporary evidence-based parenting support programs (also called 'parent training' or 'parenting intervention'), based on social learning, cognitive behaviour therapy and developmental principles, are considered effective first-line interventions for the management of behavioural problems in childhood (Sanders, 2019). Parenting support programs see the parent, rather than a therapist, as the agent of change, and aim to help parents develop the knowledge, skills, competencies and confidence to prevent and manage problem behaviours and support their child's development.

Although children with more complex clinical behavioural disorders (e.g. Oppositional Defiant Disorder (ODD), Attention Deficit Hyperactivity Disorder (ADHD) and Conduct Disorder) will typically require multidisciplinary assessment, diagnosis and management planning by a specialist service (see Chapter 8), parenting support typically remains a key component of the management plan. Despite this, most common child behavioural problems – for example, tantrums, oppositional behaviour, aggression, non-compliance, fighting, school refusal, sleep and mealtime difficulties – can be managed successfully with evidence-based parenting support that targets modifiable risk factors for the development and maintenance of child behaviour difficulties at the family level. This can be delivered in a variety of healthcare settings by appropriately trained providers, and is effective in treating child behaviour problems early and preventing the development of more serious behaviour disorders (Sanders, 2019).

The Triple P – Positive Parenting Program (Sanders, 2019) is an example of a public health approach to evidence-based parenting support. Developed in Australia and New Zealand, Triple P is a multilevel system of parenting support that has been widely disseminated internationally and used in paediatric and child health settings (Sanders, 2019). It incorporates five broad evidence-based principles to supporting healthy development for children: (1) ensuring a safe, nurturing and engaging environment; (2) creating a positive learning environment; (3) using consistent, assertive discipline; (4) having reasonable expectations of children and oneself; and (5) taking care of oneself (as a parent) (Sanders, 2019). It has demonstrated short- and long-term effects on child behaviour, and parenting and efficacy, across the spectrum of child behavioural problems.

Clinical practice guidelines and research evidence (e.g. Kaminski et al., 2008) reveal effective approaches to managing difficult child behaviours that can be summarised by the following principles.

Principles for managing behaviour

1. Have realistic expectations

Normalising child behaviours and providing guidance to parents about normal child development can help parents to maintain realistic expectations about their child's behaviour, and better prepare parents to respond to problems in a way that supports their child's development. Helping parents to establish and communicate clear expectations for children's behaviour, with age-appropriate ground rules, boundaries and limits, and the use of daily routines, provides certainty and predictability for children. Likewise, helping parents to have realistic expectations of themselves helps to reduce parenting stress and anxiety when challenges arise.

2. Build positive parent–child relationships

As described earlier in the chapter, a strong, affectionate bond with an adult caregiver helps children to feel safe and secure, and lays the foundation for healthy development and future relationships. Parents can build a strong relationship with their child by paying attention and being available to them, helping them to feel understood and accepted, spending quality time together, maintaining positive and open communication, and creating an environment where children feel comfortable to play and explore.

3. Encourage desirable behaviours

Social attention from parents and caregivers is a powerful shaper of child behaviour. Child behaviour that attracts parental attention – whether positive or negative – is more likely to be repeated. Paying attention to desirable behaviour through verbal or non-verbal reinforcement (e.g. a smile, verbal or non-verbal encouragement, praise, or use of rewards) and giving children positive feedback on their behaviour are powerful ways to reinforce desirable behaviour. These types of reinforcers are also extremely effective when helping children to learn new skills – for example, sleeping in their own bed or staying at the table at mealtimes.

4. Use effective discipline strategies

When behaviour problems do occur, the calm, decisive and consistent use of effective discipline strategies will help children learn to accept necessary rules and limits. Planned ignoring can be effective in reducing frequent but harmless misbehaviour (e.g. whining, interrupting) that is designed to get parents' attention. For more problematic behaviour, consequences that fit the situation, are brief and can be implemented immediately can be effective. For serious misbehaviour, such as physical aggression, fighting or repeated disobedience, the strategic use of time-out has demonstrated efficacy (Kaminski et al., 2008). Time-out is a non-punitive strategy that involves calmly removing the child from the space in which the problem behaviour occurred and limiting parental attention for a brief period of time before returning the child to the space, providing the child with an opportunity to demonstrate appropriate behaviour and then promptly reinforcing the child's appropriate behaviour. Time-out is designed primarily to break the cycle of parental reinforcement of unwanted behaviours (that is, where negative attention from the parent actually reinforces problem behaviours), but can also provide time and space for child and parent to calm down and develop self-regulatory capacity.

Nurses can help parents to develop the knowledge and skills required to manage child behaviour difficulties effectively and in a way that is respectful and non-hurtful, and that supports their child's development. Parents may need support with identifying contextual and other factors that may be contributing to the onset or maintenance of behaviour problems. It can be useful to take a broad approach to assessment, including family and developmental history, the parent–child relationship, and the severity and context of specific behaviours (e.g. timing, duration, precipitating factors) to gather clues about why the child may be behaving in this way at this time. Parents will often also benefit from supportive coaching in coping strategies to help them remain calm, in control and consistent with their own behaviour in the face of difficulties.

Positive parenting approaches are designed to actively teach and guide children's behaviour and are non-punitive. Importantly, there are lots of steps that parents can take (principles 1–3) to reduce the likelihood of behaviour difficulties occurring in the first place, and a focus on using assertive discipline should never overtake the importance of establishing physical and social environments that are conducive to preventing behaviour problems and supporting healthy development. In fact, the success of non-punitive behaviour-management strategies (such as planned ignoring and time-out) depends on parents establishing a usual style of interaction with their child that is high in positive reinforcement – that is, where parents normally provide plenty of attention, praise, affection and stimulation. Only then will withdrawal of parental attention be effective in shaping children's behaviour. Unfortunately, many parents attempt time-out without a sufficient understanding of how and why it works. If parents report having tried planned ignoring or time-out with limited effect, it is worth carefully reviewing how the strategies were implemented to check that essential elements have been implemented correctly, and facilitate education and skill-building as needed.

Sleep

Healthy sleep is essential to support optimal health, growth and development in childhood. It requires that children regularly get a sufficient amount of sleep that is of good quality and with regular sleep routines. However, sleep difficulties rank among the most frequent health complaints among children (Redmond et al., 2016), and concerns about child sleep are among the earliest and most common reasons for parents to consult a healthcare professional.

CASE STUDY 6.2 ZACK

As a practice nurse working in a GP clinic, you meet Zack, a 13-year-old boy who has been referred for assessment of sleep concerns. His mother, Anna, reports that Zack is difficult to rouse in the morning and often late to school. Although he is still enjoying extracurricular activities, his grades have dropped over the past semester, and he is having difficulty concentrating on his schoolwork. He has started drinking caffeinated beverages to stay awake in the afternoons. Zack reveals that he enjoys online chatting and gaming with friends in the evenings, and usually goes to bed when he starts feeling tired at around 1.00 am. Anna is concerned about this recent change in Zack's sleep patterns. She has tried to enforce earlier bedtimes but this only lasts a night or two before Zack slides back into old habits.

Sleep in childhood

Normal sleep patterns vary enormously in the first few months and years of life. From birth to around 8 weeks of age, there is often little difference between daytime and night-time sleep patterns; however, over the first few months infants start to develop the circadian rhythm that governs sleep/wake patterns, and begin to sleep for longer stretches, particularly at night. By 6 months, infants have their longest sleeps at night. Sleep patterns continue to evolve during the first year of life, with the number of daytime naps gradually decreasing, although afternoon naps may be needed until around 3 to 5 years of age.

Sleep patterns remain comparatively stable through the primary school years. Although some children fall asleep quickly, a latent period of 20 to 30 minutes is not uncommon. Although changes in sleep from childhood to adolescence are less dramatic than those from infancy to childhood, later-evening secretion of melatonin in adolescence temporarily resets the adolescent's circadian rhythm, prompting later bedtimes and later morning waking.

Sleep problems are under-recognised and under-reported in childhood, and can contribute to developmental problems if left untreated. Although some parents recognise that their child's sleep is problematic, and seek assessment and advice, others may be unsure about whether their child's sleep and sleep patterns are adequate or normal for their age. Some children with underlying sleep problems may present with more general behavioural problems, such as lack of concentration, irritability, hyperactivity and generally disruptive behaviour, and sleep problems are more common among children with medical, neurodevelopmental or psychiatric disorders.

Approaches to managing sleep

International guidelines provide general recommendations regarding the amount of sleep needed by children at different ages and stages of development (see Table 6.2). Getting the recommended hours of sleep on a regular basis is associated with better attention, learning and memory; behavioural and emotional regulation; and physical and mental health and quality of life (Matricciani et al., 2019). Conversely, consequences of inadequate, disrupted or poor-quality sleep include difficulties with emotional and behavioural self-regulation; poorer performance in cognitive, organisational and creative tasks; poorer academic performance; accidents and injuries; delayed growth; and adverse physical and mental health outcomes including hypertension, obesity, diabetes and depression (Matricciani et al., 2019).

Table 6.2 Recommendations for sleep in childhood

Age	Recommended sleep per 24-hour period
4 to 12 months	12 to 16 hours (including naps)
1 to 2 years	11 to 14 hours (including naps)
3 to 5 years	10 to 13 hours (including naps)
6 to 12 years	9 to 11 hours
13 to 18 years	8 to 10 hours

Note. There are no recommendations for infants less than 4 months of age, due to broad variation in sleep patterns and limited evidence linking infant sleep patterns and health outcomes.
Source: Adapted from Partuthi et al. (2016).

Sleep assessment is indicated during routine child health checks and/or when families present with sleep-related concerns or emotional/behaviour problems. In general, a sleep history should include sleep and activity patterns, including bedtime routines, amount and quality of sleep (including regularity of bedtimes and waking times, sleep duration, night-time awakenings, daytime sleepiness and snoring). Validated instruments that screen for common child and adolescent sleep problems are widely available, and sleep diaries (over a two-week period) can be a useful starting point to track children's bedtime, sleep onset time, rise time and number of night-time awakenings.

Sleep-related problems, even those that are developmentally normative, can be frustrating for parents, who are often exhausted themselves. It is common for children's sleep to go through periods of disruption during even relatively minor changes to their social or physical environment or activities – for example, when starting school or being away from home. These are normal reactions, and typically will resolve with a calm, systematic approach to supporting development or redevelopment of good sleep patterns. Importantly, parents will differ in their personal values and goals for their child's sleep. For example, while some parents aim for their child to sleep in their own bed, others may prefer to co-sleep with their child. The nurse's role is to promote safe sleeping practices and support families in making informed choices about sleep that meet the needs of their child and family.

Most childhood sleep problems are behavioural in origin, and behavioural interventions are considered the first line of therapy. Evidence from clinical guidelines and systematic reviews of the research evidence (Zhang et al., 2020) supports the following principles for healthy sleep in childhood.

Principles for supporting healthy sleep

1. Establish a regular sleep pattern

Setting and consistently reinforcing fixed bedtimes and waking times (including on weekends and on holidays) supports circadian rhythms and reduces the likelihood of sleep dysregulation. Morning waking time is an especially powerful reinforcer of the sleep–wake cycle. Exposure to sunlight, particularly in the early morning, helps to regulate the circadian rhythm and can make it easier to fall asleep at night.

2. Have a consistent bedtime routine

Bedtimes should be age-appropriate – that is, with bed- and wake-times set to ensure that the child receives an appropriate amount of sleep for their age – and with an established routine that provides the necessary behavioural cues for transition to sleep. Having a consistent bedtime routine from the earliest months can help infants and children to settle and prepare for sleep. A typical pre-bedtime routine might include a warm bath, brushing teeth and a bedtime story. Doing the steps in the same order each evening helps children to feel safe and secure, and reduces the likelihood of bedtime difficulties.

3. Provide a comfortable sleep environment

Families should ensure their child's night-time sleep environment is dark, quiet and comfortable. Children need to feel safe and secure at sleep time, and may settle better with a dim nightlight. Exposure to bright light or the blue light from screen devices can reduce melatonin levels and make sleep more difficult, and should be avoided in the hour or two before bedtime.

4. Time daily activities to promote sleep

Feeling hungry, anxious or worried, being engaging in vigorous physical activity in the hour before sleep and the effects of caffeine and other stimulants can make it harder for children to fall asleep. Timing children's food and fluid intake, encouraging quiet play and relaxation in the hour before sleep and avoiding caffeine can support healthy sleep.

5. Use positive parenting strategies to manage problem behaviours

General principles for managing child behaviour are effective in the management of sleep behaviour problems. In particular, having realistic expectations for the child's age and stage of development, staying consistent with expectations (e.g. bed time routines, staying in bed), encouraging and rewarding desirable behaviour (e.g. praise, behaviour charts) and ignoring undesirable behaviour (e.g. complaining, whining and bargaining) can be effective.

Healthy lifestyle

It is hard to over-state the importance of good nutrition and physical activity for healthy child development; however, the vast proportion of children don't meet current recommendations in these areas. Nutrition, physical activity and sedentary behaviour are important yet modifiable determinants of child health and development. From a clinical perspective, it is important to recognise that these behaviours may cluster together, with subsets of children experiencing concurrent problems across multiple domains (Leech, McNaughton & Timperio, 2014). Although the mechanisms by which these different health behaviours are linked are complex and still being uncovered, it is clear that aspects of children's diet, physical activity and sedentary behaviour are of concern to parents, clinicians and policy-makers alike, and that rapid changes to children's physical and social environments over the past few decades have presented new challenges.

Nutrition and physical activity

CASE STUDY 6.3 JACOB

As a paediatric nurse working in a children's hospital, you meet Jacob, a 2-year-old who has been admitted with gastroenteritis. He has had a history of multiple viral infections since starting daycare six months ago. Despite having a good variety of foods in his diet from an early age, he started showing picky eating behaviours after his first major bout of gastro. His picky eating has gotten worse over time, and his mother, Sarah, says he is now 'living on toast, chicken nuggets and crackers'. Jacob usually refuses to eat the same meal as the rest of the family, and Sarah ends up making him a special meal of his own to avoid yet another mealtime battle. She is frustrated and worried about the impact of Jacob's diet on his growth and development, but doesn't know what else to do.

There is a mountain of evidence demonstrating the importance of good nutrition and physical activity to healthy growth and development during childhood. This evidence guides policy and practice via national and international evidence-based guidelines, which provide recommendations for increasing fruit and vegetable intake, reducing consumption of energy-dense, low-nutrient discretionary (treat) foods, increasing physical activity and limiting sedentary activity (Department of Health, 2017a, 2017b; NHMRC, 2013).

Children are considered nutritionally vulnerable up to 5 years of age, so ensuring that children consume a balanced, nutritious diet with a good variety of foods from the earliest years is important to support optimum growth and development and pave the way for good eating habits in adulthood. However, the vast majority of children don't meet nutritional guidelines for vegetable intake (see Table 6.3); almost half of pre-schoolers eat discretionary (treat) foods on most days of the week; and parents report uncertainty about how to choose healthy foods for their family (Rhodes, 2017a).

Table 6.3   Minimum recommended daily serves of fruit and vegetables, legumes/beans by child age

Child age (years)	Fruit	Vegetables and legumes/beans
2–4	1	2.5
4–8	1.5	4.5
9–11	2	5
12–18	2	5 (girls) to 5.5 (boys)

Source: Adapted from NHMRC (2013).

Physical activity likewise has positive effects on almost all aspects of children's physical development, including musculoskeletal, cardiovascular and immune functioning, and developing good habits around physical activity in childhood increases the likelihood of being physically active in later years. However, children in most countries, including Australia and New Zealand, are not meeting recommended targets (Tremblay et al., 2014) (see Table 6.4). Data suggest that fewer than one in four Australian children engage in sufficient physical activity, with older children (10–14 years) even less likely to meet physical activity guidelines compared with younger children (5–9 years) (AIHW, 2020a).

Table 6.4   Physical activity and sedentary behaviour recommendations by child age

Child age (years)	Physical activity	Sedentary behaviour
Under 1	Supervised interactive floor-based play; 30 minutes of tummy time (total) per day for those not yet mobile	Not restrained for more than one hour at a time (e.g. in a stroller, car seat or highchair)
1–2	At least three hours per day, including energetic play (e.g. running, jumping, twirling)	Not restrained for more than one hour at a time (e.g. in a stroller, car seat or highchair) or sitting for extended periods
3–5	At least three hours per day with at least one hour of energetic play (e.g. running, jumping, kicking, throwing)	Not restrained for more than one hour at a time (e.g. in a stroller or car seat) or sitting for extended periods

Table 6.4 *(cont.)*

Child age (years)	Physical activity	Sedentary behaviour
5–18	At least one hour of moderate to vigorous physical activity (mainly aerobic); several hours of light physical activity; incorporate activities that strengthen muscles and bones at least three days per week	Break up long periods of sitting

Source: Adapted from Department of Health (2017a, 2017b).

Less consumption of fruit and vegetables, greater consumption of discretionary food items, and less physical activity in childhood are associated with higher body mass index (BMI), overweight and obesity, and unhealthy eating and physical activity patterns that can persist into adulthood and contribute to worse physical health (e.g. overweight/obesity, metabolic dysregulation and type 2 diabetes, hypertension, hyper-cholesterolaemia, cardiovascular disease, many cancers) and mental health (e.g. depression, anxiety) later in life (Craigie et al., 2011). In contrast, good nutrition and physical activity have positive effects on children's physical, cognitive and psychosocial development, including motor skills, coordination, balance, posture and flexibility, neurophysiology, concentration and academic performance, mental health and well-being, emotional and behavioural regulation, self-image, confidence, peer relationships and sleep (Rodrigues-Ayllon et al., 2019).

Numerous social and environmental factors have combined to create the 'obeso-genic' environment in which we now live. These include increased availability of energy-dense, nutrient-poor foods and drinks; reliance on convenience and takeaway foods; urban design that reduces daily energy expenditure (e.g. increased reliance on cars and labour-saving devices); concerns about child safety when playing outdoors; and loss of food literacy and cooking skills. However, another factor recently impli-cated in the rise of overweight and obesity among children is screen use.

Screen use

Rapid increases in children's exposure to screen devices have prompted urgent explor-ation of impacts on child health and development. Large-scale studies reveal links between excessive screen use and worse psychological health, including internalising and externalising behaviour problems; poorer self-esteem, wellbeing and quality of life; poorer cognitive development, academic outcomes and sleep; and greater adiposity/BMI (LeBlanc et al., 2012; Stiglic & Viner, 2019). Greater screen use is also associated with increased intake of high-energy foods and less fruit consumption and physical activity (Salmon, Campbell & Crawford, 2006).

National and international guidelines (see Table 6.5) (Department of Health, 2017a, 2017b) provide recommendations for screen use by children at different ages; however, less than a third of children meet these recommendations (AIHW, 2020a).

Parents are concerned that their children spend too much time using screen devices and report family conflict, child behaviour difficulties, lack of physical activity and sleep problems related to children's use of screens (Rhodes, 2017b). However, parents also report using screen devices to manage their child's behaviour (Rhodes, 2017b), and links between excessive screen use and children's psychosocial wellbeing may be at least partially explained by reduced parent–child interaction (Zhao et al., 2018).

Table 6.5 Recommended screen use limits by child age

Child age (years)	Recommendation
Under 2	No screen time – no time watching TV or using other electronic media (DVDs, computer, electronic games)
2–5	Maximum of one hour (total) screen time per day
5–18	Maximum of two hours of sedentary recreational screen time per day, encouraging positive social interactions and experiences when using screen-based electronic media

Source: Adapted from Department of Health (2017a, 2017b).

Principles to support a healthy lifestyle

Developing healthy habits from the earliest years is likely to be more efficient and effective than attempting to change established health behaviours in adulthood, and parents are in a prime position to help children develop the knowledge, skills, attitudes and confidence needed to make healthy choices that support their ongoing development (Baker, Morawska & Mitchell, 2019).

Parents' beliefs and behaviours are modifiable factors that are associated with and influence children's health behaviours. For example, parents' physical activity is correlated with children's activity levels, and children may engage in more physical activity when parents are more physically active themselves (Trost & Loprinzi, 2011). Likewise, high screen use by children is associated with parents' own behaviours and attitudes towards screen use and a lack of confidence with limit-setting (Lauricella, Wartella & Rideout, 2015), whereas less screen use is associated with parental monitoring, limit-setting and a more authoritative parenting style (Veldhuis et al., 2014).

In terms of nutrition, early parental feeding practices strongly influence children's dietary intake. Non-responsive feeding – that is, when parents pressure a child to eat, use food as a reward for behaviour (including eating behaviour) or restrict foods – is associated with poorer child self-regulation of eating behaviour, over- and underweight, picky eating, a limited variety of tolerated foods and reduced vegetable intake (Cole et al., 2017; Hurley, Cross & Hughes, 2011). Non-responsive feeding practices, such as insisting a child eat all their dinner to 'earn' dessert, are detrimental to children's natural capacity to self-regulate their food intake, with effects persisting into adulthood.

Young children who are offered a new food will typically approach it with hesitation and avoidance, and neophobic reactions are common at this young age. Children may need around 10 to 15 exposures to a new food before they are willing to accept it (Cooke, 2007; Williams et al., 2008). When parents stop offering new foods after a few initial refusals and offer only those foods for which their children show a preference, children lose the opportunity to learn to appreciate new foods, show less preference for fruit and vegetables, and are less likely to try new foods and accept them (Russell, Worsley & Liem, 2014).

Past approaches to intervention largely focused on improving children's and parents' knowledge of the benefits of good nutrition and physical activity from a biomedical perspective. We now know that improving knowledge is rarely enough to produce long-term behavioural change. Families need to know not only *what* to do, but *how* to do it. For this reason, family-focused child health education should routinely be accompanied by evidence-based parenting support to ensure that families have the skills as well as the knowledge to put child health and development recommendations into practice.

Evidence from clinical guidelines and systematic reviews of the research evidence (e.g. Black et al., 2017; Dallacker, Hertwig & Mata, 2018; Robson et al., 2020; Schmidt et al., 2012; Wu et al., 2016) support the following principles for supporting healthy lifestyle in childhood.

1. Set realistic goals and identify obstacles

Parents may need support with identifying their values around healthy lifestyle behaviours, establishing realistic goals and priorities, and identifying potential obstacles to healthy lifestyle behaviours or behaviour change. Involving children in establishing goals and expectations around health behaviours and developing and consistently enforcing clear ground rules (e.g. screen time limits) can help children feel involved and know what is expected of them. Identifying potential obstacles and planning ahead to overcome these gives families the best chance of meeting their health behaviour goals and getting back on track after disruptions (e.g. illness, holidays).

2. Provide plenty of opportunities to engage in healthy behaviours

Parents can take simple, practical steps to modify their children's environment to support healthy lifestyle behaviours – for example, ensuring that plenty of healthy food options are available at home and that discretionary food items are only purchased as an occasional treat; offering a variety of nutritious foods at mealtimes and allowing children to choose what and how much to eat; and providing opportunities for physical activity throughout the day – for example by encouraging standing rather than sitting, walking rather than driving, encouraging outdoor play and engaging in physical activity as a family.

3. Work together as a family

Incorporating healthy lifestyle choices into day-to-day family life allows parents to role-model positive attitudes and behaviours and teach children about the benefits of lifestyle choices that support health and development. Families can experiment to find physical activities and healthy foods that children enjoy. Although regular vigorous physical activity is important, not all physical activity needs to be beneficial. Swimming, dancing, skipping, jumping in puddles or flying a kite are all forms of moderate physical activity that support healthy development. Likewise, encouraging children to try new foods by providing a variety of healthy food options at mealtimes will help children to broaden their repertoire of foods; however, it is important to allow children to control what and how much they eat without pressuring them to eat or restricting food intake. Co-viewing or co-use of screens with children can help parents to monitor what children are accessing and increases the chance of children deriving educational and other benefits from screen time.

REFLECTION POINT 6.2

- Many parents of children with unhealthy behaviours around nutrition, physical activity or screen use have unhealthy habits in these areas themselves. The most successful approaches to improving children's health behaviours tend to be those that involve parents. From a social learning perspective, why might parental involvement be so important to improving children's health behaviours?

SUMMARY

- Changes to children's physical and social environments in recent decades have contributed to increases in child health problems, with the potential to affect long-term developmental outcomes.
- Almost anything in a child's immediate or wider physical and social environment can affect their development. Social ecological models can provide useful frameworks for planning and testing approaches to optimising child development.
- Strong parent–child relationships provide the basis for healthy child development. Family-centred approaches to supporting optimal child development focus on helping parents to develop the knowledge, skills and confidence to help their child flourish.
- Evidence-based strategies to manage children's behaviour, sleep, nutrition, physical activity and screen use directly and indirectly support children's physical, cognitive and psychosocial development, and have the potential to improve health and developmental trajectories across the lifespan.

LEARNING ACTIVITY

6.1 Read *Epigenetics and Child Development: How Children's Experiences Affect their Genes* (Center on the Developing Child, 2020), https://developingchild.harvard.edu/resources/what-is-epigenetics-and-how-does-it-relate-to-child-development and explore the related resources. Early life experiences directly affect gene expression and child development. What can you do to support children's developmental potential in your own clinical practice?

FURTHER READING

The following is a series of short, practice-relevant articles that build on the foundational knowledge provided in this chapter regarding common behavioural and developmental problems of childhood:

Hannan, K & Hiscock, H 2015, Sleep problems in children, *Australian Family Physician*, 44(12), pp. 800–83.

Jarman, R 2015, Finetuning behaviour management in young children, *Australian Family Physician*, 44(12), pp. 896–9.

Marks, K 2015, Infant and toddler nutrition, *Australian Family Physician*, 44(12), pp. 886–9.

REFERENCES

Australian Institute of Health and Welfare (AIHW) 2020a, *Australia's children*, AIHW, Canberra.

—— 2020b, *Australia's health 2020 data insights*, AIHW, Canberra.

—— 2020c, *Australia's health 2020: In brief*, AIHW, Canberra.

Australian Medical Association (AMA) 2010, *Developmental health and wellbeing of Australia's children and young people: AMA position statement*, AMA, Canberra.

Baker, S, Morawska, A & Mitchell, A 2019, Promoting children's healthy habits through self-regulation via parenting, *Clinical Child and Family Psychology Review*, 22, pp. 52–62.

Baumrind, D 1967, Child care practices anteceding three patterns of preschool behavior, *Genetic Psychology Monographs*, 75, pp. 43–88.

Berzinski, M, Morakwska, A, Mitchell, AE & Baker, S 2019, Parenting and child behaviour as predictors of toothbrushing difficulties in young children, *International Journal of Paediatric Dentistry*, 30, pp. 75–84.

Bijur, PE, Stewart-Brown, S & Butler, N 1986, Child behavior and accidental injury in 11,966 preschool children, *American Journal of Disease in Childhood*, 140, pp. 487–92.

Black, AP, D'Onise, K, McDermott, R, Vally, H, & O'Dea 2017, How effective are family-based and institutional nutrition interventions in improving children's diet and health? A systematic review, *BMC Public Health*, 17(818), pp. 1–19.

Bronfenbrenner, U 1979, *The ecology of human development*, Harvard University Press, Cambridge, MA.

—— (ed.) 1992, *Six theories of child development: Revised formulations and current issues*, Jessica Kingsley, London.

Center on the Developing Child 2020, *Epigenetics and child development: How children's experiences affect their genes*, Harvard University, Cambridge, MA, viewed 21 February 2021, https://developingchild.harvard.edu/resources/what-is-epigenetics-and-how-does-it-relate-to-child-development

Chen, E, Miller, GE, Kobor, MS & Cole, SW 2011, Maternal warmth buffers the effects of low early-life socioeconomic status on pro-inflammatory signaling in adulthood, *Molecular Psychiatry*, 16(7), pp. 729–37.

Cicchetti, D, Handley, ED & Rogosch, FA 2015, Child maltreatment, inflammation, and internalizing symptoms: Investigating the roles of C-reactive protein, gene variation, and neuroendocrine regulation, *Development and Psychopathology*, 27(2), pp. 553–66.

Cole, NC, An, R, Lee, S-Y & Donovan, SM 2017, Correlates of picky eating and food neophobia in young children: A systematic review and meta-analysis, *Nutrition Reviews*, 75(7), pp. 516–32.

Cooke, L 2007, The importance of exposure for healthy eating in childhood: A review, *Journal of Human Nutrition and Dietetics*, 20(4), pp. 294–301.

Craigie, AM, Lake, AA, Kelly, SA, Adamson, AJ & Mathers, JC 2011, Tracking of obesity-related behaviours from childhood to adulthood: A systematic review, *Maturitas*, 70(3), pp. 266– 84.

Dallacker, M, Hertwig, R & Mata, J 2018, The frequency of family meals and nutritional health in children: a meta-analysis, *Obesity Reviews*, 19, pp. 638–53.

Department of Health 2017a, *Australian 24-hour movement guidelines for children and young people (5 to 17 years),* Department of Health, Canberra.

—— 2017b, *Australian 24-hour movement guidelines for the early years (birth to 5 years),* Department of Health, Canberra.

Department of Health and Ageing 2011, *National framework for universal child and family health services,* Australian Government, Canberra.

Hurley, KM, Cross, MB & Hughes, SO 2011, A systematic review of responsive feeding and child obesity in high-income countries, *The Journal of Nutrition*, 141(3), pp. 495–501.

Kaminski, JW, Valle, LA, Filene, JH & Boyle, CL 2008, A meta-analytic review of components associated with parent training program effectiveness, *Journal of Abnormal Child Psychology*, 36, pp. 567–89.

Lauricella, AR, Wartella, E & Rideout, VJ 2015, Young children's screen time: The complex role of parent and child factors, *Journal of Applied Developmental Psychology*, 36, pp. 11–17.

LeBlanc, AG, Spence, JC, Carson, V, Connor Gorbor, S, Dillman, C, Jansset, I et al. 2012, Systematic review of sedentary behaviour and health indicators in the early years (aged 0–4 years), *Applied Physiology, Nutrition, and Metabolism*, 37(4), pp. 753–72.

Leech, RM, McNaughton, SA & Timperio, A 2014, The clustering of diet, physical activity and sedentary behavior in children and adolescents: A review, *International Journal of Behavioral Nutrition and Physical Activity*, 11(4), doi:10.1186/1479-5868-11-4

Maccoby, EE & Martin, JA 1983, Socialization in the context of the family: Parent-child interaction, in PH Mussen & EM Hetherington (eds), *Handbook of child psychology, Vol. 4,* Wiley, New York, pp. 1–101.

Matricciani, L, Paquet, C, Galland, B, Short, M & Olds, T 2019, Children's sleep and health: A meta-review, *Sleep Medicine Reviews*, 46, pp. 136–50.

Ministry of Health 2018, *Social, emotional and behavioural difficulties in New Zealand children: Summary of findings,* Ministry of Health, Wellington.

—— 2019. *Annual update of key results 2018/19: New Zealand Health Survey,* viewed 1 November 2020, www.health.govt.nz/publication/annual-update-key-results-2018-19-new-zealand-health-survey

Morawska, A, Calam, R & Fraser, J 2015, Parenting interventions for childhood chronic illness: A review and recommendations for intervention design and delivery, *Journal of Child Health Care*, 19(1), pp. 5–17.

Morawska, A & Mitchell, AE 2018, Children's health, physical activity, and nutrition, in *Handbook of parenting and child development across the lifespan*, Springer, Cham, pp. 289–311.

National Health and Medical Research Council (NHMRC) 2013, *Australian dietary guidelines*, NHMRC, Canberra.

National Scientific Council on the Developing Child 2010, *Early experiences can alter gene expression and affect long-term development*, Center on the Developing Child, Harvard University, Cambridge, MA.

O'Connor, TG et al. 2015, Observed parent–child relationship quality predicts antibody response to vaccination in children, *Brain, Behavior, and Immunity*, 48, pp. 165–273.

Partuthi, S et al. 2016, Recommended amount of sleep for pediatric populations: A consensus statement of the American Academy of Sleep Medicine, *Journal of Clinical Sleep Medicine*, 12(6), pp. 785–6.

Redmond, G et al. 2016, *Are the kids alright? Young Australians in their middle years. Final report of the Australian Child Wellbeing Project*, Flinders University, Adelaide, viewed 21 February 2021, https://doi.org/http://australianchildwellbeing.com.au/sites/default/files/uploads/ACWP_Final_Report_2016_Full.pdf

Rhodes, A 2015, *What the public thinks: Top ten child health problems*, Royal Children's Hospital, Melbourne.

—— 2017a, *Kids and food: Challenges families face*, Royal Children's Hospital, Melbourne.

—— 2017b, *Screen time: What's happening in our homes?*, Royal Children's Hospital, Melbourne.

—— 2018, *Child behaviour: How are Australian parents responding?*, Royal Children's Hospital, Melbourne.

Robson, SM, McCullough, MB, Rex, S, Munafo, MR & Taylor, G 2020, Family meal frequency, diet, and family functioning: A systematic review with meta-analyses, *Journal of Nutrition Education and Behavior*, 52(5), pp. 553–64.

Rodrigues-Ayllon, M et al. 2019, Role of physical activity and sedentary behavior in the mental health of preschoolers, children and adolescents: A systematic review and meta-analysis, *Sports Medicine*, 49, pp. 1383–1410.

Russell, CG, Worsley, A & Liem, DG 2014, Parents' food choice motives and their associations with children's food preferences, *Public Health and Nutrition*, 18(6), pp. 1018–27.

Salmon, J, Campbell, KJ & Crawford, DA 2006, Television viewing habits associated with obesity risk factors: A survey of Melbourne schoolchildren, *Medical Journal of Australia*, 184(2), pp. 64–7.

Sanders, MR 2019, Harnessing the power of positive parenting to promote wellbeing of children, parents and communities over a lifetime, *Behaviour Change*, 36, pp. 56–74.

Schmidt, ME et al. 2012, Systematic review of effective strategies for reducing screen time among young children, *Obesity*, 20(7), pp. 1338–54.

Slopen, N, Chen, Y, Priest, N, Albert, MA & Williams, DR 2016, Emotional and instrumental support during childhood and biological dysregulation in midlife, *Preventive Medicine*, 84, pp. 90–6.

Steinberg, L 2001, We know some things: Parent–adolescent relationships in retrospect and prospect, *Journal of Research on Adolescence*, 11(1), pp. 1–19.

Stiglic, N & Viner, RM 2019, Effects of screentime on the health and well-being of children and adolescents: A systematic review of reviews, *BMJ Open*, 9, p. e023191.

Tremblay, MS et al. 2014, Physical activity of children: A global matrix of grades comparing 15 countries, *Journal of Physical Activity and Health*, 11(Suppl. 1), pp. S113–S125.

Tremblay, RE, Masse, B, Perron, D, Leblanc, M, Schwartzman, AE & Ledingham, JE 1992, Early disruptive behavior, poor school achievement, delinquent behavior, and delinquent personality: Longitudinal analyses, *Journal of Consulting and Clinical Psychology*, 60(1), pp. 64–72.

Tremblay, RE et al. 2004, Physical agression during early childhood: Trajectories and predictors, *Pediatrics*, 114(1), pp. e43–e50.

Trost, SG & Loprinzi, PD 2011, Parental influences on physical activity behavior in children and adolescents: A brief review, *American Journal of Lifestyle Medicine*, 5(2), pp. 171–81.

Veldhuis, L, van Grieken, A, Renders, CM, HiraSing, RA & Raat, H 2014, Parenting style, the home environment, and screen time of 5-yer-old children: The 'Be Active, Eat Right' study, *PLOS One*, 9(2), p. e88486.

Whittle, S et al. 2016, Observed measure of negative parenting predict brain development during adolescence, *PLOS One*, 11(1), p. e0147774.

World Health Organization (WHO) 2020, *Improving early childhood development: WHO guideline*, WHO, Geneva.

Williams, KE, Paul, C, Pizzo, B & Riegel, K 2008, Practice does make perfect: A longitudinal look at repeated taste exposure, *Appetite*, 51(3), pp. 739–42.

Woo Baidal, JA, Locks, LM, Cheng, ER, Blake-Lamb, TL, Perkins, ME & Taveras, EM 2016, Risk factors for childhood obesity in the first 1,000 days, *American Journal of Preventive Medicine*, 50(6), pp. 761–79.

Wu, L, Sun, S, He, Y, & Jiang, B 2016, The effect of interventions targeting screen time reduction, *Medicine*, 95(27), pp. 1–8.

Zhang, Z, Sousa-Sa, E, Rereira, JR, Okely, AD, Feng, X & Santos, R 2020, Correlates of sleep duration in early childhood: A systematic review, *Behavioral Sleep Medicine*, 19(3), pp. 407–25.

Zhao, J et al. 2018, Excessive screen time and psychosocial wellbeing: The mediating role of body mass index, sleep duration, and parent–child interaction, *The Journal of Pediatrics*, 202, pp. 157–62.

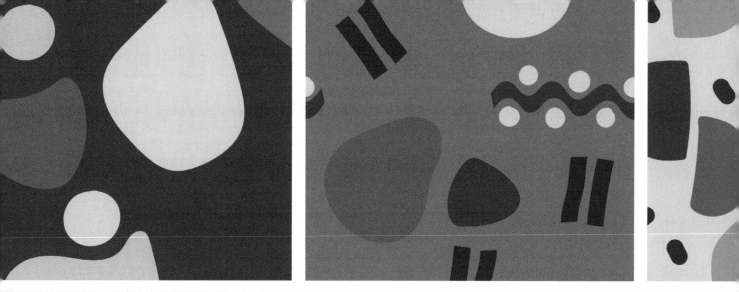

PART C

Nursing children and young people

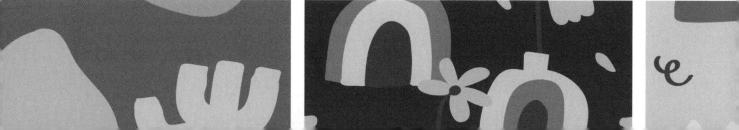

School health, health promotion and health education

Lisa Hutchinson

7

LEARNING OBJECTIVES

In this chapter you will:

- Be introduced to the variable roles and responsibilities of school nurses and frameworks that underpin school nursing practice
- Gain an understanding of a settings-based approach to health promotion with children, young people and families
- Learn strategies to promote and support health literacy development within school communities
- Recognise priority health and wellbeing issues for children and young people, and strategies to promote optimal growth and development
- Consider the role school nurses may play in arresting increasing rates of childhood overweight and obesity

Introduction

Nurses play an important role in promoting the health and wellbeing of children and families within a variety of community settings. Schools are an ideal setting through which to access school-aged children and their families and offer prevention and early intervention services. Nurses may achieve this by working with individual children and their families, as well as through advocacy for a settings-based approach to health promotion that cultivates a supportive school environment as a means of optimising children's growth and development.

This chapter will focus on the role of the school nurse. It will begin by exploring conceptual frameworks underpinning school nursing practice, and the range of factors that influence the target and scope of their role activities. Readers will then learn how the Health Promoting Schools Framework may be used to guide nursing activities to create a health-promoting environment that encourages and supports healthy behaviours. This will include an examination of how nurses work with children and families to promote their health literacy through both formal and informal health education.

The chapter will conclude with an overview of the priority health and wellbeing issues for children and adolescents, and evidence-based strategies required to address these concerns and optimise children's healthy growth and development. This will entail a close examination of the impacts of childhood overweight and obesity, and consideration of the primary, secondary and tertiary prevention activities that may be used by school nurses to help arrest this alarming epidemic.

School nursing

Social determinants of health and wellbeing – Factors that impact health, such as income or social status, housing, transportation, employment and working conditions, social support networks, education/literacy, neighborhood safety and physical environment, access to health services, and culture. Social determinants are identified to be the cause of 80 per cent of health problems (NASN, 2016).

School nurses play a significant role in delivering primary healthcare to children, young people and families in community settings. Working at the nexus of the education and healthcare systems, school nurses are uniquely positioned to build a culture of health in school communities by championing health and wellbeing; fostering health-promoting environments and behaviours; building health literacy; and serving as a conduit to other appropriate health services (Atkins, 2018; NASN, 2016). The intrinsic link between health and education underscores the value of this cross-sectoral alliance (Langford et al., 2017). A child or young person's health may directly influence their school attendance and engagement, which are essential for academic success, while educational outcomes are in turn a critical **social determinant of health and wellbeing** (AAP Council on School Health, 2016; Birch, 2017; Fleming, Hogan & Graf, 2018; Kolbe, 2019). Consequently, school nurses may not only influence the health outcomes of children and young people, but may also help to remove barriers to learning that will support their educational trajectories.

Variable role responsibilities

The role of the school nurse varies considerably, both internationally and across jurisdictions within Australia, with role activities being influenced by a wide range of factors (ANMF, 2019). The employing institution has a major bearing on the type of duties required of school nurses. Nurses work for both the health and education sectors, and are found in every type of educational setting, including government, independent and Catholic schools, boarding schools and special education facilities. They work across the age continuum, tailoring their role to the health and developmental needs of students within preschools, primary and secondary schools, and vocational and tertiary education settings. They also adapt their service delivery to meet the needs of urban, regional, rural and remote communities (ANMF, 2019).

The diversity of student populations within a given school community may also influence the focus of school nursing activities. For example, in addition to providing **universal prevention** activities for a school community, school nurses may employ a **selective** or **indicated prevention** approach to address the disparate health and wellbeing needs of students and families from minority groups (NASN, 2016). Other factors that influence the heterogeneity of school nursing practice include the conceptual framework under which the nursing service is delivered, and relevant stakeholder expectations, governmental and institutional priorities, the funding model under which the service is delivered and the support provided for the service within the school community. The expertise of individual school nurses and their educational preparation for the role will further shape service delivery (ANMF, 2019; Schaffer, Anderson & Rising, 2016).

Conceptual frameworks for school nursing practice

School nursing within Australia and New Zealand is predominantly conceptualised within a primary healthcare framework and underpinned by a social model of health that recognises health is contingent upon the socio-ecological environment in which one is born, lives, works and plays (ANMF, 2009; Buckley et al., 2012). Health equity, service accessibility, client empowerment and partnership development at the individual, family and community levels are central to this model of healthcare, with the promotion of health and the prevention of illness and injury being fundamental elements of the school nurse role (ANMF, 2009; NASN, 2016). Under this conceptual framework, school nurses may work across the spectrum of primary, secondary and tertiary prevention approaches to reduce risks or threats to health and wellbeing, integrating both individual and population-focused strategies within their school communities (Maughan et al., 2015).

Prevention level approach

Primary prevention is focused on reducing the incidence of disease and disability within a given population. Within a school setting, nurses may foster a positive school environment that is conducive to health and wellbeing. This may include advocacy and support for the development of relevant policies, such as those addressing sun safety, or hand hygiene and social distancing during the COVID-19 pandemic. It may also involve the use of social marketing strategies to raise awareness of health-promoting behaviours, such as the importance of staying virtually connected with others during mandated school closures relating to the pandemic to mitigate the mental health impact of social isolation, and promoting in the use of mindfulness to help to deal with psychosocial stressors during lockdown (Rothstein & Olympia, 2020). School nurses may also conduct individual and group health education sessions to promote

Universal prevention – Targeting services towards a whole population, or a particular cohort within that population (such as an age group), rather than a selected group/s within the population. For example, school nurse Danielle supports the delivery of universally accessible child and adolescent immunisation programs within her assigned schools, and provides health education to all students surrounding effective handwashing to help prevent the spread of novel coronavirus.

Selective prevention – Targeting services for those who have a greater than average risk of developing a disease. For example, school nurse Michael conducts hearing screening with Aboriginal students at schools within his region due to the higher prevalence of middle ear disease for this student cohort.

Indicated prevention – Targeting services for individuals at high risk of an illness or particular health concerns. For example, school nurse Saskia works collaboratively with the local community child and youth mental health service to implement early intervention strategies within her school for adolescents demonstrating early signs and symptoms of depression.

and support health literacy development to empower school community members with knowledge to minimise health risks and strategies to promote and support their health and wellbeing (ANMF, 2019; NASN, 2016; Schaffer, Anderson & Rising, 2016).

Secondary prevention involves activities to promote early detection and/or intervention to prevent or minimise the progression of illness and disease, and optimise health outcomes. In the school setting, this may involve the conduct of population-level or targeted screening and surveillance programs, such as screening for hearing and vision deficits or for sexually transmitted illnesses, and referring students for follow-up care once a health issue is detected (NASN, 2016; Schaffer, Anderson & Rising, 2016). It may also entail the delivery of first aid treatment or the emergency management of chronic health conditions such as asthma (ANMF, 2019). **Motivational interviewing** to assist students with smoking cessation, to help them avoid short- and long-term health consequences, is a further example (Maughan et al., 2015).

Tertiary prevention is focused on arresting the progression and reducing the consequences of established disease, and seeking to improve the quality of a person's life. Examples include the provision of education and support for students' self-management of chronic diseases such as diabetes, facilitating professional development for school staff to implement students' health-management plans and delivering counselling support to assist with managing symptoms of a mental health concern (ANMF, 2019; NASN, 2016; Schaffer, Anderson & Rising, 2016). It can also involve care coordination and case-management support for students' timely access and engagement with other relevant support providers, or liaison with health professionals to support a student's rehabilitation back into the school community following hospitalisation (Anderson et al., 2018).

Motivational interviewing – A counselling approach that supports a person to modify their health behaviours by encouraging them to explore factors that may be influencing their ambivalence towards making the required changes, and collaboratively developing strategies to address them.

Professionalising school nursing practice

The importance of advancing the professionalism of school nursing practice in Australia has been recognised through the National School Nursing Standards for Practice: Registered Nurse (the Standards), developed by the ANMF (2019). The second version of the Standards is structured within the domains of Professional Practice, Provision of Care, Collaborative Practice and School Nursing Environment. The comprehensive Standards provide a best-practice framework for nurses working in the school setting and promote clarity surrounding the scope of practice and the broad range of role expectations for school nurses. They also articulate nurses' professionally legislated obligations while working within the school setting and provide a means by which nurses may promote awareness of these obligations within their school communities (ANMF, 2019).

In New Zealand, there is a Child Health Nursing Knowledge and Skills Framework and a National Youth Health Nursing Knowledge and Skills Framework (College of Child and Youth Nurses, NZNO, 2014); however, there is currently no dedicated school nursing framework that clearly delineates the scope of practice and minimum qualification for school nurses. Buckley et al. (2012) have called for a national-level policy with regard to the provision of school nursing services in New Zealand, particularly in view of the country's focus on nurses leading change in the provision of primary healthcare. The New Zealand Nurses Organisation (NZNO) has been undertaking research to inform the development of a school nursing framework, which may lend support to a strategy to introduce school nurses into every secondary school in New Zealand (Cookson, 2018).

School nurse expertise

The dynamic nature of school nursing and the diversity of role activities can necessitate a broad repertoire of knowledge and skills, including:

- an understanding of the interconnecting principles of primary healthcare, and how to work with school communities to promote equity, access, empowerment, community self-determinism and inter-sectoral collaboration
- familiarity with a settings-based approach to health promotion and appropriate strategies to build capacity for health within the school environment
- knowledge of child and/or adolescent growth and development, and specific health risks for the targeted lifespan stage to inform appropriate prevention activities. Competence is also required in building rapport and effectively communicating with children and/or young people to optimise their access and engagement with service activities.
- understanding of the legislation that underpins healthcare delivery to children and adolescents in a cross-sectoral environment, particularly relating to privacy and confidentiality, medication management, students' capacity for informed decision-making and autonomous service access, and child safety obligations
- skills in the delivery of health education to children and/or young people, and an ability to facilitate educational sessions for parents and school staff
- contemporary knowledge of evidence-based resources to support health education delivery and build health literacy within school communities
- stakeholder engagement skills to work collaboratively with school staff, parents and community agencies to facilitate a partnership approach to the promotion of health and wellbeing within school communities
- health-counselling, case-coordination and advocacy skills, as well as knowledge of relevant local services and access criteria, to ensure children and young people receive timely and appropriate support for their identified health and wellbeing needs
- social marketing capabilities as a means of influencing the knowledge, values and attitudes of school community members to promote health and wellbeing
- a willingness to champion good health and wellbeing and serve as a credible wellness role model within the school community (Anderson et al., 2018; ANMF, 2019; Maughan et al., 2015; Schaffer, Anderson & Rising, 2016; Walker, 2014).

REFLECTION POINT 7.1

School nursing roles vary across school communities and are influenced by a range of factors, including the employing institution, the diversity of the student population and the framework underpinning service delivery.

- In light of these disparities, how might nurses prepare effectively for a career in school nursing?

Health promotion in the school setting

Health promotion is a fundamental responsibility of school nurses. The Ottawa Charter for Health Promotion (WHO, 1986, p. 1) defines health promotion as the 'process of enabling people to increase control over, and to improve their health'. This not only encompasses actions directed at strengthening the skills and capabilities of individuals and communities, but recognises the importance of healthy public policy and the need for supportive environments to make it easier for people to make healthier choices. This involves actions to reorient social, environmental and economic conditions to reduce their impact on both individual and population level health and wellbeing (Hung et al., 2014).

An emphasis on health-promoting environments is central to a settings-based approach to health promotion. This involves the comprehensive integration of health-promotion activities across all areas of a targeted setting to minimise risk factors and create an environment that supports optimal health (John-Akonola & Nic-Gabhainn, 2014). Schools represent an ideal setting for this approach to health promotion, as facilitating a supportive school environment can help cultivate knowledge, attitudes and behaviours in children and adolescents that are conducive to both their short- and long-term positive health and wellbeing (Langford et al., 2015).

Health Promoting Schools Framework

The World Health Organization's 'Health Promoting Schools' (HPS) Framework is an internationally recognised settings-based approach to health promotion which takes an ecological approach to creating school environments which encourage and support health and healthy behaviours (Banfield, McGorm & Sargent, 2015). The HPS framework (see Figure 7.1) comprises three interconnected domains, which are predominantly focused on:

1. effective health education integrated throughout the formal school curriculum (and underpinned by appropriate professional development for teaching staff)

2. fostering a supportive physical and social environment that is conducive to health and promotes a sense of belonging (underpinned by relevant school health and wellbeing policies), and

3. promoting partnerships and engagement with staff, families, agencies and the wider community (Banfield, McGorm & Sargent, 2015; Turunen et al., 2017).

Various terminologies have been used to describe the HPS framework since it was introduced in the 1980s, including the 'whole-school approach', 'comprehensive school health' and 'coordinated school health'; however, the underlying

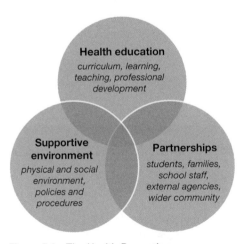

Figure 7.1   The Health Promoting Schools Framework
Source: Adapted from WHO (1996).

concepts of HPS have endured and are focused on facilitating an integrated, whole-of-community approach to the promotion of health and wellbeing (Brown et al., 2018).

CASE STUDY 7.1 TRACEY

Tracey has just commenced working as a school nurse in a secondary public school located in a large metropolitan suburb. To learn more about the school community, Tracey reviews census data to determine the suburb's sociodemographic profile. To glean information about the school's culture, Tracey reviews the school's website and peruses its latest strategic plan, recent annual reports and school policies. She discerns high rates of absenteeism, a minimal focus on health and wellbeing, and limited community engagement.

Tracey conducts a **windshield survey** as she drives to the school, noting numerous fast food outlets in the immediate vicinity of the school grounds. She observes many students entering the school eating hot chips with gravy for breakfast, and with large bottles of cola and energy drinks protruding from their backpacks. She also notes a higher than average proportion of students who are overweight or obese. A preliminary discussion with the canteen convenor reveals that the menu does comply with the school's nutrition and healthy eating policy requirements. However, the convenor admits there are limited fresh food options and a predominant use of pre-packaged food items, which she attributes to a lack of volunteer support. She also cites this as the key barrier to providing a breakfast service.

How might the HPS framework underpin initiatives to promote health and wellbeing within this school community, and what role might Tracey play in supporting this?

Windshield survey – A systematic observation of a community made from a moving vehicle.

School nursing within the HPS Framework

To promote a sense of ownership and engender participation in health and wellbeing initiatives, school nurses should facilitate a bottom-up approach, encouraging school community members to identify priority issues and work collaboratively to address these issues. This may be achieved through the formation of a HPS committee, comprising a representative sample of all key stakeholders within the school community, including parents, students, teaching and non-teaching staff, and relevant community groups such as the parents and citizens (P&C) association. The committee may identify priority health and wellbeing issues through the conduct of a school health audit. This will help to establish how the school is currently addressing key health and wellbeing issues, the available resources, and gaps that need to be addressed. The audit may be aided by the conduct of surveys and focus group interviews, and the use of suggestion boxes to garner input and promote involvement of school community members. Collected data will not only inform relevant initiatives, but will also provide a benchmark to help gauge the impact of initiatives on the perceptions of health and wellbeing within the school community (WA Health Promoting Schools Association, 2020).

The next step involves the HPS committee's development of an action plan, which outlines strategies relating to each domain of the HPS framework, as success relies on a comprehensive approach to implementation. The action plan may be informed by relevant evidence-based initiatives, and should delineate realistic and measurable goals as well as suitable methods of evaluating the achievement of these goals (Hagell, Rigby & Perrow, 2015). A cyclical and collaborative approach to planning, implementation and evaluation of initiatives is needed to ensure these are tailored to the specific needs of the school community (Darlington, Violon & Jourdan, 2018; Hung et al., 2014).

To promote the sustainability of a settings-based approach to health promotion, school nurses may champion the use of the HPS Framework and support school communities in the implementation process, but they should be mindful not to drive health-promotion and prevention programs within their schools. Instead, they should assume a facilitative role and catalyse change by building capacity within school communities and fostering a sense of ownership among community members (Eckerman et al., 2014; Langford et al., 2017). Examples of how school nurses may support activities within each of the HPS domains are listed in Table 7.1.

Table 7.1 Supportive HPS activities

Health education	Supportive environment	Partnerships
• Liaising with curriculum coordinators to promote integrated and sequential delivery of health and wellbeing content across year levels • Signposting suitable curriculum resources and co-facilitating lessons with a health and wellbeing focus • Promoting professional development opportunities for school staff to assist in the delivery of the school curriculum surrounding identified health issues	• Advocating for school environments that are conducive to health – for example, providing adequate shade, healthy canteen menus and breakfast programs • Supporting school communities to recognise the intrinsic links between health and education, and the importance of promoting health and wellbeing • Promoting the development and implementation of supportive school health policies • Collaborating on the development of protocols and procedures relating to the identification and support of students at risk of specific health concerns • Rallying and empowering champions within the school to facilitate the progression of health-focused interventions • Contributing expertise in the assessment, implementation and evaluation of initiatives, including the provision of support to develop relevant funding applications • Utilising social marketing principles and tools to promote change in awareness, attitudes and health-related behaviours	• Promoting partnership development with relevant community agencies to enhance the support available for identified health needs within the school community • Supporting the coordination of health expos to promote awareness of relevant community services and their access criteria • Facilitating parent education sessions addressing strategies to promote child and adolescent health and wellbeing • Promoting the involvement of P&C committees and student councils in fundraising and support for health-promoting initiatives in the school setting

Australian Student Wellbeing Framework

A further framework that may guide nurses in their health-promotion endeavours within schools, and one that complements the comprehensive HPS Framework, is the Australian Student Wellbeing Framework. This was introduced by the federal government in 2018 to help to build safe, supportive learning environments that optimise inclusion and promote student resilience and wellbeing (Department of Education, Skills and Employment, 2020). An online Student Wellbeing Hub has been created (www.dese.gov.au/student-resilience-and-wellbeing/student-wellbeing-hub), which outlines the five key elements of the framework: leadership, inclusion, student voice, partnerships and support. It also provides a school wellbeing audit tool that aids schools in assessing their performance against these key elements. The site also houses a plethora of curriculum resources, professional development activities and information for students and parents/caregivers to support a comprehensive approach to the promotion of student resilience and wellbeing, including strategies and resources to combat bullying, which is a serious problem within schools and has a deleterious impact on student wellbeing (Australian Institute for Teaching and School Leadership, 2017).

Fundamentals of health education

Health education is an integral component of a comprehensive approach to health promotion in the school setting. It also represents a pivotal role activity for school nurses, as it underpins all three levels of prevention (Duff, 2015). Nurses may engage in informal health education through opportunistic health teaching with students during one-on-one consultations. They may also share health information and promote health and wellbeing with school community members through newsletters, bulletin board notices and web pages, or via health expos (Conway, 2015; Duff, 2015; Hagell, Rigby & Perrow, 2015). A more formal approach to health education may involve their structured work with small groups of students, the delivery of professional development with school staff and parent information sessions, and the co-facilitation of classroom-based lessons with a health and wellbeing focus (Loschiavo, 2015).

Health literacy promotion

An important concept underlying all types of health education is the promotion of health literacy. This encapsulates the knowledge, attitudes and capabilities of individuals to understand and engage with health-related information in order to promote and maintain their health and wellbeing (Hagell, Rigby & Perrow, 2015; Loschiavo, 2015). According to Nutbeam, a leading health literacy expert (cited in Hagell, Rigby & Perrow, 2015), the effective promotion of health literacy involves more than facilitating the acquisition of health information. It encompasses a tri-level hierarchy of health literacy promotion that addresses an individual's functional, interactive and critical health literacy needs. This entails empowering them to:

• assess and evaluate health information, manage risk and make appropriate lifestyle choices

- effectively navigate the health system and seek timely support, and
- actively contribute to strategies to improve the social determinants of health (Hagell, Rigby & Perrow, 2015).

When working with individuals, it is important to consider the stages of health behaviour change a person goes through as they prepare to modify their behaviour, and the variable information and support needs they may have at these different stages, which may influence the approach to health literacy promotion (Hagell, Rigby & Perrow, 2015). A further consideration is the importance of taking an assets- or skills-based approach to health literacy promotion, supporting individuals to build skills in decision-making and providing them with an opportunity to practise and apply their learning rather than just imparting information about what they 'should' or 'should not' do to maintain health (Hagell, Rigby & Perrow, 2015).

Effective communication

School nurses need to be well versed in health literacy principles to optimise the impact of their health-education activities (Pontius, 2013). This not only includes tailoring delivery to the age and developmental stage of children and young people, but also adapting verbal and written communication with parents/caregivers when they are the targets of health education to accommodate their variable health literacy needs. Box 7.1 outlines the key factors to consider when verbally communicating health information.

BOX 7.1 CONSIDERATIONS WHEN VERBALLY COMMUNICATING HEALTH INFORMATION

- Limit the content to three to five key health messages that they need to know 'right now' to address the health concern, and withhold information that is 'nice' to know.
- Repeat key messages at least three times in different ways, ensuring the information imparted is both specific and concrete.
- Chunk information into manageable portions.
- Avoid 'yes', 'no' and closed-ended questions, and ask them to paraphrase and repeat back the key messages to ensure they have been adequately explained.
- Employ the teach-back method, asking how they would explain this to others as a means of assessing their comprehension.
- Avoid the use of medical jargon, and simplify terms and phrases into plain, everyday, concrete language.
- Use graphics to explain concepts and to reinforce messaging.
- Enlist the support of an interpreter when necessary to ensure that messages are relayed appropriately to people for whom English is a second language

Source: Based on Pontius (2013).

Promoting health literacy with adults through written communication requires similar considerations. According to the 2012 Survey of Adult Skills, 44 per cent of Australians aged between 16 and 65 years are functionally illiterate (OECD, 2012). This means that they do not have the reading and writing skills to manage daily living and employment tasks that require reading skills beyond a basic level. This has huge ramifications for their health literacy, and particularly their capacity to understand and act on health information. Health education materials targeting parents and correspondence regarding their child's health must therefore be written in a manner that supports their engagement and understanding. Tips on how to achieve this are outlined in Box 7.2.

BOX 7.2 TIPS ON EFFECTIVELY COMMUNICATING WRITTEN HEALTH INFORMATION

- Limit content to include only necessary (rather than 'nice-to-know') information, include the most important information upfront, and bold key words for emphasis.
- Use short sentences (15 to 20 words), limit the use of punctuation and use headings, subheadings and bulleted lists to break up complex topics.
- Use conversational, everyday language with shorter, unambiguous words, no medical jargon and limited use of statistical information.
- Use the 'active voice', starting sentences with a verb and personalising content by using the terms 'you' and 'your'.
- Clearly alert them to what needs to be done and why it is important to them. This may be facilitated by a question-and-answer format, or using analogies familiar to the intended audience.
- Promote readability by using an uncomplicated font style (such as a serif font), a body text font size of between 12 and 14 points, left line justification with right ragged text and well-spaced lines.
- Use graphics that contribute meaningfully to the message being imparted, such as demonstrating simple steps of a procedure. These should be adult-oriented rather than childish images; however, avoid overly realistic anatomical images and ensure cultural relevance.

Source: Based on Pontius (2014).

REFLECTION POINT 7.2

More than two in five Australian adults are functionally illiterate (OECD, 2012). This has significant ramifications for their health literacy, influencing their ability to comprehend and evaluate health information and navigate the health system. It is therefore vital for school nurses to use appropriate strategies to accommodate the health literacy needs of parents/caregivers during informal health education delivery.

- What strategies might the school nurse use to determine the effectiveness of their communication?

Adult-focused health education and professional development sessions

School nurses may be called upon to deliver health education sessions to parents/caregivers, as well as professional development sessions for school staff and community members. When delivering group sessions to adults, nurses should not only be mindful of the communication strategies outlined above, but also consider adult learning principles to optimise their engagement and their learning outcomes. There are numerous theories relating to the determinants of learning, which may guide the school nurse in using appropriate instructional strategies; however, a relatively simplistic approach is the VARK model developed by Fleming and Mills (1992, cited by Kitchie, 2020). VARK is an acronym denoting visual, aural, read/write and kinaesthetic, and it highlights the various learning styles that may be preferred by learners. The school nurse may readily incorporate a range of teaching and learning strategies to accommodate these different styles – for example:

- presenting graphs and flowcharts for visual learners
- facilitating small-group discussions for aural learners
- providing written learning materials for read/write learners
- using role-plays or other practical learning activities for kinaesthetic learners (Kitchie, 2020).

Classroom-based health education

Formal classroom-based health education is a vital element of a comprehensive approach to school health promotion (Leahy & Simovska, 2017). In Australia, health education is delivered primarily through the Australian Curriculum: Health and Physical Education (HPE), which promotes a sequential approach to addressing selected health and wellbeing topics for all school students from Foundation level to Year 10 (ACARA, 2021). The two strands within the HPE learning area are: Movement and Physical Activity; and Personal, Social and Community Health. Within the latter strand, focus areas that span all year levels include the safe use of medicines; food and nutrition; the health benefits of physical activity; mental health and wellbeing; relationships; and safety. In the later years of schooling, it is recommended that students learn about sexuality, and alcohol and other drugs (ACARA, 2021).

Despite the relatively comprehensive coverage of focus areas within the HPE learning area, there is jurisdictional discretion to adapt content delivery relative to teachers' professional knowledge and the local school context. A crowded curriculum and competing academic priorities can also overshadow the importance of a comprehensive approach to health education (Lynch, 2015; Shackleton et al., 2016). The quantity and quality of health education are imperative to support the development of health-enhancing behaviours (Barwood, Cunningham & Penney, 2016), and therefore nurses can serve as key advocates within their schools to champion and support appropriate content delivery that advances health literacy development and equips students to address contemporary health and wellbeing issues (Conway, 2015).

Effective advocacy requires school nurses to understand where topics are addressed within the curriculum and how they are sequenced across the learning continuum. It also requires a working knowledge of the underpinning aims and propositions of health education delivery, the anticipated learning outcomes and the **pedagogical approach** required to facilitate these learning outcomes. This will not only support nurses to source appropriate curriculum resources and suitable professional development activities for teaching staff; it will also equip them to effectively contribute to health education delivery through the co-facilitation of relevant lessons.

Pedagogical approach – Refers to the style of interaction between the teacher and students as well as the teaching and learning methods that are used, and the resultant impact on students' capacity to learn.

CASE STUDY 7.2 GABI

Gabi is the school nurse for a small rural secondary school. She is approached by the year-level coordinator to support the delivery of sexual health education to Year 9 students, as the HPE teacher has reportedly expressed his discomfort in addressing this topic. Gabi meets with the coordinator and the HPE teacher to plan a suitable approach. She first assesses the relationships and sexuality content that has been delivered to students in previous years and maps this to recommendations outlined in the HPE curriculum. She identifies suitable evidence-based teaching resources published by the state's family planning organisation, and clarifies how these may be tailored to build on the existing knowledge base of the student cohort and the time-frames for the lessons allocated to this topic. Gabi seeks the teacher's input into other pedagogical considerations, including the differentiation of learning activities to accommodate students' specific learning needs.

Gabi discusses the need to establish ground rules with each class at the beginning of the lessons in view of the sensitive nature of the topics being addressed, and discusses other strategies to promote an inclusive learning environment. She also flags the need for the teacher's active co-facilitation of these lessons, and highlights the availability of professional development resources to support him to upskill in the topics under consideration.

Pedagogical considerations

Effective health education utilises skills-based participatory pedagogies that correlate knowledge and skills with the actions needed to achieve health and wellbeing. This includes the provision of opportunities for students to critically engage with health knowledge, and to develop and apply skills such as reasoning, problem-solving, informed decision-making, refusal and reflection (Barwood et al., 2016; Fairbrother, Curtis & Goyder, 2016; Matthews, 2014). For example, a relevant activity might require secondary school students to critique a health-related app or website to determine the credibility and accessibility of health information, or a primary school cohort might be asked to view food items and assign them to certain food groups.

Health education should also be delivered sequentially through a scaffolded learning approach that builds on prior learning, and content and resources should have personal and community relevance to the targeted students. It is also important to differentiate learning activities to accommodate students' identified learning needs, and employ strategies to promote a safe, supportive and inclusive learning environment (Matthews, 2014). The school nurse should discuss appropriate strategies with classroom teachers prior to co-facilitating health education lessons, as they will understand the learning needs of their student cohort.

Differentiated instruction and a safe and inclusive learning environment

Promoting a safe and inclusive learning environment involves catering to the diversity of need within the classroom, and may entail strategies such as:

- the deliberate placement of students to accommodate sensory deficits
- the use of visual aids to support those with English as a second language
- avoiding the use of ethno-centric images in presentations and learning resources
- assigning activities relative to differing abilities
- utilising inclusive language to combat stereotypes based on race, ability, gender or sexuality, such as the use of gender-neutral titles like 'partner' instead of boyfriend or girlfriend, and positive terms to refer to people with disabilities (Department of Education, Tasmania, 2012, 2014).

A further means of promoting an inclusive environment is to collaboratively establish ground rules with students to guide behavioural expectations throughout the lesson, particularly when addressing sensitive topics such as sexual health. Appropriate ground rules may include acknowledgement that students may have variable levels of experience with the lesson content, and as such they should not tease one another for asking questions, displaying embarrassment or discomfort, or responding to questions posed to the class. Students should also agree to demonstrate respect for others' opinions and values; utilise respectful language and appropriate terms rather than slang words; and agree to maintain privacy by not sharing personal stories or information with the group, or asking others personal questions (Schroeder, Goldfarg & Gelperin, 2015).

It is not appropriate to agree with students that 'what is said in the room, stays in the room' in the event of a disclosure of abuse, as this would need to be reported in accordance with child safety legislation (Schroeder, Goldfarg & Gelperin, 2015). Instead, school nurses should utilise the ground rules exercise to advise students where they may seek support should they wish to discuss matters of a private nature. In the event that a student does begin to disclose a private matter during the lesson, they should be protectively interrupted and redirected to the ground rules, highlighting that these issues are best discussed in private following the lesson.

Promoting student participation

Building upon students' existing knowledge is a key strategy to promoting their engagement in learning. Introducing the learning objectives at the outset of the lesson and asking students to articulate what they already know about a topic can help to consolidate this learning and provide 'coat hangers' upon which to hang new knowledge acquired in the present lesson. Posing questions prior to presenting information promotes critical inquiry and helps to keep students interested in a presentation. Working from simple to more complex concepts is also recommended, as is providing information in manageable chunks and interspersing didactic presentations with activities to keep them focused and engaged (Conway, 2015). Learning materials that are relevant to students' context, such as relatable case studies or technology-based activities, will optimise their participation and learning. Peer-to-peer learning is an effective means of knowledge transfer and a further means of facilitating student participation. Offering students choices about elements of the lesson can also promote a sense of agency and foster participation (Conway, 2015).

Utilising an activity such as a short quiz during the lesson and inviting questions can allow students to gauge their progress with their learning and clarify their understanding of content delivery. Depending on the age of the targeted student cohort, a question box is an ideal means through which to promote safety and inclusion. Request that all students write their answers on a piece of paper and place it in the box to avoid embarrassment or stigmatisation (Splendorio & Reichel, 2013). If they do not wish to ask a question, then request that they record a key learning that they have gleaned from the lesson. Respond to the questions in a brief and factual manner, particularly with respect to provocative questions. If the student has used slang terms, paraphrase the question utilising appropriate terminology, and reword the question from first person to third person so as not to personalise the response. If students ask values-based questions such as an appropriate age to engage in a certain behaviour, it is helpful to redirect the question and seek a response from the class, as this will help to highlight the range of attitudes and values associated with an issue (Splendorio & Reichel, 2013).

Healthy growth and development

Healthy growth and development entail the promotion of physical, mental, emotional and social wellbeing (Ontario Ministry of Health and Long-Term Care, 2018). Preventative programs that foster the development of knowledge, skills and resources can help to mitigate risk and optimise protective factors to improve health and developmental outcomes, particularly through the more vulnerable periods of transition. Early childhood through to school transition is a particularly crucial period, which sets the stage for health and developmental outcomes (Peterson, Loeb & Chamberlain, 2018). Adolescence represents a further vulnerable life stage, which can have a positive or negative influence on an individual's longer-term health outcomes (Department of Health, 2019). School nursing services should therefore ensure a 'proportionate universalism' approach to service delivery, which involves supplementing universally available services with targeted support activities for parents and families during these crucial lifespan stages.

CASE STUDY 7.3 JUDY

Judy works as both a community child health and a school nurse in a regional community. In addition to providing parenting support, and growth and developmental checks for babies and toddlers, Judy conducts universal hearing and vision screening with prep children at local primary schools. This service model has been offered to the

(cont.)

community for the past 30 years. Judy has become increasingly aware of the importance of promoting children's readiness for school in order to optimise their educational outcomes. She reviews the Australian Early Development Index (AEDI) data, a national progress measure for childhood development, and notes that the children in her community are developmentally vulnerable on most of the reported domains. Judy also reviews the grey and peer-reviewed literature to determine the evidence base behind universal school screening activities.

In line with her findings, Judy advocates with key stakeholders to reorient the service model to include a focus on supporting children's school readiness, and gains approval to spearhead these service revisions. In lieu of vision screening activities, she collaborates with schools and local optometrists to promote comprehensive eye assessments as a prerequisite for children's school entry. In view of the national newborn hearing screening program, which successfully identifies children with sensorineural hearing loss, Judy also negotiates for a selective approach to hearing screening in schools and establishes suitable referral criteria.

Judy then engages with local early childhood education and care services and pre-schools to support the implementation of developmental screening using the validated Parents' Evaluation of Developmental Screening (PEDS) tool. She works with educators to upskill them in supporting parents' completion of this tool, and imparts health teaching strategies they may use to empower parents to support their children's development. She also supports the educators to understand the importance of adapting their approach to accommodate parents' health literacy. Judy encourages the referral of children identified with concerns to community child health services for a comprehensive secondary developmental screen and timely referral to early intervention services as indicated. She is confident that this approach will contribute to addressing the alarming rates of childhood developmental delay in her local area.

Priority health and wellbeing concerns

As evidenced in the above case study, being familiar with priority health and wellbeing concerns for Australian children and adolescents can inform school nurses' implementation of appropriate preventative health activities with parents/caregivers and school communities. Box 7.3 provides an overview of statistics drawn from the Australian Institute of Health and Welfare (AIHW, 2020), which underscore the need for focused efforts to redress other alarming trends.

BOX 7.3 ALARMING CHILD AND ADOLESCENT HEALTH AND WELLBEING STATISTICS

- Approximately one in four children aged 5 to 14 years is overweight or obese.
- Just over 4 per cent of children consume the recommended daily intake of vegetables, and nearly 27 per cent of children have inadequate fruit consumption.

- Nearly 30 per cent of children aged 2 to 17 years do not engage in sufficient activity in line with recommended guidelines.
- Children aged from 5 to 14 years spend an average of two hours per day on screen-based activities (with only 3.5 minutes of this devoted to homework), while the recommended screen time for this age group is less than two hours per day.
- Approximately one in five children aged 8 to 12 years reports negative experiences such as unwanted contact and content while using social media.
- Approximately one in seven children aged 4 to 17 years meets the criteria for a medical diagnosis of a mental disorder, while one in five aged 15 to 19 years meets the criteria for a probable serious mental illness.
- Around three in five Year 4 students and two in five Year 8 students experience bullying on a weekly or monthly basis.
- The number of deaths from suicide for young people is higher now that it was a decade ago.
- Around 1.5 per cent of children aged 0 to 14 years are hospitalised for injury each year, with falls accounting for nearly half of these injuries.
- An estimated 43 per cent of children are reported to have at least one chronic health condition, and 20 per cent have two or more conditions.
- One in ten children aged between 0 and 14 years suffers from asthma.
- Over 7 per cent of children aged 0–14 years have some level of disability, with intellectual and sensory/speech impairments being the most common types of disability experienced.
- Almost 35 per cent of children live in families with poor family functioning.
- Over half of parents who have experienced partner violence said their children had seen or heard the violence, while nearly 4000 assaults against children each year are related to family violence.
- Approximately 0.4 per cent of children aged 0 to 14 years are homeless.
- Around 20 per cent of children are not developmentally ready for school, which can have a detrimental impact on their long-term wellbeing.
- Around 10 per cent of children are not fully immunised at 2 years of age, which negatively impacts herd immunity.
- Nearly one quarter of children aged 6 to 14 years have experienced decay in their permanent teeth and over 10 per cent have untreated decay.

Source: AIHW (2020).

Addressing priority health and wellbeing concerns

The National Action Plan for the Health of Children and Young People (Department of Health, 2019) outlines broad strategies to address priority health and wellbeing concerns. These strategies may guide school nurses in their approach to working with families and school communities to improve health and wellbeing outcomes for children and young people. They include the following approaches:

- Supporting families to understand how crucial the first 2000 days of a child's life are to their long-term developmental outcomes, and working to improve parental engagement in the early years of child development. This may be achieved by:

- routinely reading with children to stimulate their cognitive development and their language and literacy skills, and to strengthen parent–child relationships
- encouraging conversation, asking them questions, playing games with them, promoting independence in toileting and dressing, and providing opportunities to draw and develop their fine motor skills
- promoting regular engagement in preschool programs to build children's social and emotional competence and help to prepare them for school entry.

- Continuing to build parenting skills during children's middle years and adolescence, especially supporting them to understand how to respond appropriately to behaviours relating to different developmental stages, and how to parent proactively and protectively.

- Advocating for effective anti-bullying strategies within schools, and upskilling families in how to respond appropriately to children's reports of bullying and promote their development of resilience and social and emotional coping skills, particularly during the middle years of childhood.

- Promoting awareness of the high rates of mental ill-health among children and young people, and the strong correlation between mental ill-health and engagement in risky behaviours such as substance misuse. Also helping to break down barriers to help-seeking such as stigma and poor mental health literacy, and promoting protective factors such as adequate sleep and good sleep hygiene, a nutritious diet, and physical activity.

- Ensuring that schools are equipped with effective age-appropriate and culturally sensitive suicide-prevention strategies. Supporting families to understand risk and protective factors, how to broach the issue of suicide with children and young people, and how to respond appropriately to admissions of suicidality.

- Advocating for the delivery of sequential respectful relationships education across all school year levels, and disseminating resources to families to initiate safe and supported conversations around family and domestic violence and sexual abuse.

- Promoting the importance of consistently high rates of immunisation for infectious diseases to achieve herd immunity and interrupt disease transmission, and disseminating myth-busting information to facilitate informed decision-making surrounding childhood immunisation.

- Raising awareness of the avenues of support available for families with children with chronic conditions to optimise effective self-management, and implementing best practice frameworks to enable continued engagement in learning and social connection during periods of hospitalisation.

- Promoting oral health literacy, such as the need to decrease consumption of sugary foods and drinks and brush twice daily, and increasing awareness of dental service accessibility via school oral health programs and community-based clinics.

- Helping to redress high rates of overweight and obesity through preventative health strategies to improve nutrition and physical activity. (In view of the significant and increasing rates of childhood overweight and obesity, the next section of this chapter is devoted to this topic.)

Tackling childhood obesity

The World Health Organization (WHO, 2016) describes childhood obesity as a global epidemic and one of the most serious public health challenges of the twenty-first century. The condition has both short- and long-term multi-systemic health consequences. Children suffering from obesity are at increased risk of experiencing a range of health concerns as outlined in Box 7.4.

BOX 7.4 HEALTH ISSUES EXPERIENCED BY CHILDREN SUFFERING OBESITY

- Asthma and other breathing problems such as obstructive sleep apnoea
- Abnormal blood glucose levels potentiating type 2 diabetes
- Elevated blood pressure and triglycerides
- Musculoskeletal problems
- Gastrointestinal problems
- Dental caries and periodontal disease
- Accelerated pubertal maturation, as well as menstrual and reproductive problems
- Mental health problems associated with negative self-image, low self-esteem, disordered eating, and teasing and bullying
- Nutritional deficiencies and inadequate bone health, increasing the risk of osteoporosis later in life

Source: CDCP (2011); WHO (2016).

In addition to the burden of disease that may be suffered during childhood, approximately 80 per cent of overweight children become overweight or obese adults (PHAA, 2016). The following list outlines the types of chronic conditions that may be experienced by adults who suffer from obesity. Overweight and obesity during adulthood not only decrease quality of life but also significantly increase the risk of premature death (CDCP, 2011; WHO, 2016). Chronic conditions that may be experienced by adults suffering obesity include:

- type 2 diabetes
- high blood pressure
- metabolic syndrome
- heart disease
- kidney disease
- fatty liver disease
- osteoarthritis
- stroke
- sleep apneoal
- several types of cancer.

The key determinants of childhood obesity are unhealthy eating and physical inactivity (Day, Sahota & Christian, 2019; Langford et al., 2015), although genetic predisposition and inadequate sleep are recognised as contributing factors (WHO, 2016). Poor community and neighbourhood design and safety negatively impact on children's physical activity levels, as does their increasing exposure to screen-based, sedentary leisure activities (CDCP, 2011). The obesogenic environment in which children are raised also negatively influences their food choices and intake, with a bombardment of advertisements for unhealthy foods and increasingly large portion sizes offered through fast food outlets (Schroeder, Travers & Smaldone, 2016; WHO, 2016).

Pivotal role of schools

Due to the extended contact that children have with schools and the symbiotic relationship between health and education, schools play a pivotal role in positively influencing healthy eating and physical activity to prevent childhood obesity (Day et al., 2019; Schroeder et al., 2016; Stylianou & Walker, 2018; Williams & Mummery, 2015). School nurses are ideally positioned within schools to advocate for and/or support health-promoting initiatives to address childhood obesity through primary, secondary and tertiary prevention activities (AAP Council on School Health, 2016; Baker Powell, Keehner Engelke & Neil, 2018).

Primary prevention

A coordinated whole-school approach to obesity prevention can positively impact the factors that contribute to the onset of this condition. This involves building healthy literacy within the school community, capitalising on community partnerships and providing a supportive school environment that enables healthy food choices and engagement in physical activity (Day et al., 2019; Langford et al., 2015).

The promotion of a supportive school environment should begin with an assessment of current school-based healthy eating and physical activity policies. All Australian public schools are mandated to adhere to the national school canteen guidelines, which outline a traffic light system to inform the selection of foods and drink that may be supplied in schools. The guidelines have been incorporated into state and territory policies, and when implemented with appropriate monitoring and accountability strategies have proven effective in reducing children's intake of energy-dense foods and drink and positively influencing the attitudes of parents (Stylianou & Walker, 2018). National legislation also mandates the provision of two hours of physical activity each school week for students in primary and junior secondary education settings, with most states and territories reflecting this requirement in relevant policies (Stylianou & Walker, 2018). School nurses may work with school staff and P&C associations to assess their understanding of relevant school nutrition and physical activity policy requirements, and to encourage the effective implementation of these policies within individual schools.

Further activities by school nurses to promote a supportive school environment could include:

- advocating for well-maintained water fountains to facilitate students' ready access to fresh water

- initiating school newsletter items to increase parental health literacy surrounding healthy food and drink choices, and recommended daily physical activity requirements to optimise healthy growth and development
- championing students' increased access to physical activity opportunities through the provision of safe spaces, facilities and equipment.

The last of these may entail the progression of grant applications for funding for school resources; enhancing student access to equipment during school break periods; ensuring appropriate supervision during structured and unstructured physical activity programs; and collaborating with community agencies to increase the availability of exercise and sporting activities outside of school hours (CDCP, 2011). Positive role modelling by school staff also contributes to a supportive school environment. To this end, school nurses may support the development of a staff wellness program to promote healthy eating, physical activity and weight management among school staff as a further strategy to combat childhood obesity (Williams & Mummery, 2015).

Building the health literacy of students surrounding healthy eating and physical activity is another important component of a whole-school approach to obesity prevention (WHO, 2016). Various stand-alone health-education programs have been introduced to encourage healthy eating, such as the nationally funded Stephanie Alexander Kitchen Garden Program (Eckerman et al., 2014). To instil a sense of ownership and promote the sustainability of such programs, research evidence has demonstrated the importance of embedding them within the curriculum and building them into the core business of the school (Day, Sahota & Christian, 2019; Eckerman et al., 2014; Langford et al., 2015). School nurses may play an instrumental role in supporting schools to source suitable health education programs and advocating for their inclusion in the curriculum. For adolescents, this should include media literacy programs that target the prevention of both obesity and negative body image, due to the propensity for young people to adopt unhealthy and dangerous behaviours to control their weight (Durocher & Gauvin, 2019). Nurses may also help to build the capacity of school staff through support for the coordination of appropriate professional development to facilitate the effective implementation of selected programs (Day, Sahota & Christian, 2019).

A further strategy to build students' health literacy involves a 'seize the moment' approach, whereby school nurses incorporate a rapid assessment of dietary intake and physical activity into their routine interaction with students for other health concerns. This facilitates the provision of relevant information and resources, and provides opportunities for brief motivational interviewing to encourage behavioural changes to improve their diet and physical activity levels (Baker Powell, Keehner Engelke & Neil, 2018; CDCP, 2011).

Secondary prevention

In some jurisdictions throughout the world, school nurses conduct **body mass index (BMI)** screening programs and refer overweight and obese children to intervention services to address their weight concerns (Turner, Owen & Watson, 2016). There is insufficient evidence of the impact of BMI screening on preventing and reducing childhood obesity – particularly screening programs that are conducted in isolation from other preventative strategies focused on improving nutrition and physical activity

Body mass index (BMI) – The most common measure of overweight or obesity, calculated by dividing a person's weight in kilograms by the square of their height in metres i.e. BMI = weight (kg)/height (m^2). BMI levels of children and adolescents are expressed relative to others of the same age and sex.

within the school setting (Thompson & Madsen, 2017). However, as the pervasiveness of this condition can lead to desensitisation, it is thought that BMI screening may serve as a means of correcting parent and student misperceptions about weight status and encouraging their adoption of healthy lifestyle choices (CDCP, 2011). To avoid stigmatisation of students, nurses must take care to maintain children's privacy and confidentiality when conducting BMI screening activities. They should communicate the results sensitively and without judgement to students and parents, to discourage harmful weight-loss practices, and highlight that the BMI result is considered within a range relative to other children of the same height and age. They should also ensure that screening programs are underpinned by appropriate intervention support available within the community for children identified with weight concerns (CDCP, 2011).

Tertiary prevention

Some studies have explored the potential for school nurses' involvement in the delivery of obesity intervention programs within schools, which involve the use of behavioural strategies and counselling support to help students overcome barriers to healthy eating and physical activity (Høstgaard Bonde, Bentsen & Lykke Hindhede, 2014; Schroeder, Goldfarb & Gelperin, 2015; Turner, Owen & Watson, 2016). A variety of practice challenges have reportedly impeded school nurses in these endeavours, including time pressures and competing priorities, inadequate training in obesity management and a lack of parental willingness for children to participate in such programs (Baker Powell, Keehner Engelke & Neil, 2018; Johnson et al., 2018; Turner, Owen & Watson, 2016).

Considering the strong influence that families have on children's food intake, family-centred counselling is paramount for any real change to be realised, so obesity intervention programs should ideally involve both children and their parents (Yubik & Lee, 2014). Supporting children to shift from overweight or obese to a healthy weight also requires more intensive intervention than can be provided exclusively in a school setting (Schroeder, Goldfarb & Gelperin, 2015; Turner, Owen & Watson, 2016). Further, singling out individual students for school-based intervention activities increases their risk of stigmatisation, which may detrimentally impact their emotional wellbeing (Høstgaard Bonde, Bentsen & Lykke Hindhede, 2014; Schroeder, Goldfarb & Gelperin, 2015). Consequently, school nurses may be better served by focusing their efforts on primary prevention activities, and working with their school communities to help combat the onset of childhood obesity (Day, Sahota & Christian, 2019).

REFLECTION POINT 7.3

School nurses may help to redress alarming rates of childhood obesity through support for a whole-school approach to preventing this condition. However, the obesogenic environment and society's increasing desensitisation to obesity may pose some challenges.

- Considering the importance of a bottom-up approach to health-promoting initiatives to facilitate ownership and sustainability, how might school nurses advocate for the prioritisation of this issue within school communities and engender support for primary prevention activities?

SUMMARY

- Working at the nexus between the health and education sectors, school nurses play a crucial role in promoting the health and wellbeing of children, young people and their families, and advancing both health and educational outcomes. The role activities they undertake to achieve this depends on a variety of factors, including the expectations of their employer and the conceptual framework within which they work.
- School nursing practice that is underpinned by a coordinated, whole-school approach to health promotion is focused on partnership development and the cultivation of a school environment that promotes and enables healthy choices.
- Utilising formal and informal health education to build the health literacy of students, families and school community members empowers them with knowledge and skills to optimise their health and wellbeing.
- Understanding priority health and wellbeing issues for children and young people, and implementing evidence-based strategies to optimise their healthy growth and development, enable nurses to target their efforts appropriately and utilise effective primary, secondary and tertiary prevention activities to achieve positive outcomes.
- Overweight and obesity represent a significant health concern for children and adolescents, which can impact their health and wellbeing into adulthood. School nurses can contribute to strategies to arrest increasing rates of obesity, particularly through health-promotion efforts to prevent the onset of this condition.

LEARNING ACTIVITIES

7.1 Review the Australian Guide to Healthy Eating (Department of Health, 2013) and answer the following questions:
- What is the recommended number of daily serves of vegetables for girls aged 4 to 8 years?
- What is the recommended number of daily serves of vegetables for boys aged 12 to 13 years?
- Only 4 per cent of children consume the recommended daily intake of vegetables. How could this issue be addressed using a whole-of-school approach?

7.2 Refer to the Australian Curriculum: Health and Physical Education (ACARA, 2021) and undertake the following exercises:
- Explore the 'Personal, Social and Community Health' strand for Years 9 and 10. Consider the sub-strand entitled 'Communicating and Interacting for Health and Wellbeing' by clicking on the Elaborations tab. Then click on the 'RS' tab for each of the threads within this sub-strand to determine the recommended content coverage for Relationships and Sexuality.
- Consider how knowledge of the Australian Curriculum may support school nurses to contribute effectively to health education.

FURTHER READING

Australian Government 2014, *National healthy schools canteens guidelines,* viewed 20 February 2021, www.health.gov.au/sites/default/files/documents/2021/03/national-healthy-school-canteens-guidelines-for-healthy-foods-and-drinks-supplied-in-school-canteens.pdf

Australian Government Department of Education and Training 2018, *Australian Student Wellbeing Framework,* viewed 20 February 2021, https://studentwellbeinghub.edu .au/media/9312/aswf_flyer.pdf

Australian Government Department of Health 2019, *National action plan for the health of children and young people 2020–2030*, viewed 20 February 2021, www1.health.gov.au/internet/main/publishing.nsf/Content/ 4815673E283EC1B6CA2584000082EA7D/$File/FINAL%20National%20Action% 20Plan%20for%20the%20Health%20of%20Children%20and%20Young% 20People%202020-2030.pdf

Australian Institute of Health and Welfare (AIHW) 2020, *Australia's children,* viewed 20 February 2021, www.aihw.gov.au/getmedia/6af928d6-692e-4449-b915-cf2ca946982f/aihw-cws-69-print-report.pdf.aspx?inline=true

Australian Nursing and Midwifery Federation (ANMF) 2019, *National School Nursing Standards for Practice: Registered Nurse*, viewed 20 February 2021, http://anmf.org .au/documents/reports/ANMF_National_School_Nursing_Standards_for_Practice_ RN_2019.pdf

REFERENCES

AAP Council on School Health 2016, Role of the school nurse in providing school health services, *Pediatrics,* 137(6), p. e20160852.

Anderson, L, Schaffer, M, Hiltz, C, O'Leary, S, Luehr, R & Yoney, E 2018, Public health interventions: School nurse practice stories, *The Journal of School Nursing,* 34(3), pp. 192–202.

Atkins, R, 2018, Four lessons learned from school nurses in New Jersey about building a culture of health, *NASN School Nurse,* March, pp. 106–8

Australian Curriculum, Assessment and Reporting Authority (ACARA) 2021, *Health and Physical Education*, viewed 22 March 2020, https://australiancurriculum.edu.au/f-10-curriculum/health-and-physical-education/

Australian Institute for Teaching and School Leadership (AITSL), 2017, *Spotlight: Bullying in Australian schools*, viewed 20 September 2020, www.aitsl.edu.au/docs/default-source/research-evidence/spotlight/spotlight_bullying.pdf?sfvrsn=613bf73c_6

Australian Institute of Health and Welfare (AIHW) 2020, *Australia's children,* cat. no. CWS 69, AIHW, Canberra, viewed 19 April 2020, www.aihw.gov.au/getmedia/6af928d6-692e-4449-b915-cf2ca946982f/aihw-cws-69-print-report.pdf.aspx?inline=true

Australian Nursing and Midwifery Federation (ANMF) 2009, *Primary health care in Australia: A nursing and midwifery consensus view*, Australian Nursing and Midwifery Federation, Canberra.

—— 2019, *National School Nursing Standards for Practice: Registered Nurse*, viewed 20 February 2021, http://anmf.org.au/documents/reports/ANMF_National_School_ Nursing_Standards_for_Practice_RN_2019.pdf

Baker Powell, S, Keehner Engelke, M & Neil, J 2018, Seizing the moment: Experiences of school nurses caring for students with overweight and obesity, *The Journal of School Nursing,* 34(5), pp. 380–9.

Banfield, M, McGorm, K & Sargent, G 2015, Health promotion in schools: A multi-method evaluation of an Australian school youth health nurse program, *BMC Nursing,* 14(1), p. 21.

Barwood, D, Cunningham, C & Penney, D 2016, What we know, what we do and what we could do: Creating an understanding of the delivery of health education in lower secondary government schools in Western Australia, *Australian Journal of Teacher Education (Online)*, *41*(11), pp. 15–30.

Birch, C 2017, Improving schools, improving school health education, improving public health: The role of SOPHE members, *Health Education & Behaviour*, 44(6), pp. 839–44.

Brown, K, Elliott, S, Robertson-Wilson, J, Vine, M & Leatherdale, S 2018, Can knowledge exchange support the implementation of a health-promoting schools approach? Perceived outcomes of knowledge exchange in the COMPASS study, *BMC Public Health*, 18(1), p. 351.

Buckley, S, Gerring, Z, Cumming, J, Mason, D, McDonald, J & Churchward, M 2012, School nursing in New Zealand: A study of services, *Policy, Politics & Nursing Practice*, 13(1), pp. 45–53.

Centers for Disease Control and Prevention [CDCP] 2011, School health guidelines to promote healthy eating and physical activity, *Morbidity and Mortality Weekly Report*, 60(5), viewed 10 February 2020, www.cdc.gov/healthyschools/npao/strategies.htm

College of Child & Youth Nursing, New Zealand Nurses Organisation 2014, Resources, viewed 19 September 2020, www.nzno.org.nz/groups/colleges_sections/colleges/college_of_child_youth_nurses/resources

Conway, S 2015, Health education: Leading the way to a healthy future, *NASN School Nurse,* January, pp. 10–12.

Cookson, D 2018, What is the role of a school nurse? *Kai Tiaki: Nursing New Zealand*, 24(2), p. 8.

Darlington, E, Violon, N & Jourdan, D, 2018, Implementation of health promotion programmes in schools: An approach to understand the influence of contextual factors on the process? *BMC Public Health*, 18(163), pp. 1–7.

Day, R, Sahota, P & Christian, M 2019, Effective implementation of primary school-based healthy lifestyle programs: A qualitative study of views of school staff, *BMC Public Health,* 19(1239), doi:10.1186/s12889–019-7550-2

Department of Education, Skills and Employment 2020, *The Australian Student Wellbeing Framework*, viewed 20 September 2020, www.education.gov.au/national-safe-schools-framework-0

Department of Education, Tasmania 2012, *Department of Education learners first – connected and inspired: Guidelines for inclusive language (version 2)*, viewed 6 January 2020, https://documentcentre.education.tas.gov.au/documents/guidelines-for-inclusive-language.pdf

—— 2014, *Learners first – good teaching guide: Differentiated Classroom Practice – learning for all*, viewed 6 January 2020, https://documentcentre.education.tas.gov.au/Documents/Good-Teaching-Differentiated-Classroom-Practice-Learning-for-All.pdf

Department of Health 2013, *The Australian guide to healthy eating*, viewed 6 January 2020, www1.health.gov.au/internet/publications/publishing.nsf/Content/nhsc-guidelines~aus-guide-healthy-eating

—— 2019, *National action plan for the health of children and young people 2020–2030*, viewed 13 April 2020, www1.health.gov.au/internet/main/publishing.nsf/Content/4815673E283EC1B6CA2584000082EA7D/$File/FINAL%20National%20Action%

20Plan%20for%20the%20Health%20of%20Children%20and%20Young%
20People%202020-2030.pdf

Duff, C 2015, Health education: A school nurse role, *NASN School Nurse,* January, pp. 8–9.

Durocher, E & Gauvin, L 2019, Adolescents' weight management goals: Healthy and unhealthy associations with eating habits and physical activity, *Journal of School Health*, 90(1), pp. 15–24.

Eckerman, S, Dawber, J, Yeatman, H, Quinsey, K & Morris, D 2014, Evaluating return on investment in a school based health promotion and prevention program: The investment multiplier for the Stephanie Alexander Kitchen Garden National Program, *Social Science & Medicine*, 114, pp. 103–12.

Fairbrother, H, Curtis, P & Goyder, E 2016, Making health information meaningful: Children's health literacy practices, *SSM - Population Health,* 2, pp. 476–84.

Fleming, L, Hogan, J & Graf, K 2018, Healthy communities – the role of the school nurse: Position statement, *NASN School Nurse,* 33(3), pp. 189–91.

Hagell, A, Rigby, E & Perrow, F 2015, Promoting health literacy in secondary schools: A review, *British Journal of School Nursing,* 10(2), pp. 82–7.

Høstgaard Bonde, A, Bentsen, P & Lykke Hindhede, A 2014, School nurses' experiences with motivational interviewing for preventing childhood obesity, *The Journal of School Nursing,* 30(6), pp. 448–55.

Hung, T, Chiang, V, Dawson, A & Lee, R 2014, Understanding of factors that enable health promoters in implementing health-promoting schools: A systematic review and narrative synthesis of qualitative evidence, *PLOS ONE,* 9(9), p. e108284

John-Akinola, Y & Nic-Gabhainn, S 2014, Children's participation in school: A cross-sectional study of the relationship between school environments, participation and health and well-being outcomes, *BMC Public Health,* 14(964), pp. 1–10.

Johnson, R, Oyebode, O, Walker, S, Knowles, E & Robertson, W 2018, The difficult conversation: A qualitative evaluation of the 'Eat Well Move More' family weight management service, *BMC Research Notes,* 11, p. 325.

Kitchie, S 2020, Determinants of learning, in S. Bastable (ed.), *Nurse as educator: Principles of teaching and learning for nursing practice* (5th ed.), Jones & Bartlett Learning, Burlington, MA.

Kolbe, L 2019, School health as a strategy to improve both public health and education, *Annual Review of Public Health*, 40, pp. 443–63.

Langford, R, Bonnell, C, Jones, H & Campbell, R 2015, Obesity prevention and the Health Promoting Schools Framework: Essential components and barriers to success, *International Journal of Behavioural Nutrition and Physical Activity, 12*(15), pp. 1–17.

Langford, R, Bonnell, C, Komro, K, Murphy, S, Magnus, D, Waters, E, Gibbs, L & Campbell, R 2017, The Health Promoting Schools Framework: Known unknowns and an agenda for future research, *Health Education & Behaviour,* 44(3), pp. 463–75.

Leahy, D & Simovska, V 2017, Critical perspectives on health and wellbeing education in schools, *Health Education,* 117(5), pp. 430–3.

Loschiavo, J 2015, *Fast facts for the school nurse: School nursing in a nutshell* (2nd ed.), Springer, New York.

Lynch, T, 2015 Health and Physical Education (HPE): Implementation in primary schools, *International Journal of Educational Research,* 70, pp. 88–100.

Matthews, C 2014, Critical pedagogy in health education, *Health Education Journal,* 73(5), pp. 600–9.

Maughan, E, Bobo, N, Butler, S, Schantz, S & Schoessler, S 2015, Framework for 21st Century School Nursing Practice: An overview, *NASN School Nurse,* 30(4), pp. 220–31.

National Association of School Nurses (NASN) 2016, *The role of the 21st century school nurse (position statement)*, NASN, Silver Spring, MD.

Ontario Ministry of Health and Long-Term Care 2018, *Healthy growth and development guidelines, 2018,* viewed 19 April 2020, www.health.gov.on.ca/en/pro/programs/publichealth/oph_standards/docs/protocols_guidelines/Healthy_Growth_and_Development_Guideline_2018.pdf

Organisation for Economic Co-operation and Development (OECD) 2012, *Australia: Survey of adult skills (PIACC),* viewed 6 January 2020, www.gpseducation.oecd.org

Peterson, J, Loeb, S & Chamberlain, L 2018, The intersection of health and education to address school readiness of all children, *Pediatrics,* 142(5), p. e20181126.

Pontius, D 2013, Health literacy part 1: Practical techniques for getting your message home, *NASN School Nurse,* September, pp. 247–52.

—— 2014, Health literacy part 2: Practical techniques for getting your message home, *NASN School Nurse,* January, pp. 31–42.

Public Health Association of Australia (PHAA) 2016, *Public Health Association of Australia: Policy-at-a-glance – prevention and management of overweight and obesity in Australia policy*, viewed 31 May 2020, www.phaa.net.au/documents/item/1701

Rothstein, R & Olympia, R 2020, School nurses on the frontlines of healthcare: The approach to maintaining student health and wellness during COVID-19 school closures, *NASN School Nurse,* September, pp. 269–75.

Schaffer, M, Anderson, L & Rising, S 2016, Public health interventions for school nursing practice, *The Journal of School Nursing,* 32(3), pp. 195–208.

Schroeder, E, Goldfarb, E & Gelperin, N 2015, *Rights, respect, responsibility: A K–12 sexuality education curriculum*, viewed 6 January 2020, https://advocatesforyouth.org/wp-content/uploads/2018/10/teachers-guide-1.pdf

Schroeder, K, Travers, J & Smaldone, A 2016, Are school nurses an overlooked resource in reducing childhood obesity? A systematic review and meta-analysis, *Journal of School Nursing*, 86(5), pp. 309–21.

Shackleton, N, Jamal, F, Viner, R, Dickson, K, Patton, G & Bonnell, C 2016, School-based interventions going beyond health education to promote adolescent health: Systematic review of reviews, *Journal of Adolescent Health,* 58, pp. 382–96.

Splendorio, D & Reichel, L (2013), *Tools for teaching comprehensive human sexuality education,* John Wiley & Sons, Hoboken, NJ.

Stylianou, M & Walker, J 2018, An assessment of Australian school physical activity and nutrition policies, *Australian and New Zealand Journal of Public Health,* 42, pp. 16–21.

Thompson, H, & Madsen, K 2017, The report card on BMI report cards, *Current Obesity Reports,* 6, pp. 163–7.

Turner, G, Owen, S & Watson, P 2016, Addressing childhood obesity at school entry: Qualitative experiences of school health professionals, *Journal of Child Health Care,* 20(3), pp. 304–13.

Turunen, H, Sormunen, M, Jourdan, D, von Seelen, J & Guijs, G 2017, Health promoting schools: A complex approach and a major means to health improvement, *Health Promotion International,* 32, pp. 177–84.

WA Health Promoting Schools Association 2020, *Health promoting schools toolkit,* viewed 24 May 2020, http://wahpsa.org.au/resources/health-promoting-schools-toolkit-2

Walker, J 2014, Wellness promotion – school nurses as models of health, *NASN School Nurse,* May, pp. 128–9.

Williams, S & Mummery, K 2015, We can do that! Collaborative assessment of school environments to promote healthy adolescent nutrition and physical activity behaviours, *Health Education Research*, 30(2), pp. 272–84.

World Health Organization (WHO) 1986, *Ottawa Charter for Health Promotion. First International Conference on Health Promotion Ottawa*, 21 November 1986 – WHO/HPR/HEP/95.1, viewed 6 January 2020, www.healthpromotion.org.au/images/ottawa_charter_hp.pdf

—— 1996, *Regional guidelines: Development of health-promoting schools – a framework for action,* viewed 6 January 2020, https://apps.who.int/iris/bitstream/handle/10665/206847/Health_promoting_sch_ser.5_eng.pdf?sequence=1&isAllowed=y

—— 2016, *Consideration of the evidence on childhood obesity for the Commission on Ending Childhood Obesity*, report of the Ad Hoc Working Group on Science and Evidence for Ending Childhood Obesity, Geneva, Switzerland, viewed 10 February 2020, https://apps.who.int/iris/bitstream/handle/10665/206549/9789241565332_eng.pdf;sequence=1

Yubik, M & Lee, J 2014, Parent interest in a school-based, school nurse-led weight management program, *The Journal of School Nursing,* 30(1), pp. 68–74.

Mental healthcare for children and adolescents

Jennifer Fraser, Lindsay Smith and Julia Taylor

8

LEARNING OBJECTIVES

In this chapter you will:

- Gain an understanding of mental disorders and mental health problems experienced in childhood and adolescence
- Become familiar with factors that may negatively or positively influence mental health in children and young people
- Learn how good mental health and resilience can be influenced in children and young people
- Develop an understanding of how to help children and young people experiencing an eating disorder
- Consider the role digital technology can play in the mental health of children and young people
- Learn nursing skills that help promote good mental health in children and young people

Introduction

Child and youth mental health –
A state of mental wellbeing in
which children and young people
can realise their abilities and reach
optimal growth and development.

The focus of this chapter is the role of the nurse in optimising **child and youth mental health**. An overview of mental disorders experienced during childhood and adolescence is followed by a discussion of mental health promotion for children and young people. A section on eating disorders is also included. Although the lifetime prevalence of eating disorders is very low, they are common, and nurses play an important role in the care of those affected children and young people admitted to hospital for treatment. The importance of working closely with the parents and families of children and young people disabled by mental illness and the services available to them is emphasised throughout the chapter.

Mental health problems and mental disorders

The Australian Institute of Health and Welfare (AIHW) published the first national survey of child and adolescent mental health and wellbeing in Australia in 1998. The second survey was published in 2015 (Lawrence et al., 2015); it includes data on the use of mental health services by children, young people and their families. The survey provides valuable information on the prevalence of **child and youth mental disorders** in Australia. The AIHW also publishes a list of services that exist for people living with a mental disorder and makes recommendations for services that are needed. The latest survey indicates that while the prevalence of mental health disorders for children and young people remained stable between 1998 and 2015, there was a significant increase in the use of mental health services for Australians aged 4–17 years. In summary, 14 per cent of children aged 4–17 years in Australia experienced mental health problems – 16.3 per cent of boys and 11.5 per cent of girls (Lawrence et al., 2015).

Child and youth mental disorder – A mental disorder, as distinct from a mental health problem, is characterised by a clinically recognisable set of symptoms or behaviours that interfere substantially with social, academic or occupational functioning. Different types of mental disorders consist of a different combination of symptoms that may differ in severity (Sawyer et al., 2000).

Using a similar survey design, the prevalence of social, emotional and behavioural difficulties in New Zealand children aged from 3 to 14 years has been measured by the Ministry of Health (2018). Parents were asked to complete the Strengths and Difficulties Questionnaire (SDQ). The survey indicated that almost 8 per cent (57 000) of New Zealand's children experienced social, emotional and/or behavioural difficulties at concerning levels and an additional 7 per cent reported some concerns. Statistically significant differences between boys and girls were found, with boys more likely than girls to live with mental health concerns. Māori children were more likely than non-Māori children to have been identified by their parents as having problems. The report emphasises that while these children and their families need extra support, the majority of New Zealand's children are developing without any significant social, emotional or behavioural problems (Ministry of Health, 2018).

The extent to which children and young people experience symptoms and/or behaviours that cause disruption to parents, teachers, peers and society in general varies. Assessment over time is necessary to distinguish the type, frequency and severity of disruption. Many children who are referred for treatment do not have symptoms that meet the criteria for a mental disorder; however, this does not mean that the symptoms and behaviour may not meet the criteria at another point in time. The cutoff point between those who receive a formal diagnosis and those who do not is arbitrary, and children move above and below the threshold in meeting the *Diagnostic and Statistical Manual of Mental Disorders* (5th edition) (DSM-5) (APA, 2013) criteria for mental disorders.

Disorders are presented in DSM-5 according to age, gender and developmental characteristics. The first section of this chapter focuses on those childhood conditions commonly experienced in healthcare settings in which paediatric nurses practise. While not an exhaustive list of the conditions experienced in childhood, they are the conditions that experienced the most intense research and scrutiny during the period leading up to the release of DSM-5. These are Autism Spectrum Disorder (ASD) and Attention Deficit Hyperactivity Disorder (ADHD).

To better understand these changes, the first section of this chapter summarises selected mental disorders of children and young people. How children's social, behavioural and emotional symptoms are categorised and diagnosed is important to how they are treated. Diagnosis is complex, and the child's development and its trajectory must be considered. For example, some behaviours demonstrated by a 14-month-old infant are acceptable, whereas if the same behaviours continue through to the child's second or third birthday, this may be reconsidered and the behaviours could indicate a mental disorder.

General paediatric nurses in Australia are not responsible for the diagnosis of mental disorders in children, but understanding is crucial. **Child and youth mental health services** are offered within hospitals and other community settings, but children with mental disorders also present to paediatric services for a range of reasons other than their mental healthcare. For this reason, it is important to understand disorders of children and young people, and how they are best managed for optimal care in the paediatric environment.

Child and youth mental health services – Provide specialist mental health services for children and young people, and assistance to their families or carers.

Attention Deficit Hyperactivity Disorder (ADHD)

ADHD is the most prevalent child mental disorder, not only in Australia and New Zealand, but worldwide (Riglin et al., 2016). Children present with inattention, hyperactivity and impulsivity and, compared with their normative peers, have poor learning ability, low academic outcomes and social incompetence. There are three sub-types of ADHD: inattentive; hyperactive impulsive; and combined. Symptoms can persist into the adult years (Riglin et al., 2016).

ADHD is a complex disorder that is difficult to manage well. Management needs to be based on comprehensive neuropsychological and psychoeducational assessments. This not only determines the diagnosis, but also establishes the existence of any potential comorbid conditions (Feldman & Reiff, 2014). Comorbidity is common with this disorder and occurs in as many as two-thirds of children with ADHD. Comorbid conditions include learning disabilities, Conduct Disorder, Oppositional Defiant Disorder (ODD) and anxiety (Sawyer et al., 2016). Almost half (45 per cent) have learning disabilities, placing them at risk of poor educational achievement and potentially low socioeconomic status (Grizenko et al., 2013). Furthermore, poor academic self-concept is associated with the development of anti-social behaviours. Children with the inattentive type of ADHD tend to have the greatest academic failure rates, and do poorly at mathematics in particular (Grizenko et al., 2013).

Nursing assessment and interventions

Parenting interventions that focus on child behaviour management have proven to be somewhat successful. If implemented correctly, these have been reported to reduce the main symptoms of ADHD in both the short and longer term (Hoath & Sanders, 2002). Importantly, they can improve parenting satisfaction and confidence. At the same time, it is important to emphasise that behaviour management is not as effective as medication, and medication is especially successful in raising the likelihood of academic success and school completion (Grizenko et al., 2013). These outcomes bode well for the child's trajectory into adult life.

The safety and effectiveness of non-stimulant drugs and long-acting methylphenidate and amphetamine medications have been demonstrated in research conducted over the past two decades (Feldman & Reiff, 2014). Parents do remain reluctant to medicate their children for ADHD, despite obvious behavioural and academic improvements when treated with psychostimulants (Grizenko et al., 2013). Longer-term effects of medication for ADHD are not well understood at present.

REFLECTION POINTS 8.1

- A high proportion of children and young people – boys and girls – report mental health problems in Australia.
- Behavioural and emotional changes and changes in function should be referred immediately and appropriately.
- Ongoing monitoring of the medication regimens is encouraged, and augmentation with behaviour-management strategies is recommended.

What do you think are the factors that act as barriers to children and their families receiving assistance with childhood mental health problems?

Autism Spectrum Disorder (ASD)

ASD is a lifelong developmental disability featuring deficits in social communication and social interaction with repetitive patterns of behaviour, interests or activities (APA, 2013). The prevalence rate is estimated to be from 5.7 to 21.9 per 1000, with boys more commonly affected than girls (CDCP, 2014). In the fourth edition of the *Diagnostic and Statistical Manual of Mental Disorders* (APA, 2000), DSM-IV, children with ASD were categorised as having one of: autistic disorder; Asperger's Disorder; or pervasive developmental disorder not otherwise specified (PDD-NOS). With the release of DSM-5, these are all now referred to as a single condition, ASD. This is an important change because, for some children, one of the former categories may still be used. As previously mentioned, DSM-5 relates to diagnoses made since its release in 2013, meaning that children will continue to have a diagnosis of Asperger's Syndrome. ASD also has a severity rating of

1, 2 or 3, depending on how much support the person needs. Some people have mild symptoms, while others have more severe and pervasive disability (APA, 2013).

ASD is characterised by the child having difficulties in each of two areas: deficits in social communication; and fixated interests and repetitive behaviours. Deficits in social communication include poor social interaction and limited use of language to communicate. Some children will not speak at all, not respond when spoken to and not join in with others' actions and activities. The second area – fixated interests and repetitive behaviours – can obviously only be observed as the child grows and certain developmental milestones are not met. Having narrow and intense interests is more obvious as the child goes to school and is expected to become involved in others' interests and games. Sensory sensitivities are also characteristic. The child may choose to wear only one type of fabric, may dislike labels on clothes or have particular bedding preferences. One of the most difficult manifestations is the desire to eat only certain foods with a specific texture or colour.

It is critical to be able to diagnose ASD in early childhood so that early intervention can be implemented. There are a number of successful evidence-based programs available, targeted to the way ASD presents in the individual child. Critical decisions about schooling need to be made early, as adequate mechanisms of support are required to optimise learning ability in children with ASD. These decisions should be revised regularly, with reflection on the most appropriate context for learning.

Transition to high school – and indeed to adult health and educational services – needs to be planned carefully in advance.

Nursing assessment and interventions

Be sensitive to the way the child is experiencing the world. For example:

- Listen to the parents' concerns and provide accurate information.
- Acknowledge that the clinic setting is unfamiliar and therefore potentially highly stressful to the child.
- If the child becomes an inpatient, work closely with the parents to establish structure and routine.
- Understand the ways in which the child communicates discomfort and anxiety.

REFLECTION POINTS 8.2

- Because nurses will encounter children and young people with ASD across a wide range of services, it is essential to become familiar with what ASD is, to understand how to identify children with ASD and to understand how a formal diagnosis is made.
- Anxiety, depression and dissociative responses to stress are comorbid conditions to ASD.

In the hospital setting, how can the nursing staff assist in reducing the risk of children becoming overwhelmed with emotions such as anger and frustration?

Externalising disorders: Oppositional Defiant Disorder (ODD) and Conduct Disorder (CD)

Conduct Disorder (CD) is a formal term used to identify a subset of disruptive children who present with severe and persistent behaviour problems (APA, 2013). Oppositional Defiant Disorder (ODD) is diagnosed when the child is repeatedly argumentative, loses their temper easily and has issues with anger and resentment. These behaviours vary in frequency and severity, and diagnosis tends to be arbitrary. The problems they cause can affect parents, teachers, peers and society in general. CD is much more extreme and features a child who violates the rights of others, is aggressive and is deliberately cruel to other people or animals.

Until recently, the research conducted in this field was gender biased because of the high rates of CD found in boys. However, this has now been reversed, and the trajectory for girls' mental health and wellbeing is starting to attract attention. Adolescent onset of CD in girls shares a similar trajectory towards adult psychopathology and criminal activity to childhood onset CD – that is, that early onset of CD is associated with a poorer prognosis. On the other hand, adolescent onset of CD in boys tends to be adolescent limited – that is, they are likely to grow out of their conduct problems (Kjeldsen et al., 2016). This is an important finding because it points to the need to pay more attention to CD that develops in the adolescent years, especially for girls.

Not all children who meet the criteria for CD will become chronic offenders as adults, but the risk is high. Parents need to be motivated and engaged to contribute to the parenting interventions available. This requires regular feedback and consultation to keep them on track with a tailored program that meets the needs of their child. Institutionalisation and other forms of group-based treatments are not advised due to the strengthening of deviant behaviours through group pressure. Parents may feel that they need respite, but if possible the best approach is to modify their interactions with the child to reduce the severity of the child's conduct problems (Dadds & Fraser, 2003).

REFLECTION POINTS 8.3

- Family interventions show the most promise of success.
- Disruptive behaviour patterns become more resistant with age.
- Early intervention and prevention are needed.

How can parents be reassured that their parenting style did not cause the child's behaviour problems when modifying the parenting style succeeds in treating the behaviour problems?

Internalising disorders: Anxiety and depression

There are similar explanations for both child and adult depression. These include loss, learned helplessness, negative cognitions, and low serotonin and norepinephrine activity in the brain. Young children are likely to have comorbid separation anxiety, phobias, somatic complaints and behaviour problems. The diagnosis for paediatric depression relies on the ability of the child or their parent to report on the internal affect of the child. Depressed mothers may also over-report depressive symptoms in their child, although a transactional approach to child development suggests that the child's characteristics exacerbate the maternal psychopathology (Sameroff & MacKenzie, 2003) – that is, a mother is more likely to be depressed if her child exhibits symptoms of mental health problems. Moreover, a healthy father appears to mediate the relationship between maternal depression and child psychopathology, whereas a child with both parents affected by mental illness is at high risk of childhood depression and other disorders (Goodman et al., 2011).

A number of adverse outcomes may result from childhood mental disorders and poor mental health. These include general suffering, functional impairment, stigma, discrimination and even premature death (McLaughlin et al., 2012). Given the importance of community-based early intervention and prevention approaches to developmental disruption, and children's and young people's mental health and wellbeing, this chapter will now focus on the importance of promoting mental health.

REFLECTION POINTS 8.4

- Nurses work with children and young people in a range of settings, including the mental health and youth justice systems.
- Promotion of mental health and wellbeing for children and young people has a place in all settings, not only child and adolescent mental health services or the youth justice system.
- Children and young people's mental health problems affect the health and wellbeing of their families and communities.
- A number of developmental factors contribute to the onset of mental disorders in children.

What strategies can be used to incorporate mental health nursing skills into general paediatric nursing?

Risk and protective factors

A number of developmental characteristics or events are associated with the onset of mental problems in children and young people. The worst outcomes result from the cumulative effects of multiple **risk** factors acting on a single child. These risk factors overlap and place the child at risk for both internalising (anxiety and depression) and externalising (CD, ODD) disorders. Thus, the same risk factors can be identified for each (McLaughlin et al., 2012). Risk and protective factors are presented in Table 8.1.

Risks – Disturbances to mental health that threaten system function, viability or development.

Table 8.1 Risk and protective factors for mental health problems in childhood and adolescence

Types of factors	Risk factors	Protective factors
Child factors	Genetic risk	High intelligence
	Brain damage	Good general health
	Low intelligence	Engaging temperament
	Difficult temperament	Good social skills
	Poor social skills	High self-efficacy
	Low self-esteem	High self-esteem
Parenting and family factors	Poor-quality relationship with parents	Warm and positive relationship with parents
	Insecure attachment style	Secure attachment style
	Harsh, inflexible or inconsistent discipline	Fair, consistent discipline with clear boundaries for behaviour
	Inadequate supervision	Strong involvement with child
	Parental conflict	Domestic harmony
	Parental psychopathology	Good mental health of parents
School factors	Bullying	Strong school culture of support
	Poor resources	Good supervision
	Peer problems, such as social exclusion and excessive teasing	Effective social relationship with peers
	Teacher factors, such as lack of inclusivity skills, poor communication skills	Strong sense of inclusivity, use of strengths-based communication
Societal factors	Low socioeconomic status	Child's rights upheld
	Discrimination	

Sources: Goodman et al. (2011); Loeber & Hay (1997); McLaughlin et al. (2012); Rutter (2005); Sameroff & MacKenzie (2003); Scott et al. (2011).

Promoting mental health in children and young people

Optimal health and development across the lifespan are supported by mental health and resilience that develops from the early years of life. The foundation of early life is built through generations – supporting one generation to thrive supports the next. Paediatric nursing may thus have an intergenerational impact when promoting mental health in children and young people.

CASE STUDY 8.1 JASON

As a paediatric nurse in an acute care setting, you meet Jason, a 16-year-old male admitted for investigations related to recurring abdominal pains and weight loss. Jason has recently been discharged from hospital following an appendicectomy. His previous admission was uneventful; however, Jason now discloses to you that he has been feeling down lately and has been 'having trouble' at school. Until recently, Jason would have been described as an enthusiastic school student. Now he is noticeably withdrawn, increasingly alone at lunchtime and not participating in class or after-school and weekend activities. There are concerns that Jason is being bullied.

Jason is an only child and lives with his mother, who is employed mainly after hours as a cleaner. His father left the family when he was a baby and Jason has had no contact with him since. Jason and his mother have always been close, but recently Jason has seemed more distant to her. You notice that during the admission procedure Jason's mother reported leaving dinner prepared for Jason when she goes to work. Lately she has been finding most of it in the bin when she gets home late. She has also noticed that Jason seems startled and anxious when he receives notifications on his mobile phone. She has tried to talk to Jason about these issues but he refuses to discuss them.

When you meet with Jason, he spends some time telling you about his life up to this point. Over the next few days, you develop a rapport with Jason and see from his body language and conversation that he is becoming more comfortable. You speak to him about his concerns and allow him to talk about what he believes has been happening. He says he has always been bullied at school and it hasn't really bothered him. Lately, though, this bullying has intensified, and he has been getting threats via social media. He feels he has no break from the bullies as since they got his phone number and found him online, they torment him day and night. You gently ask Jason about his eating habits and his mother's concern that he is not eating enough. Jason appears uncomfortable and says he just doesn't feel like eating much anymore, especially in the evenings, as this is when his bullies harass him most, which causes him to feel stressed and anxious.

The spectrum of child and youth mental health

Procter et al. (2017: 5) define mental health as

> the ability to cope with and bounce back from adversity, to solve problems in everyday life, manage when things are difficult and cope with everyday stressors. Good mental health is made possible by a supportive social, friendship and family environment, good work–life balance, physical health and, in many instances, reduced stress and trauma.

These authors also define mental illness as

> a clinically diagnosable condition that significantly interferes with an individual's cognitive, emotional and/or social abilities. The diagnosis of mental illness is

generally made according to the classification systems of the *Diagnostic and Statistical Manual of Mental Disorders* (DSM) (APA, 2013) or the International Classification of Diseases (ICD). (Procter et al., 2017, p. 5)

It is important to understand that mental health and mental disorders are not mutually exclusive or the opposite of each other. Children and young people do not display the characteristics of only one or the other at any point in time. Such a binary misunderstanding fosters stigmatisation and a reduced outcome of care and wellbeing (Williams, 2020). Rather, mental health and mental health conditions can best be understood as being on a continuum (see Figure 8.1). Likewise, the nursing response to mental health is best understood as being on a continuum of care.

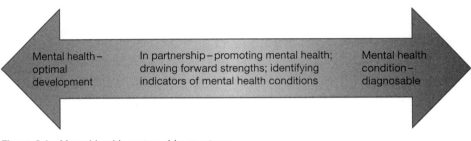

Figure 8.1   Mental health partnership spectrum

REFLECTION POINTS 8.5

The paediatric nurse's collaborative role in supporting child and youth mental health includes:

- identifying indicators of possible mental health conditions
- utilising referral services when a diagnosable mental health condition is considered
- partnering with children and young people in mental health condition treatment plans.

Paediatric nurses can also implement independent nursing actions in the promotion of mental health based on a deep understanding of the determinants of mental health. These nursing actions may include:

- fostering health literacy related to mental health and mental health conditions
- partnering with children and young people in mental health and wellbeing plans.

Where on the mental health partnership spectrum (Figure 8.1) would you place the collaborative and independent paediatric nurse actions listed here to promote child and youth mental health?

Understanding paediatric nurses' engagement with the mental health of children and young people as being on a spectrum highlights the importance of a holistic understanding of the bioecological factors of mental health and how they coalesce to promote an adaptive response to life challenges and resilience across the lifespan.

Recent advances in understanding the determinants of health and neuroplasticity have led to an awareness that much can be done to promote positive mental health in children and adolescents, resulting in a positive impact on life outcomes. Through enhancing early life experiences, reducing deprivation and strengthening the supportive pathways during childhood and adolescence, many determinants that challenge mental health development can be reduced substantially (Fox et al., 2015; Sollis, 2019).

The Dunedin Multidisciplinary Health and Development Study, a longitudinal study of New Zealanders, also demonstrates a significant association between early childhood experiences and reduced later life outcomes and mental health (Caspi et al., 2017). The Dunedin Study demonstrates that life experience tends to reflect movement along the mental health partnership spectrum. Schaefer et al. (2017) report that most participants in the Dunedin Study experience short periods of diagnosable mental health condition/s at some point in their life, so mental health history reflects movement along the mental health partnership spectrum as the norm. Some people experience enduring mental health throughout their childhood and adult life; however, there is currently limited evidence to indicate what factors strongly support enduring mental health across the lifespan. Childhood family experience appears to demonstrate the strongest relationship with enduring mental health. Paediatric nurses' efforts to foster mental health literacy in families may make an important contribution to enduring mental health and decreased periods of diagnosable mental health conditions.

Across Australia and New Zealand, there is a strong move towards a child and youth wellbeing outcomes approach in policy and services. However, child and youth wellbeing is not synonymous with mental health, and the two constructs are not interchangeable. Rather, a holistic promotion of child and youth wellbeing fosters enhanced mental health in a reciprocal, or bidirectional, relationship. Values-based paediatric nursing can also enhance the development of mental health. These values and attitudes are seen in paediatric nurses' practice when the presence of parents at the bedside of their hospitalised child, along with engagement in care and decision-making, is facilitated (O'Connor, Brenner & Coyne, 2019). In paediatric nursing, gaining age-appropriate consent for family involvement and decision-making conveys respect for the child or young person, recognises the uniqueness of the person and promotes self-determination and participation in decision-making (Gottlieb & Gottlieb, 2017).

Promoting child mental health literacy among parents and carers is another example of an effective strategy that paediatric nurses can independently implement during every admission to the hospital or healthcare service, which improves early recognition of mental health conditions and promotes timely intervention (Rhodes et al., 2018). In promoting mental health literacy, language matters. Consider reframing a deficit-based medically orientated approach to a wellbeing, strengths-based outcomes approach (Babington, 2020). Strengths are found in the child, in their family, in their community and in the healthcare system. Supporting mental health requires strengthening the attributes of each. Nurses engaging with families, drawing on the strengths of the child and their family, is an emerging approach to increasing family participation in healthcare and creating a strengths-based approach to supporting the mental health of children and young people requiring healthcare. For example, nurses engaging in family strengths-oriented therapeutic conversation with children, young people and their parents/caregivers is a powerful independent nursing strengths-based action. Following such a family–nurse conversation, families report enhanced well-being outcomes (Svavarsdottir et al., 2020). Practice frameworks such as the Common Approach® (see Box 8.1) help to guide quality conversations

BOX 8.1 THE COMMON APPROACH®

The Common Approach®, developed by the Australian Research Alliance for Children & Youth (ARACY) (Goodhue, 2015), is a flexible framework to help all professionals have quality conversations with young people and families about all aspects of their wellbeing, including aspects that fall outside the professional's usual area of work (see Figure 8.2). It aims to support children and young people at a universal, preventative level, and to be accessible to everyone who interacts with young people. It is designed not only to be adaptable to a wide range of situations, but also to provide a common language and approach that can support collaboration across sectors.

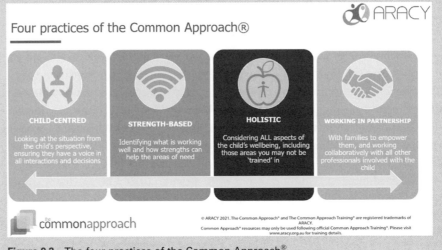

Four practices of the Common Approach®

CHILD-CENTRED	STRENGTH-BASED	HOLISTIC	WORKING IN PARTNERSHIP
Looking at the situation from the child's perspective, ensuring they have a voice in all interactions and decisions	Identifying what is working well and how strengths can help the areas of need	Considering ALL aspects of the child's wellbeing, including those areas you may not be 'trained' in	With families to empower them, and working collaboratively with all other professionals involved with the child

© ARACY 2021. The Common Approach® and The Common Approach Training® are registered trademarks of ARACY.
Common Approach® resources may only be used following official Common Approach Training®. Please visit www.aracy.org.au for training details.

Figure 8.2   The four practices of the Common Approach®
Source: ARACY (2021). Reproduced with permission.

At the centre of the Common Approach® is a useful tool for use in practice: the Wellbeing Wheel (see Figure 8.3). The Wellbeing Wheel provides a visual and holistic view of a child or young person's life, based on The Nest (ARACY, 2013). ARACY's work is focused around The Nest, a wellbeing framework for children and young people developed by ARACY from the voices of around 4000 children, young people and experts. The Nest shows that for a child or young person to thrive, their needs must be met in six key, interlocking domains of child and youth wellbeing:

1. Being valued, loved and safe
2. Having material basics
3. Being healthy (physically, mentally, emotionally)

4. Learning (in formal and informal environments)
5. Participating (in decisions, groups, community)
6. Having a positive sense of identity and culture

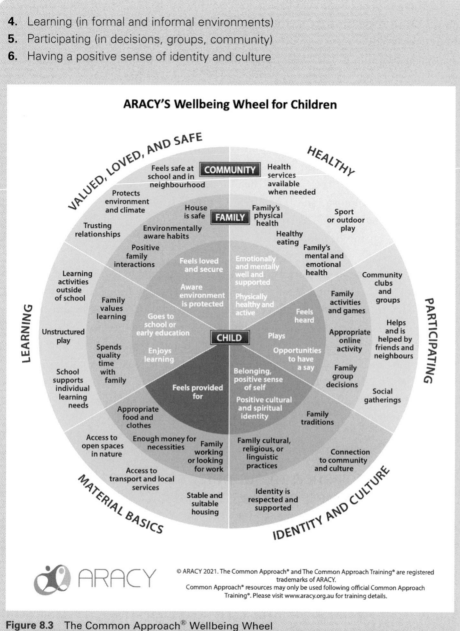

ARACY'S Wellbeing Wheel for Children

© ARACY 2021. The Common Approach® and The Common Approach Training® are registered trademarks of ARACY.
Common Approach® resources may only be used following official Common Approach Training®. Please visit www.aracy.org.au for training details.

Figure 8.3 The Common Approach® Wellbeing Wheel
Source: ARACY (2021). Reproduced with permission.

The six domains of child and youth wellbeing in The Wellbeing Wheel are evidence based (ARACY, 2013), and together promote holistic wellbeing and mental health.

The Wellbeing Wheel includes discussion prompts in each of the six domains of child and youth wellbeing, based on common indicators of areas of potential strength or need (see prompts in Figure 8.3). Practitioners are required to be trained in the Common Approach®, to apply the method and to access the resources (see www .aracy.org.au for details).

The majority of children progress into adulthood well. Their mental health is a foundation of their capacity to thrive throughout life. They have experienced a life without deprivation across multiple domains of wellbeing, and they have discovered the keys to adapting to the challenges and stresses that face all children and adolescents. Unfortunately, far too many children exposed to toxic stress – chronic over-stimulation of the stress-response system – and deprivation across more than one of the six domains of child and youth wellbeing are at risk of declining mental health, being disengaged from learning, disconnected from their family identity and culture and/or participating in their community (NSCDC, 2012a; Sollis, 2019). It is well recognised that children can and do experience mental health conditions. Sollis (2019, p. 46) identifies that 'mental health concerns are starting early in a young person's life, with almost 1 in 10 children aged 6–7 having a low score on the social emotional problems scale'. Early intervention and support can have a significant positive effect on the development of future mental health and resilience (NSCDC, 2012b, 2015).

Understanding what concerns children and young people can help guide discussions exploring their mental health and signify where mental health promotion may be required. Paediatric nurses can contribute to promoting mental health by asking young people how satisfied they are with their achievements in each of the six domains of child and youth wellbeing in their life. Paediatric nurses can promote child mental health through embedding holistic nursing care with child and family partnerships in child-centred, strengths-based paediatric nursing care practices. Supporting families of children who require paediatric nursing care allays their distress, increasing the family's capacity to care for their child (Tallon, Kendall & Snider, 2015).

Promoting resilience to support mental health in children and young people

Resilience is defined as 'the capacity of a dynamic system (such as a child or family) to adapt successfully to disturbances that threaten system function, viability or development' (Masten & Barnes, 2018, p. 99). Child and youth mental health is dependent on adaptive capacity, which is fundamental for resilience. Adaptive capacity skills can be learnt especially well during childhood, while the brain has a strong capacity for plasticity (Masten & Barnes, 2018). Paediatric nurses can also help cultivate supportive adult–child relationships, such as the nurse–child relationship, that help children build resilience. Resilience programs for children and young people have been linked to improved mental health (Khanlou & Wray, 2014).

Across New Zealand and Australia, there is a strong move towards a wellbeing approach to policy and services. In a ground-breaking Australian first, ARACY developed a national plan for child and youth wellbeing, The Nest action agenda (ARACY, 2013). The Nest action agenda strives to provide a framework for promoting child and youth wellbeing, including the mental health of children and young people. New Zealand has established the Child and Youth Wellbeing Strategy to enhance the wellbeing of all New Zealand children (Department of the Prime Minister and Cabinet, 2019). Examples of how a child and youth wellbeing approach is translated to practice include the Common Approach® discussed above; the New Zealand Child Wellbeing whole-of-government approach (Department of the Prime Minister and Cabinet, 2020); and It Takes a Tasmanian Village (Tasmanian Government, 2021). The focus on holistic child and youth wellbeing includes targeted strategies to promote mental health.

Being valued, loved and safe

A positive relationship with parents or caregivers is the first step towards children and youth being valued, loved and safe, and maintaining mental health. However, the need for children and youth to be valued, loved and safe is a whole-of-community responsibility. The past failure of Australian institutions involved in child and youth services to protect children and young people from abuse has been documented extensively (see the Royal Commission into Institutional Response to Child Sexual Abuse website, www.childabuseroyalcommission.gov.au). The testimonies of child abuse victims provide examples of the magnitude of mental, physical, emotional and spiritual distress that can result from children and youth not being valued, loved and safe in the community. When abuse occurs – in the family or in the community – the shattering of love and safety can pervade the child's life and substantially reduce mental health. Noble-Carr, Barker and McArthur (2013, pp. 19–20) report that young people who had experienced abuse

> most often [struggled with] long-lasting emotional pain, disillusionment and a negative view of the world, which sometimes resulted in shutting oneself off from the world . . . [they] experienced feeling alone, or even suffering from agoraphobia . . . leaving them alone to overcome very negative perceptions of themselves and the world around them.

Their mental health is compromised by the abuse. The first strategy used to promote mental health is fostering a respectful, loving and safe ecology for children and adolescents, both in the home and in all forms of community care. Paediatric nursing may include early notification and referral of families in need of support. Such nursing action demonstrates a commitment to the rights of the child (see the responsibility to report child maltreatment section in Chapter 2).

Developing child and youth mental health is everyone's responsibility, and begins during the antenatal period. The first 1000 days of life is an important period with an impact on life outcomes such as mental health. For example, a child's interactions with parents and those around them from birth establish the foundation for mental health through responsive caregiving, stimulating healthy neurodevelopment during this period (Rubenstein, 2020). Investing in services that support parents' wellbeing is also an investment in the mental health of children and adolescents. Nurses caring for children also have a role to play in caring for the family. If the child's experience includes maternal/familial deprivation and toxic stress, the healthy development, mental health and life chances of the child can be adversely affected. The experience that appears to have the most potent influence on promoting mental health for children and youth, and that promotes the development of neural pathways and functioning, is being involved in a positive, loving and safe relationship with others from birth and throughout early childhood.

Promoting positive participation

During childhood, positive participation is fundamental to positive learning experiences and personal development, with significant benefits such as increased confidence and self-esteem in young people (ARACY, 2013). Positive family, peer, classroom and community engagement can be encouraged by including children and youth in decision-making, especially regarding matters that affect their health and any healthcare they may require (see the section on participation rights in Chapter 2). Participation through technology for social connection is an emerging area that requires further research to determine the relationship with positive mental health outcomes. Higher rates of mental health conditions in children and youth during times of stress and community-wide disasters, such as the COVID-19 pandemic, have been reported (Singh et al., 2020). Early COVID-19 responses globally included mandatory physical distancing, and at times strict isolation measures and school closures, reducing regular social connections for children and young people. The impact of social deprivation on mental health is likely to be seen over the life course of these young people (Orben, Tomova & Blakemore, 2020). Whittle et al. (2020) researched how parenting and family factors related to COVID-19 had an impact on child and adolescent mental health. Their research concluded that when parents/carers had difficulty communicating about COVID-19 with children, child mental health decreased. Paediatric nurses can support parents and families to talk with their children and include their participation during stressful events, such as pandemics, natural disasters and hospital admissions, to help maintain the mental health of children and adolescents. Youth participation in decision-making and activities that develop personal skills, along with institutions (such as hospitals and healthcare services) that offer opportunities for positive experiences, have a positive effect on young people and promote mental health.

Fostering a positive sense of identity and culture

Paediatric nursing and the requirements of healthcare should not hinder the development of a positive sense of identity and culture in children and young people, especially when they are experiencing long admissions and living with chronic conditions. Children and young people develop a positive sense of identity and culture through:

- having good relationships with family and friends
- undertaking activities they enjoy
- undertaking activities that have meaning to them, their family and their community
- having knowledge of and making meaning out of personal, family and social history
- using language
- sharing food
- having shared ideas of what makes a good life (i.e. values, morals and religious beliefs)
- being distinct/special/unique
- showing respect
- being well regarded by others
- being proud (Renshaw, 2019, p. xi).

Some ways in which paediatric nurses can foster a positive sense of identity and culture during times of healthcare include: exploring with families ways of facilitating connections; being inclusive of families during healthcare; encouraging ongoing participation in enjoyable and meaningful activities such as sharing favourite food; and using culturally sensitive communication (Minnican & O'Toole, 2020).

A strength of the New Zealand Child and Youth Wellbeing Strategy is its powerful recognition, support and valuing of cultural identity, as seen in the Guiding Principles of the Framework (Department of the Prime Minister and Cabinet, 2019, and see above). The New Zealand Children's Commissioner recognised that:

> We know cultural identity is important for people's sense of self, belonging and how they relate to others. A strong cultural identity can contribute to people's overall wellbeing. For children and young people, developing a positive cultural identity is linked to protective factors against risks to their wellbeing, and resilience from adverse situations. (Becroft, 2017, p. 1)

In Australia and New Zealand, many factors impact the success of passing on traditional beliefs, and result in young people not forming a connection with their culture, community and family; this can potentially impact mental health development.

Managing disordered eating and eating disorders experienced by children and young people

Disordered eating is an emerging challenge. This term encompasses both the concepts of body image – including conformity to cultural standards and body dissatisfaction – and body weight management – including nutrition, obesity, restrained and binge eating. At the centre of disordered eating is the child or young person, as well as their biological growth requirements and their relationship with their context or environment, which influences their eating behaviour. Nurses caring for children and young people experiencing disordered eating must move beyond considering individual factors and encompass multiple contextual influences (Harris, 2015). The *Child and Youth Health Practice Manual* identifies 'the difference between disordered eating and eating disorders is the frequency and severity of the associated behaviours' (Queensland Hospital and Health Service, 2014, p. 242). The Butterfly Foundation (2020, p. 1) explains that

> Eating disorders are a group of mental health conditions associated with high levels of psychological distress and significant physical health complications. They involve a combination of biological, psychological and sociocultural factors. Left unaddressed, the medical, psychological and social consequences can be serious and long term.

Paediatric nurses may encounter children and young people with disordered eating and undiagnosed eating disorders. Appropriate specialist nursing actions, identified in the discussions on Anorexia Nervosa and Bulimia Nervosa below, are applicable in the context when any nurse considers that undiagnosed disordered eating and eating disorders may be presenting. In responding to concerns, it is important to maintain a trusting relationship and seek consent for referral and further assessment.

Eating disorders can quickly become life-threatening, and need to be taken very seriously once identified in children and young people. Management requires an individualised approach to treatment and nursing care. Eating disorders are not exclusive to childhood or adolescence, nor are they one-dimensional. Indeed, eating disorders may be experienced across the lifespan. For children and young people, the best evidence available indicates that family-based treatments should be applied to prevent the very serious mental and physical health outcomes that can result from eating disorders (Jewell et al., 2016).

Anorexia Nervosa (AN) and Bulimia Nervosa (BN) are two common eating disorders seen in paediatrics. They are also the eating disorders that have attracted the most research and treatment attention to date. AN features extremely low weight for age, distorted body image and fear of weight gain. BN features binge eating/purging cycles with the intense fear of weight gain (APA, 2013). Treatments for both include family therapy and multi-family therapy. According to Jewell et al. (2016), key elements of treatment are:

- an inclusive, family approach
- a parents as therapist approach
- externalisation of the disorder.

Treatment is complex, requiring specialist skills. Paediatric nurses knowledgeable about disordered eating and eating disorders can significantly help promote healthy eating in children and adolescents. Key health-promotion strategies recommended in the Queensland *Child and Youth Health Practice Manual* for body dissatisfaction and disordered eating include promoting positive cultural and social messages, addressing personal characteristics of the individual and promoting self-esteem and strong family/social relationships to strengthen resilience. However, evidence does not support simply talking about causes, symptoms and outcomes as being effective prevention or treatment technique (Queensland Hospital and Health Service, 2014, pp. 242–3). Paediatric nurses' relationship with children and young people diagnosed with AN is itself health promoting, and is one key aspect of the recovery process (Salzmann-Erikson & Dahlén, 2016).

Mental health and technology: Nursing children and young people in the technological age

Children and young people born in the twenty-first century have grown up with digital technology as part of their daily lives to a degree not experienced by any previous generation. In Australia in 2016, 97 per cent of households with children aged under 15 years had access to the internet at home, with a mean number of 7.8

internet-connected devices per household (ABS, 2018). Australian adolescents between 15 and 17 years of age have the highest internet use of any age group, with 98 per cent reporting regular internet usage (ABS, 2018). There is a similar statistical story in New Zealand, with 91 per cent of teenagers reporting that they spend more than one hour online every day and over half stating that they use three or more devices to access the internet (Netsafe, 2018).

This integration of technology into young people's lives can have both positive and negative ramifications for their mental health and overall wellbeing. Technology can enhance young people's connections with their friends, family and broader communities; it has broadened the educational landscape with new and emerging educative tools being implemented in school systems; it can increase accessibility to education and service provision for young people living in rural and remote areas; and it can be fun! Unfortunately, there are also some downsides to technology use among children and young people: a more sedentary lifestyle; vulnerability to online predators; internet/cyber addictions; and exposure to potentially challenging or even traumatising content and cyberbullying (RANZCP, 2018). These negative aspects of technology use can have serious and deleterious impacts on the mental and physical wellbeing of children and young people (RANZCP, 2018).

In the paediatric nursing context, clinicians need to understand the role of technology in the lives of the children and young people for whom they are providing care. An understanding of the types of technologies used by this cohort and the benefits and dangers associated with their use can assist paediatric nurses to build rapport, conduct thorough clinical assessments and even provide clinical care. In recent years, the high rates of technology use and literacy occurring among young people have led to new and innovative ways of engaging with and supporting the health and wellbeing of this group. Several e-health apps and web-based programs are now in use in Australia and New Zealand, often aimed at improving mental health, with many showing positive outcomes (Punukollu & Marques, 2019; RANZCP, 2018). For example, Aunty Dee is an online tool for Pacific and Māori young people that provides guided support to work through a self-identified mental health issue (Le Va, 2021). Beyond Blue in Australia developed The Check-in app to help young people support a friend who may be struggling with their mental health (Beyond Blue, 2020).

Twelve practical strategies for promoting mental health in children and young people

Evidence-based strategies for promoting the mental health of children and youth have been identified recently through extensive reviews. These strategies can be summarised in a list that provides guidance for promoting mental health through paediatric/child health nursing care in a facility or the community:

1. Be encouraging and focus on strengths, both initially and throughout the care, with a focus on skills development. For example, encourage the young person to

identify personal strengths and discuss how these strengths might be used to enhance their mental health. Identify existing barriers to good mental health, and introduce specific skills that may help to avert the potential detrimental impacts of those barriers.

2. Focus your paediatric nursing on relationship-building and be committed to the child or young person and their family's needs and wants. Use a communication style that respects the rights of the child and the family, building their trust as partners in healthcare and not simply as recipients of your service.

3. Be mindful of, and assess, the expressed needs and wants of the child or young person and their family (if possible) before engaging in mental health support. This engages the child or young person and helps build a positive sense of self. Empower children and young people to feel that they are participating fully in the process and the decision-making, both initially and throughout their care. For example, seek the child or young person's ideas on strategies to implement.

4. Gather information about the child or young person directly from them equally with other sources. Ask what the issue is and why they may be acting the way they are in response. For example, on admission ask the child why they think they are with you and what they would like to achieve. Be collaborative in all care.

5. Focus on outcomes of care, such as developing behaviours that are known to be protective and that build resilience. For example, assist the child or young person to identify existing support networks within their life, and encourage aspiration-building and community engagement.

6. Identify and meet immediate needs such as practical support, safety and access to other services. Be practical in the provision of support by providing concrete acts in response to real needs. For example, provision of school breakfast programs can support both learning and behaviour, leading to building self-esteem and resilience characteristics.

7. Have multiple gateways into the support service, and be inclusive by reducing eligibility criteria. Universality of service avoids stigmatisation of mental health services. Ensure a quick response to initial referrals and inquiries for service, and follow up on any absence multiple times. Such actions help to build trust.

8. Research has identified protective factors, stresses and circumstances that are strongly predictive of outcomes for children and young people. Many of these factors are malleable, especially when identified early. Paediatric nurses are in a position to identify and respond to promote positive outcomes for children and young people. Families are especially open to change and support when in contact with paediatric nurses implementing family-focused nursing and family partnerships.

9. Multicultural services are a great starting point; however, they are often unable to adequately meet the specific and complex mental health needs of refugee children and youth. For example, specialist programs and counselling for young people who have experienced torture and trauma should be developed specifically for the needs of young refugees, and bicultural and bilingual services should be available through referral.

10. Child and adolescent mental health conditions are recognised as an indicator that the child/family is in possible need of targeted support to prevent or address child abuse and neglect. The best way to promote mental health and protect at-risk children is to prevent child abuse and neglect from occurring through assisting the family before problems escalate into crises.

11. Be aware of the positive and negative aspects of technology use among children and young people when providing care. Be alert to possible problematic use and cyberbullying that might be impacting the mental health of this group. Stay informed about new and emerging technologies that can assist and support young people to be mentally and physically healthy. Integrate appropriate evidence-based technologies into your care of young people where appropriate.

12. Developing a context where children and families are empowered to engage in healthcare and decision-making is supported by shared care planning with a focus on strengths – what is going well, what needs to improve and what we are going to do in partnership.

These 12 practical strategies have been collated from the following evidence-based reports: Fox et al. (2015), Sollis (2019) and Renshaw (2019), and supported with examples from Julia Taylor's nursing experience with children and youth.

CASE STUDY 8.2 JASON RESOLUTION

You plan to gain further insight into Jason's mental health by asking whether there have been any changes in his sleeping patterns, concentration or ability to enjoy and maintain his usual activities. You also assess his safety by asking Jason whether he feels he is at risk of self-harm, and he says he would never hurt himself. You give Jason the number for Kids Helpline and encourage him to call it at any time if he needs someone to talk to. During discharge planning, you ask Jason whether it would be okay with him if you sent a referral letter to his school's counselling support team. You check that Jason consents to you sharing information about his experience of bullying and the disruption this is causing to his normal eating habits. Jason agrees to this plan.

During a post-discharge paediatric clinic visit, Jason states that he is feeling happier and that the bullying has lessened. His relationship with his mother is improving. He says that his school counsellor has helped him a lot and that he and his mother have now changed their routine to eat together before she goes to work. You ask Jason whether he has adult support other than his mum, and Jason states that he is close to his aunt and that she is aware of the issues he has been experiencing. You encourage Jason to talk to her if he needs to and also remind him of Kids Helpline if he needs support in the future.

This case study raises numerous issues and potential paediatric nursing interventions. Outcomes may vary and new stressors may arise for Jason. Other nursing interventions and strategies beneficial for promoting positive outcomes are not discussed. Can you identify what other essential paediatric nursing care you could instigate and why?

SUMMARY

- Being valued, loved and safe; having strong relationships, positive experiences and supportive environments; actively participating in community and social activities; and fostering a positive sense of culture and identity all help to build adaptive capacity in children and young people.
- Building an adaptive capacity allows the child or young person to manage the transitions and stresses they will experience in childhood and throughout life. This is the foundation of mental health and a resource for recovery from mental health conditions.
- Mental health can be promoted most effectively using a strengths-based approach, enhancing resilience in children, young people and families.
- All nursing interactions have the potential to build on the determinants of mental health.

LEARNING ACTIVITY

This activity enables you to apply your learning to a practical independent paediatric nursing action. Refer to Case study 8.2. Maintaining Jason's holistic wellbeing will help to maintain and strengthen his mental health. Remember, the chapter discussed how the two are not interchangeable; rather, they are interdependent.

Children who experience bullying are more likely to display mental health concerns, including feelings of anxiety and depression (AIHW, 2020, p. 371). It is important to recognise that bullying should not be ignored and that 'children who chronically bully may also have mental health issues that require specialist intervention' (Lodge, 2014, p. 2). A positive sense of connection to his family, school and community is an important strategy to promote mental health. Partnering with Jason to consider his holistic and his mental health may promote Jason's resilience.

Using the information in Jason's case study, develop a wellbeing plan with a focus on promoting mental health across the six domains of child and youth wellbeing using the Child and Family Wellbeing Plan (Communities Tasmania, 2018) available online.

FURTHER READING

Bale, J, Grové, C & Costello, S 2020, Building a mental health literacy model and verbal scale for children: Results of a Delphi study, *Children and Youth Services Review*, 109, viewed 20 March 2021, https://doi.org/10.1016/j.childyouth.2019.104667. This article provides an evidence-base for mental health literacy and offers practical strategies for nurses to include in their daily practice.

Procter, N, Baker, A, Baker, K Hodge, L & Ferguson, M 2017, Introduction to mental health and mental illness: Human connectedness and the collaborative consumer narrative, in N Procter, H Hamer, D McGarry, R Wilson & T Froggatt (eds), *Mental health: A person-centred approach* (2nd ed.), Cambridge University Press, Melbourne, pp. 1–28. A discussion of the connections between mental health and mental illness at an advanced level, building on the nursing knowledge and skill you have developed by reading Chapter 8.

United Nations Children's Fund (UNICEF) 2020, *Averting a lost COVID generation: A six point plan to respond, recover and reimagine a post-pandemic world for every child,*

UNICEF, New York, viewed 20 March 2021, www.unicef.org/reports/averting-lost-generation-covid19-world-childrens-day-2020-brief. A global holistic perspective on the international COVID-19 health issue that has the potential to impact the lives of children and young people for many years into their future.

REFERENCES

Australian Bureau of Statistics 2018, *Household use of technology: Australia 2016–17*, cat no. 8146.0, viewed 20 March 2021, www.abs.gov.au/ausstats/abs@.nsf/mf/8146.0

Australian Institute of Health and Welfare (AIHW) 2020, *Australia's children*, cat. no. CWS 69, AIHW, Canberra.

American Psychiatric Association (APA) 2000, *Diagnostic and statistical manual of mental disorders* (4th ed.) [DSM-IV], APA, Washington, DC.

—— 2013, *Diagnostic and statistical manual of mental disorders* (5th ed.) [DSM-5], APA, Washington, DC.

Australian Research Alliance for Children & Youth (ARACY) 2013, *The Nest action agenda*, ARACY, Canberra.

—— 2021, *The Common Approach®*, ARACY, Canberra, viewed 20 March 2021, www .aracy.org.au/the-nest-in-action/the-common-approach

Babington, B 2020, *Beyond 2020: Towards a successful plan for the National Framework for Protecting Australia's Children 2009–2020 final report on national consultations*, Families Australia, Canberra.

Becroft, A 2017, *Child and youth voices on their positive connections to culture in Aotearoa: Engaging children and young people in matters that affect them*, Office of the Children's Commissioner, Wellington.

Beyond Blue 2020, *The Check-in App*, viewed 20 March 2021, www.beyondblue.org.au/about-us/about-our-work/young-people/the-check-in-app

Butterfly Foundation 2020, *Eating disorders can affect anyone*, Butterfly Foundation, Sydney.

Caspi, A, Houts, R, Belsky, D, Harrington, H, Hogan, S, Ramrakha, S, Poulton, R & Moffitt, T 2017, Childhood forecasting of a small segment of the population with large economic burden, *Nature Human Behaviour*, 1, p. 0005.

Centers for Disease Control and Prevention (CDCP) 2014, *Prevalence of Autism Spectrum Disorder among children aged 8 years – Autism and Developmental Disabilities Monitoring Network, 11 sites, US, 2010*, viewed 20 February 2014, www.cdc.gov/mmwr/pdf/ss/ss6302.pdf

Communities Tasmania 2018, *The Child and Family Wellbeing Assessment Tool booklet*, Department of Communities Tasmania, Hobart.

Dadds, MR & Fraser, JA 2003, Prevention programs, in C Essau (ed.), *Conduct and Oppositional Defiant Disorders: Epidemiology, risk factors and treatment*, Lawrence Erlbaum, Mahwah, NJ, pp. 193–224.

Department of the Prime Minister and Cabinet 2019, *Child and Youth Wellbeing Strategy*, viewed 20 March 2021, https://childyouthwellbeing.govt.nz/resources/child-and-youth-wellbeing-strategy

—— 2020, *Mental Wellbeing*, viewed 20 March 2021, https://childyouthwellbeing.govt.nz/measuring-success/indicators/mental-wellbeing

Feldman, HM & Reiff, MI 2014, Attention Deficit Hyperactivity Disorder in children and adolescents, *New England Journal of Medicine*, 370, pp. 838–46.

Fox, S, Southwell, A, Stafford, N, Goodhue, R, Jackson, D & Smith, C 2015, *Better systems, better chances: A review of research and practice for prevention and early intervention,* ARACY, Canberra.

Goodhue, R (2015). *The delivery of a child and family wellbeing project using the Common Approach – final report,* ARACY, Canberra.

Goodman, SH et al. 2011, Maternal depression and child psychopathology: A meta analytic review, *Clinical Child and Family Psychology Review,* 14(1), pp. 1–27.

Gottlieb, LN & Gottlieb, B 2017, Strengths-based nursing: A process for implementing a philosophy into practice, *Journal of Family Nursing,* 23(3), pp. 319–40.

Grizenko, N, Cai, E, Claude, J, Ter-Stepanian, M & Joober, R 2013, Effects of methylphenidate on acute math performance in children with Attention-Deficit Hyperactivity Disorder, *Canadian Journal of Psychiatry,* 58(11), pp. 632–9.

Harris SM 2015, Black American female eating disorders and body image: A bioecological perspective, *The Negro Educational Review,* 66(1–4), pp. 27–54.

Hoath, FE & Sanders, MR 2002, A feasibility study of Enhanced Group Triple P Positive Parenting Program for Parents of Children with Attention-Deficit/Hyperactivity Disorder, *Behaviour Change,* 19(4), pp. 191–206.

Jewell, T, Blessitt, E, Stewart, C, Simic, M & Eisler, I 2016, Family therapy for child and adolescent eating disorders: A critical review, *Family Process,* 55, pp. 577–94.

Khanlou, N & Wray, R 2014, A whole community approach towards child and youth resilience promotion: A review of resilience literature, *International Journal of Mental Health Addiction,* 12, pp. 64–79.

Kjeldsen, A, Nilsen, W, Gustavson, K, Skipstein, A, Melkevik, O & Kareevold, EB 2016, Predicting well-being and internalising symptoms in late adolescence from trajectories of externalizing behavior starting in infancy, *Research on Adolescence,* doi:10.1111/jora.12252

Lawrence, D et al. 2015, *The mental health of children and adolescents: Report on the second Australian Child and Adolescent Survey of Mental Health and Wellbeing,* Department of Health, Canberra.

Le Va 2021, *Aunty Dee,* viewed 20 March 2021, www.auntydee.co.nz

Lodge J 2014, *Children who bully at school,* AIHW, Melbourne.

Loeber, R & Hay, D 1997, Key issues in the development of aggression and violence from childhood to early adulthood, *Annual Review of Psychology,* 48, pp. 371–410.

Masten, AS, Barnes, AJ 2018, Resilience in children: Developmental perspectives, *Children,* 5(7), pp. 98–114.

McLaughlin, KA et al. 2012, Parent psychopathology and offspring mental disorders: Results from the WHO World Mental Health Surveys, *British Journal of Psychiatry,* 200, pp. 290–9.

Minnican, C, O'Toole, G. 2020, Exploring the incidence of culturally responsive communication in Australian healthcare: The first rapid review on this concept, *BMC Health Services Research,* 20(1), p. 20.

Ministry of Health 2018, *Social, emotional and behavioural difficulties in New Zealand children: Summary of findings,* Ministry of Health, Wellington.

National Scientific Council on the Developing Child (NSCDC) 2012a, *The science of neglect: The persistent absence of responsive care disrupts the developing brain,* Center on the Developing Child, Harvard University, Cambridge, MA.

—— 2012b, *Establishing a level foundation for life: Mental health begins in early childhood*, Center on the Developing Child, Harvard University, Cambridge, MA.

—— 2015, *The science of resilience*, Center on the Developing Child, Harvard University, Cambridge, MA.

Netsafe 2018, *New Zealand teens' digital profile: A factsheet*, Netsafe, Wellington, viewed 20 March 2021, www.netsafe.org.nz/wp-content/uploads/2018/02/NZ-teens-digital-profile_factsheet_Feb-2018-1.pdf.

Noble-Carr, D, Barker, J & McArthur, M 2013, *Me, myself and I: Identity and meaning in the lives of vulnerable young people*, Institute of Child Protection Studies, Canberra.

O'Connor, S, Brenner, M & Coyne, I. 2019, Family-centred care of children and young people in the acute hospital setting: A concept analysis. *Journal of Clinical Nursing* 28, pp. 3353–67.

Orben, A, Tomova, L & Blakemore, SJ 2020, The effects of social deprivation on adolescent development and mental health, *The Lancet Child & Adolescent Health*, 4(8), pp. 634–40.

Procter, N, Baker, A, Baker, K Hodge, L & Ferguson, M 2017, Introduction to mental health and mental illness: Human connectedness and the collaborative consumer narrative, in N Procter, H Hamer, D McGarry, R Wilson & T Froggatt (eds), *Mental health: A person-centred approach* (2nd ed.), Cambridge University Press, Melbourne, pp. 1–28.

Punukollu, M. & Marques, M. 2019, Use of mobile apps and technologies in child and adolescent mental health: A systematic review, *Evidence-Based Mental Health*, 22(4), pp. 161–6.

Queensland Hospital and Health Service 2014, *Child and youth health practice manual*, Children's Health Queensland Hospital and Health Services, Brisbane.

Renshaw, L 2019, *A positive sense of identity and culture: Defining and measuring progress for children and young people in Australia – a literature and scoping review on developing better indicators*, ARACY, Canberra.

Riglin, L et al. 2016, Association of genetic risk variants with Attention-Deficit/Hyperactivity Disorder trajectories in the general population, *JAMA Psychiatry*, 73(12), pp. 1285–92.

Rhodes, A, Measey, M, O'Hara, J & Hiscock, H 2018, Child mental health literacy among Australian parents: A national study, *Journal of Paediatrics and Child Health* 54 (Suppl. 2), pp. 7–22.

Royal Australian & New Zealand College of Psychiatrists (RANZCP) 2018, *Position statement 72: The impact of media and digital technology on children and adolescents,* Royal Australian & New Zealand College of Psychiatrists, Melbourne.

Rubenstein, L. 2020, *Building children's potential: A capability investment Strategy*, ARACY, Canberra.

Rutter, ML 2005, Environmentally mediated risks for psychopathology: Research strategies and findings, *Journal of the American Academy of Child Adolescent Psychiatry*, 44, pp. 3–18.

Salzmann-Erikson, M & Dahlén, JJ 2016, Nurses' establishment of health promoting relationships: A descriptive synthesis of Anorexia Nervosa research, *Journal of Child and Family Studies*, 26(1), pp. 1–13.

Sameroff, AJ & MacKenzie, MJ 2003, Research strategies for capturing transactional models of development: The limits of the possible, *Development and Psychopathology*, 15(3), pp. 613–40.

Sawyer, M et al. 2000, *The mental health of young people in Australia*, Commonwealth Government, Canberra.

Sawyer, MG, Reece, CE, Sawyer, ACP, Johnson, S, Lawrence, D & Zubrick, SR 2016, The prevalence of stimulant and antidepressant use by Australian children and adolescents with Attention-Deficit/Hyperactivity Disorder and Major Depressive Disorder: A national survey, *Journal of Child and Adolescent Psychopharmacology*, 27(2), pp. 177–84.

Schaefer, JD, Caspi, A, Belsky, DW, Harrington, H, Houts, R, Horwood, LJ, Hussong, A, Ramrakha, S, Poulton, R & Moffitt, TE 2017, Enduring mental health: Prevalence and prediction. *Journal of Abnormal Psychology*, 126(2), pp. 212–24.

Scott, KM et al. 2011, Association of childhood adversities and early-onset mental disorders with adult-onset chronic physical conditions, *Archives of General Psychiatry*, 68, pp. 838–44.

Singh, S, Roy, D, Sinha, K, Parveen, S, Sharma, G & Joshi, G 2020, Impact of COVID-19 and lockdown on mental health of children and adolescents: A narrative review with recommendations, *Psychiatry Research*, 293, p. 113429.

Sollis, K 2019, *Measuring child deprivation and opportunity in Australia: Applying The Nest framework to develop a measure of deprivation and opportunity for children using the Longitudinal Study of Australian Children*, ARACY, Canberra.

Svavarsdottir, EK, Kamban, SW, Konradsdottir, E & Sigurdardottir, AO 2020, The impact of family strengths oriented therapeutic conversations on parents of children with a new chronic illness diagnosis, *Journal of Family Nursing*, 26(3), pp. 269–81.

Tallon, MM, Kendall, GE & Snider, PD 2015, Rethinking family-centred care for the child and family in hospital, *Journal of Clinical Nursing*, 24(9–10), pp. 1426–35.

Tasmanian Government 2021, *It Takes a Tasmanian Village: Child & Youth Wellbeing Strategy*, viewed 30 August 2021, https://hdp-au-prod-app-tas-shapewellbeing-files.s3.ap-southeast-2.amazonaws.com/4916/2950/7211/210301_Child_and_Youth_Wellbeing_Strategy_2021_wcag.pdf.

Whittle, S, Bray, K, Chu Lin, S & Orli Schwartz, O 2020, Parenting and child and adolescent mental health during the COVID-19 pandemic, viewed 20 May 2021, https://psyarxiv.com/ag2r7

Williams, AA 2020, The next step in integrated care: Universal primary mental health providers, *Journal of Clinical Psychology in Medical Settings*, 27(1), pp. 115–26.

Child and family: Psychosocial considerations and response to illness

Elizabeth Forster, Ibi Patane and Robyn Rosina

With acknowledgement to Jennifer Fraser
for the second edition

9

LEARNING OBJECTIVES

In this chapter you will:

- Be introduced to psychosocial development, and explore the ways by which paediatric nurses can promote psychosocial development in the context of childhood illness and hospitalisation
- Learn about the stages of psychosocial development according to Erikson's model
- Explore contemporary family characteristics and models of paediatric nursing care that promote family partnership and involvement
- Come to understand the Family Partnership Model and family-centred care, and their importance in paediatric nursing
- Gain an understanding of family assessment and psychosocial considerations for families when a child or young person is experiencing illness

Introduction

This chapter pays special attention to the responses of children, young people and their families to disruptions to a child's health. When a child experiences an acute or chronic illness, we can expect a number of **emotional** and **behavioural responses** exhibited by children. The paediatric nurse's knowledge of child behaviour and child development can be of great benefit in assisting parents and caregivers to promote resilience in the child or young person. In the same way, understanding the impact of a child's illness on the family can promote optimal family development, function and coping and enhance family partnership and strengths.

This chapter presents guidelines and recommendations for managing emotional and behavioural responses related to children's experiences of illness. The chapter provides an overview of psychosocial development to best illustrate the relationship between child development, and response and adaptation to illness. The relationship is bidirectional – that is, responses are shaped according to the psycho-developmental stage of the child or young person, and at the same time developmental outcomes are impacted by the experiences and challenges of both acute and chronic illness. The family is also impacted when a child or young person is experiencing illness. Families are central to the care of children – in fact, the paediatric patient and their wider family constitute the focus for care. This chapter therefore also explores what it means to be a family and family-centred care, and presents frameworks that can be used to assess and consider the psychosocial needs of families when a child is experiencing illness.

The psychosocial development of children and young people experiencing disruptions to health

Opportunities for developmental experiences that promote healthy psychosocial development may be compromised by childhood illness. The presence of chronic illness may disrupt the pace and timing of developmental milestone achievements. Indeed, regression of previously mastered milestones may be observed. Long absences from school, and limited opportunities for taking responsibility and for the experience of achievement, can compromise psychosocial developmental mastery. For some younger children, the inability to play and the absence of a playgroup can reduce opportunities for developmental progress. Feeling different from peers and the experience of interrupted peer group activity make it even more difficult for some children and young people to achieve developmental milestones.

The sequencing and progression of child development are shaped by day-to-day life experiences and interactions, both within families and with other people in the community (Erikson, 1968). Children and young people with a **chronic illness** may often require extended hospital admissions that result in the child being isolated from family members and peer groups. Periods of life-threatening crises, persistent anxiety and distress, endurance of pain and long **hospitalisations** can limit healthy experiences

Emotional response – A reaction to an internal feeling, accompanied by physiological changes that may or may not be manifested outwardly.

Behavioural response – A person's actions or reactions in response to external or internal stimuli.

Chronic illness – Any illness 'that persists over a long period and affects physical, emotional, intellectual and social functioning' (Anderson, Anderson & Glanz, 1998).

Hospitalisation – A period of medical care in a hospital.

for physical and psychosocial task experimentation and mastery. Longer-term outcomes may result, including behavioural and mental health issues, learning problems and vocational challenges.

Further challenges can emerge when the physical effects of the disease and treatments, such as pain, fatigue, limits to physical activity, physical restrictions and school absence (Pinquart & Teubert, 2012), increase the sense of difference from well peers. There are numerous environmental mediators that can act as, or become, protective factors when an individual is faced with developmental compromise. Yet environmental factors, such as child abuse, domestic violence, poverty and living with family substance abuse, can also be risk factors (Bell et al., 2016; Bellis et al., 2014). Other factors, such as the severity and visibility of the illness, acuity of current health state, duration of the illness and time since diagnosis, can also impact the developmental environment (enablers and barriers) to predispose or protect the young person from the adverse effects of illness and impact on **psychosocial development** (Falvo, 2013). However, the relationship between these factors and moderation of the environment is complex.

Psychosocial development – The acquisition of social attitudes and skills, including emotional self-regulation, and the development of the personality from infancy through maturity.

Erikson's theory of psychosocial development

Following the stages proposed by Erikson's (1968) theory of psychosocial development from infancy through to young adulthood, the chapter will now examine the impact of pain, illness and disability, and the responsiveness of nursing practice. According to Erikson (1968), the six psychosocial developmental stages are:

1. trust versus mistrust: infancy (first year of life)
2. autonomy versus shame and doubt: infancy (second year of life)
3. initiative versus guilt: early childhood – the preschool years (3–5 years)
4. industry versus inferiority: middle and late childhood (infants and primary school – 6 years to puberty)
5. identity versus identity confusion: adolescence (10–20 years)
6. intimacy versus isolation: early adulthood (twenties and thirties).

Trust versus mistrust: Infancy (first year of life) and the sick infant

Erikson's first psychosocial developmental stage, from birth to 1 year, begins with the conflict of basic trust versus mistrust. According to the theory, this conflict is resolved if the infant experiences a sense of trust about having their needs met without high levels of anxiety or distress. For example, the situation of distress may arise for infants while waiting for care in busy hospital wards or with inconsistent caregiving or the absence of parental care. Delays in the gratification of the infant's needs and persistent anxiety can induce a poor or negative resolution of the conflict of trust versus mistrust. A negative resolution of this stage can result in feelings of mistrust and anxiety about the responsiveness of the environment to meet the infant's needs in the future (Erikson, 1968).

The resolution of this first developmental stage is also important to the process of attachment to a caregiver in infancy. Bowlby (1969), a major attachment theorist, proposed that it is in fact the infant who elicits care by a series of built-in behaviours such as crying, sucking, clinging, gazing and smiling. These behaviours trigger a caregiving response – that is, rather than the parent initiating caregiving, it is the infant who initiates this responsivity to cues. The caregiver, however, needs to be sensitive to these cues in order to respond appropriately to the infant's needs. In the case of a sick infant, distance from the primary caregiver can result in separation anxiety and an anxious attachment style (Bowlby, 1969). This situation may compromise the development of trust inherent in Erikson's stage of trust versus mistrust. The post-natal stage of development is a 'sensitive period', when bonding can occur and attachment to a consistent caregiver – ideally a parent – can begin (Newman & Newman, 2011). Clearly, illness and hospitalisation during early infancy can put the quality of attachment and the developmental task to accommodate a sense of trust for sick infants at risk.

The theory of human attachment explains that child development throughout infancy and early childhood is grounded in the security of the parent–infant relationship (Ainsworth et al., 1978; Bowlby, 1951, 1969, 1988). Developmental problems among hospitalised infants and toddlers appear to relate to limited opportunities for nurturance by caregivers, as well as to how the child adapts to the developmental environment over time. These two themes of parent–infant attachment and adaptation to the developmental environment dominate the literature on the impacts of frequent hospitalisation on children's development.

Attachment theory

Attachment theory – The theory of the relationships between humans, particularly the mother (or another primary caregiver) and the child.

John Bowlby, influenced by Freud's work, was the seminal **attachment theorist**. Bowlby formulated the concept that children are born biologically pre-programmed to form attachment to people as a secure base to enable survival (Bowlby, 1969, 1988). After testing Bowlby's assumptions, Ainsworth established the concept of the attachment figure or secure base from which the infant can explore the world (Ainsworth et al., 1978). In addition, Ainsworth added to this theory the concept of maternal sensitivity to infant signals and its role in the development of the infant–mother attachment (Bretherton, 1992). The work of both Bowlby and Ainsworth continues to provide strong evidence for the key tenets of attachment theory to make sense of the needs and opportunities for developmentally responsive healthcare.

REFLECTION POINTS 9.1

- Family-centred care is based on the tenets of attachment theory, in recognition of the importance of maintaining a secure attachment relationship in infancy and childhood.
- Sick infants and toddlers need ongoing opportunities for nurturance by caregivers to prevent developmental problems associated with hospitalisation.
- What strategies would you use to promote secure attachment between a hospitalised infant and their primary caregiver?

CASE STUDY 9.1 EVIE

Evie, aged 11 months, was admitted to hospital at 4.00 am with respiratory distress and diagnosed with bronchiolitis. Her oxygen saturations go down when she gets upset. Her mother has had to go home to care for her other three young children. Evie's parents both work shifts. Her father will be able to arrange to take some time off from his job to care for Evie's siblings, but for now Evie's mother needs to be at home. Evie eats a normal family diet supplemented with bottles of formula four times a day. She has been screaming and crying out for her mother ever since she left 20 minutes ago.

Evie clearly has a strong attachment to her mother. In her mother's absence as a secure base and caregiver, Evie's distress is evidenced by her reduced oxygen saturation. Factors that can exacerbate traumatic reactions to the hospital experience for young children include prolonged response times, emotional distress, painful procedures and traumatic stress, which can have long-term consequences. Inconsistent caregivers and changes in routine can further contribute to distress in hospitalised young children. Exploring options for Evie's parents to coordinate 'rooming in' with Evie and encouraging her siblings to visit if appropriate make Evie's hospitalisation less stressful. Paediatric nurses can also maintain a regular routine of care for Evie, ensure effective pain management, and roster the same nurses to provide consistent care that is responsive to Evie's distress. Enabling healthy developmental experiences such as play could also ameliorate the potential adverse effects of hospitalisation. These are just some of the considerations a paediatric nurse might consider to mitigate the emotional and physiological impact of trauma associated with separation from parents and family while in hospital.

In order for the nurse to decide how best to care for Evie until her mother can return in the evening, the nurse needs to understand that a child's reaction to hospitalisation depends not only on the psychoemotional developmental maturity of the child, but also on:

- their previous experience of hospitals and illness
- separation and their resilience to being separated from the primary caregiver
- their innate and acquired coping skills
- the seriousness and visibility of the illness or disability
- the quality of support networks the family can access.

As mentioned previously, separation from the primary caregiver creates the greatest stress for young children in the first year of life and in the preschool age group. Separation anxiety manifests as initial protesting and crying when the caregiver leaves the infant. This is especially characteristic between 9 and 11 months of age, but can be experienced throughout childhood. This is followed by a period of despair and withdrawal, when the child will appear depressed. They may be less communicative and regress developmentally. If separated further – that is, if the parent fails to reappear – the child will become detached from the external environment and develop superficial relationships with others as they adjust to separation (Ainsworth et al., 1978). Good

(cont.)

planning and attention to the developmental needs of the child are needed to reduce Evie's risk of separation anxiety. In keeping with family-centred care, in most paediatric settings one parent is encouraged to 'room in' and stay with their hospitalised infant or child. However, as in Evie's case, parents may have competing caregiving responsibilities, or financial, transport and work-related factors that may interfere with their ability to be present continually for their hospitalised child (Lulgjuraj & Maneval, 2021). Paediatric nurses can also collaborate with members of the multidisciplinary team, such as social workers, who may be able to facilitate additional practical support to families while their infant or child is hospitalised.

Nursing assessment and interventions

Strategies to reduce the impact of separation anxiety are based on a detailed assessment of the seriousness of the child's condition, the family's previous experiences and resources, and consideration of the impacts of hospitalisation and the medical procedures that will be necessary for an optimal recovery. Where the parent is unavailable during the child's hospitalisation, there are a number of key elements of care that the nurse should know, understand and be able to implement. Importantly, the child's routines – especially their dietary requirements, play and sleep routines, and self-care abilities such as feeding, dressing and toileting – must be documented carefully. Planning care around usual activities and familiar routines may be challenging, but the benefits of having a relaxed child will outweigh the inconvenience. A favourite toy and some familiar books might assist in soothing Evie while her mother is absent. If possible, assist the mother to problem-solve so she can make staying with Evie in hospital a priority. For example, prompt her to think of responsible friends or relatives who she could trust to care for her other children. Seek advice about any other relatives familiar to Evie who might be able to stay in hospital at times when she cannot. It is well recognised that the role and bond with other family members such as grandparents, aunts/uncles and older siblings can substitute for absent parents. Maintaining these relationships, which encourage trust, autonomy and initiative, can optimise health development experiences and act as protective factors, with grandmother involvement particularly noted as a supportive and protective factor (Barnett et al., 2010). Parents, as well as their children, experience stress during times of illness and hospitalisation; supporting parental problem-solving can be very helpful and comforting.

Autonomy versus shame and doubt: Infancy (second year of life) and the sick toddler

Erikson's second stage of psychosocial development, from 1 to 3 years, involves resolving the conflict of autonomy versus shame and doubt (Erikson, 1968). The child's discovery of a will of their own marks this stage. The child begins to walk and climb, and develops the mental powers to make decisions. Autonomy begins to form during this stage, when parents or caregivers offer guided choices and do not overly restrict, force or shame the child (Erikson, 1968). Children who are restrained too much or punished too harshly may be at risk of developing a sense of shame and self-doubt (Erikson, 1968). For young children with chronic illness, the achievement of milestones such as walking and climbing may be impossible or delayed by the impact of the disease process. Incapacity and physical limitations may also compromise the attainment of a sense of competence for children with chronic illness.

The diagnosis and treatment of chronic conditions often involves multiple painful procedures that can risk traumatic stress for the child, parents and siblings (National Child Traumatic Stress Network, 2016). These experiences can result in poorer **emotional regulation** and an increased risk of anxiety and mood disorders (Pao & Bosk, 2011; Thabrew, Ruppeldt & Sollers, 2018). The hospital experience can become an extremely stressful period for both the child and the family. The anxiety and distress that a child may experience during invasive and traumatic procedures and over the course of a chronic illness can have long-term psychological consequences (Tennant et al., 2020).

A common reaction to stress in children is regression of developmental gains. The young child who was toilet trained may need to wear nappies again until they become more resilient in a stressful situation, and the toddler who was beginning to dress independently may need some assistance while in hospital. The extra attention paid to the child will assist with the adjustment to hospitalisation. Parents can become quite distressed to see their children regress in this way, and need to be reassured that this is generally a temporary and expected response to the stress of illness and hospitalisation. Patience and understanding are needed, and the nurse may use strategies such as modelling the behaviours and providing anticipatory guidance, thus preparing the parents for the extra care and attention the child will need to overcome stress (see Box 9.1).

Emotional regulation – The desired outcome of early childhood emotional development; involves being able to appropriately manage or regulate emotions – for example, to be able to cheer yourself up and calm yourself down after stress or disappointments, and to respond appropriately during social interactions.

BOX 9.1 NURSING ASSESSMENT AND INTERVENTIONS

- If possible, prepare the child and parent/family for hospitalisation.
- Prevent or minimise separation from caregivers.
- Prevent or minimise loss of control for child and family.
- Provide effective pain management.
- Provide age-appropriate play equipment.
- Provide opportunities for the child to play.
- Understand that regression may occur and support parents to accept adaptive behaviours.

Initiative versus guilt: Early childhood – the preschool years (3–5 years)

The third stage of Erikson's theory of psychosocial development explains the period from approximately 3 to 5 years. This developmental period is marked by courage and independence (Erikson, 1968). The child gains initiative and is capable of planning and problem-solving. With this stage also comes a new emotion: guilt. Children at this stage of development may experience a feeling of guilt when their initiatives are unsuccessful.

Case study 9.2 involves David, a 5-year-old boy with Down syndrome. Erikson's conflict of initiative versus guilt is a particularly important and critical stage and milestone for many children with disabilities. David's story highlights the importance of recognising developmental mastery among children with disabilities, and the key role played by nursing practice in optimising developmental opportunities within hospital experiences for this group. The case example of David highlights not only the importance of identifying anxiety, but also how difficult it is to recognise behavioural developmental cues and to ensure responsive nursing care. Getting to know David and his developmental abilities pre-illness is vital to enable his developmental progress and an awareness of regression as much as possible.

CASE STUDY 9.2 DAVID

David has been admitted to hospital for further medical management of congenital heart defects that are now impairing his cardiac function. Prior to admission to hospital, David was able to assist with dressing and, after prompting by his mother, Kath, is mostly able to use the toilet by himself. David is in his second year at preschool/pre-prep and attends two days per week. David and his family have been learning sign language to assist in his communication, although David does have a small expressive vocabulary that he uses. Early in the admission, the insertion of an intravenous cannula was required to administer antibiotics. David was very distressed, having had numerous blood tests previously and thrashed about violently and requiring some therapeutic holding for the procedure. After the procedure, David remained distressed and struggled, and was incontinent, spitting and refusing to swallow medication. He eventually pulled the cannula out. Kath became visibly distressed and later disclosed feelings of helplessness, powerlessness and an inability to protect and/or control or even influence her son's experience in the hospital. When at home, even when David was sick, she was able to control or at least soothe and make things easier for him. Kath also felt that her son was aware of her distress and her inability to protect him, which always made his behaviour worse.

The anxiety levels of mothers are reported to be a powerful predictor of anxiety among children in this age group (Smith & Kaye, 2012). There is evidence that a child's anxiety level in some way moderates the coping strategies of the mother (Burns-Nadar, Hernandex-Reif & Porter, 2014). Understanding and ameliorating maternal anxiety may potentially be a powerful environmental mediator that can in turn moderate anxiety experienced by hospitalised children and facilitate resolution of the conflict of industry versus inferiority. At the very least, it may prevent developmental regression and the loss of previously acquired or current developmental achievements. For David, it may have been a loss of previously attained skills and current developmental mastery – for example, self-care skills such as toileting, feeding himself, feeling safe and being able to control his behaviour.

Parents' and carers' perspectives and knowledge of the child's mood and behaviour, and particularly the information they can provide about premorbid developmental functioning, are extremely valuable to enable rather than compromise developmental progression. Particularly for children such as David, it could be useful to explore previous developmental achievements – specifically emotion regulation, feeding, sleeping routines, bathing or the level of support required for these activities. Young children often find it more difficult to articulate their distress in a meaningful way, which is particularly apparent in children with developmental delays. In addition, David and his family use sign language as well as verbal communication, and this can make it challenging for him to communicate his feelings and needs to health professionals who do not 'sign'. The inability to communicate can lead to further frustration and distress for David. Appropriate preparation for the traumatic proced-ures and pharmacological and non-pharmacological interventions are often needed to reduce distress associated with painful procedures (Shave et al., 2018). Consulting Kath about strategies she and nursing/medical staff have used previously to calm David (prior to and during venipuncture) may have reduced the need for restraint and the level of anxiety that ensued. Routine monitoring of mood, emotions, behaviour and functioning before and after traumatic procedures can identify rising anxiety for both parents and their children. Anticipating and identifying anxiety can create opportunities to ameliorate distress and avoid losses in developmental mastery during hospitalisation and at home after discharge.

Nursing interventions that target maternal anxiety are important when it comes to moderating the anxiety of children undergoing traumatic procedures. Parental anxiety about a procedure directly affects the child's anxiety level, and thus heightens their response to procedural pain (Beardon, Feinstein & Cohen, 2012). Nursing interventions that empower the child and/or normalise the hospital experience as much as possible – particularly for children with developmental delays – may promote developmental opportunities. Interventions that consider the challenges to optimal child development can also promote the retention of previous levels of developmental mastery. Developmental regression can weaken opportunities to resolve and master later developmental conflicts and milestones.

Numerous developmental windows of opportunity occur as a child grows and matures, and the transition from childhood to adolescence is a critical period to assist children to engage in increased responsibility for self-care. This lays the foundation for developing greater responsibility and independence in adolescence and adulthood.

Parents and caregivers are the cornerstone of their children's health decisions, experiences and behaviours. Working with parents to achieve optimal health, growth and development requires an understanding of how caring for a child with a chronic condition or disability can impact parent functioning and wellbeing. Not only are the parents responsible for the child's treatment regimen, emergency care responses and daily care routines; their responsibilities extend to the day-to-day management of the child's condition.

REFLECTION POINTS 9.2

- The nurse cares for the child, parents and family in paediatric nursing settings to optimise developmental opportunities and the child's and family's health.
- Acknowledging maternal anxiety can reduce the anxiety of hospitalised children.
- Children's development can regress due to pain, illness and isolation. Parents need to understand that some developmental progress may be lost temporarily while the child is in hospital.
- What strategies could you use to help promote a sense of initiative for David during his hospitalisation? How would you involve David's parents in these strategies?

An important consideration for nurses caring for David is the fact that children with disability are at higher risk of suffering all types of abuse, including neglect (Flynn & McGregor, 2017; Svensson, Bornehag & Janson, 2011). Children with disabilities are more than three to four times more likely than their non-disabled peers to be neglected or abused (Flynn & McGregor, 2017; Frederick, Devaney & Alisic, 2019). These estimates of higher risk may be linked to an over-representation of children with disabilities and/or social disadvantage in formal care (Flynn & McGregor, 2017). As discussed in Chapter 2, the paediatric nurse has a responsibility to detect and respond to the recognition of child abuse and neglect. Children are vulnerable due to their dependence on adults for care, for having their developmental needs met and for providing a harmonious and supportive family environment.

There is ongoing concern about the increased vulnerability of children with chronic illness and those with longer-term disabilities. Children and young people with disabilities are vulnerable for a variety of reasons, including a lack of knowledge or awareness of inappropriate behaviours, communication impairments that impede their ability to disclose abuse or neglect, the inability to flee due to physical impairments and their reliance on others for personal care (Frederick, Devaney & Alisic, 2019). The evidence for children with chronic illness and disability being at risk of emotional, behavioural and social delay, and their increased likelihood of suffering child abuse and neglect, demonstrates their overwhelming risk. This situation highlights the importance of paying attention to the family environment, family functioning and relative need for support.

Morawska, Calam and Fraser (2014) highlight that the characteristics of the family environment and the severity and chronicity of the illness, rather than the specific childhood illness, are the best predictors of adjustment to chronic illness in childhood. More recently, White et al. (2018) proposed the THRIVE Framework to describe the key ways people adjust to and cope with chronic illness. The acronym THRIVE and an explanation of what each letter stands for can be seen in Table 9.1.

These are important findings, guiding our understanding of adjustment to chronic illness for paediatric patients and their families. For example, if children with chronic illness or their families are not engaging in positive emotional responses, then paediatric nurses and the multidisciplinary healthcare team will need

Table 9.1 The THRIVE Framework

Coping factor	Description
Therapeutic interventions	These are interventions used by health professionals to promote coping, and may include education for knowledge and skills and self-care.
Habit and routine	This includes habits and routines relating to diet, exercise, hobbies and social activities.
Relational-social factors	This involves social support from friends and family, and can include emotional support, practical support or informational support, which can protect against the negative impacts of stress.
Individual differences	Individual differences need to be considered in order to promote optimal coping (e.g. age, gender, ethnicity, severity of symptoms and socioeconomic status).
Values and beliefs	This includes values, attitudes and beliefs that may promote positive physical and psychological outcomes – for example, spirituality may enhance quality of life and coping.
Emotional factors	Emotional responses can be linked to adjustment to chronic illness. Positive and expressive emotions, rather than negative, repressive or avoidant responses and emotions, are more likely to lead to positive adjustment.

Source: Adapted from White et al. (2018).

to support children and families to develop more adaptive emotional responses and coping skills.

REFLECTION POINT 9.3

How might you apply the THRIVE Framework when caring for a child with a chronic illness and their family? Use the acronym and write down some examples that address each element of the framework.

Internalising conditions such as depression and anxiety, and externalising disorders (those that feature behaviour problems and aggression) (Pinquart & Shen, 2011) can impact family relationships and adjustments (Flynn et al., 2018) and school absence and engagement (Lum et al., 2017), so they need to be acknowledged and managed. Of particular importance during hospitalisation is the risk of poor interpersonal and social skill development and self-regulation for the child or young person. Children who present with poorer social and emotional skills will find hospitalisation extremely stressful, and should receive extra attention (Lambert et al., 2013). Their limited capacity for self-regulation can result in externalising behaviours of aggression, and violence may also be experienced. Parents may commonly adopt a permissive parenting style for the child with a chronic condition, fearing that discipline may add to the stress of their life. Unfortunately, this can further contribute to poor regulation of the child's own emotional reactions. Reactions to injury and illness include crying, resistance, oppositional behaviour and aggressive outbursts. As the child develops, the concerns become more complex. The young child may fear disability and lack of privacy, and use words more effectively to describe fear and pain. School-aged children are especially vulnerable to stress as they struggle for independence and seek peer acceptance.

Industry versus inferiority: Middle and late childhood (primary school – 6 years to puberty)

Social and cultural factors also play a key role in the way children in the fourth stage of psychosocial development respond. According to Erikson (1968), this is an important stage in the development of self-confidence. Children in this stage are likely to be able to form moral values and work hard to get things right. A capacity to recognise cultural and individual differences emerges with an expression of individuality and independence.

Fine motor coordination increases during this stage, and children in this age group are capable of completing complex motor tasks. This improves their ability to play games that require hand–eye coordination, such as soccer and handball, and extends to the physical skills required to become involved in complex health procedures such as applying creams and independently managing bandaging.

Perceptual thinking moves towards conceptual thinking – that is, the child moves from a way of thinking based on what they see (perceptual) to judging a situation based on their own reasoning (conceptual). Concrete thinking matures with abstract thought and a greater understanding of their health condition. This developmental achievement means that children of this age have more agency in determining their own health behaviours. They are able to contribute more to discussion, have an opinion and make decisions for themselves. They often have a strong sense of industry and enjoy accomplishment that can be harnessed into positive health behaviours and greater responsibility. Outside the hospital context, school-aged children are usually achieving a sense of mastery in various tasks they complete at home and at school, and a stay in hospital may limit their opportunities to repeatedly engage in and complete tasks successfully (Lerwick, 2013). As young children attempt to participate in, or are strongly encouraged to take some responsibility for, selected aspects of their treatment, there are opportunities to foster this sense of mastery. The involvement in play activities that are promoted by groups such as the Starlight Foundation assists children to achieve a sense of success, mastery and therefore industry. A good example is *Juiced TV*, which is a television show at Queensland Children's Hospital that is made by hospitalised children who conduct interviews and create and help produce segments (Children's Hospital Foundation, 2021).

Children may become frustrated when they are unable to participate successfully in their own care, and parents play an important role in managing any negative behavioural responses that children may engage in and the conflicts that may arise. Interestingly, in relation to parenting style, authoritative parenting styles are associated with better management of childhood illness, and with superior child adjustment (Park & Walton-Moss, 2012; Pinquart, 2013). Higher rates of emotional and behavioural problems among children with chronic illness may be explained by their parents' expectations of behaviour, over-protection and a reluctance to discipline a sick child (Ernst et al., 2019). Understandably, parents may set different expectations for their child's behaviour, especially during hospitalisation. A high level of parenting stress and low parenting self-efficacy are known to reduce parents' ability to manage their children's behaviour, and to manage treatment regimens crucial to the management of childhood illness (Guite et al., 2018; Helgeson et al., 2011). Nursing practice can ensure or optimise parental control and decision-making in the context of healthcare. Children can then perceive that parents are more often in charge of care and safety at home and in hospital contexts of care.

REFLECTION POINTS 9.4

- The domains of physical, mental and psychosocial health, and disruptions to health are intricately linked – particularly during childhood.
- Consequently, each domain requires careful assessment and interventions to ensure good physical and mental health, and to ensure optimal psychosocial development.
- The family remains in charge of care and safety in hospital and at home, reinforcing parent and child self-efficacy and confidence in the world, despite the uncertainty of illness.
- When caring for a school-aged child who has been hospitalised for a long period, you observe that they are arguing frequently with their parents and refusing to obey their parents' directions. Given what you now understand about the developmental stage of industry vs inferiority, how might you foster psychosocial development and support the parents?

Identity versus identity confusion: Adolescence (10–20 years)

As children move from childhood into the adolescent years, different developmental issues arise. Assuming the management of their own health and treatment regimens becomes increasingly important. The impact of their illness on their physical and psychosocial development becomes more tangible and personally 'real' to the young person. For some young people and their families, this can be quite overwhelming.

Erikson (1968) marks the period of adolescence, from 10 to 20 years, as the fifth stage of human psychosocial development. This stage presents the conflict of identity versus identity confusion, and the transition from childhood to adulthood. The achievement of the earlier developmental tasks, regardless of the quality of mastery, becomes integrated into a lasting sense of identity and an emerging recognition of one's place in society. A more negative outcome is recognised by identity confusion and uncertain future occupational potential and, for some, indications of emerging mental illness.

The achievement of a sense of identity is a particularly critical stage for optimal independent functioning and mental health for young people with chronic illness.

Young people with chronic illness may spend long periods in hospital or might be confined largely to their homes. This situation limits the experience of a social context of peers and the community to work on the developmental conflict of identity versus identify confusion. Other vital experimentation with roles, normal levels of risk-taking behaviours and the development of cognitive abilities have the potential to be limited. The cumulative effect of experiencing fewer developmental experiences and poorer psychosocial development becomes apparent during adolescence. Given that some children and young people spend so much time in hospital during infancy, childhood and adolescence, nursing practice has the capacity to create opportunities for psycho-social growth and development through day-to-day hospital experiences.

Erikson believes that it is not the rapid growth and sexual impulses *per se* that disturb adolescents, but rather an acute fear of being different, or of not conforming to a peer group. Clearly, for the chronically ill young person, this situation can cause increased anxiety. Young people also worry about the future and how they will be able to lead an independent life (Erikson, 1968). The visibility of a disease, in terms of physical difference from peers and forced dependence on others for care, presents major developmental challenges to the conflict of achieving a sense of identity. More often, the developmental trajectory does not conform to the timing and tempo of peers' development. Clearly, an open-mind and astute developmental mastery skills are essential to adolescent health nursing practice.

Translation to practice and transition to adult care

The developmental environment for many young people with chronic illness is dominated by hospital experiences. These experiences have the opportunity to inhibit or facilitate developmental task mastery. Through their ongoing contact with chronically ill young people and their families, nurses are influential in the healthcare context of the young person's developmental world, and they need a thorough understanding of adolescent psychosocial development and risk assessment. Moreover, nurses are perfectly placed to identify young people struggling with psychosocial development and self-regulation, whether represented by treatment adherence challenges, emerging mental illness or difficult and/or at-risk behaviours.

Transition to adult care is another important consideration for paediatric nurses when caring for adolescents. The young person and their family need support to prepare for their increasing responsibility for self-management as they transition into adult healthcare settings. Similarly, parents will need support as they relinquish elements of care responsibilities to their teenager (Bratt et al., 2017). Preparation for this transition will normally begin in childhood, when children are encouraged to be involved in managing selected elements of their chronic illness care. Some of the issues that can arise are a poorly planned, abrupt or delayed move to adult services, or the young person ceasing engagement with health services when the paediatric service is no longer available to them. Therefore there is a need for a planned transition period as this is a time of loss for the young person who likely feels safe in the paediatric health service but at the same time strives for independence. There is no 'right age' for transition to occur, and it depends on the young person's developmental stage and available supports (Aldiss et al., 2016). Aldiss et al. (2016) also discuss the transition period being challenging for parents and often difficult for the health professionals, who have formed a strong relationship with the young person and their family. Therefore, this planned and staged process needs to be a partnership between the young person, the family and the healthcare providers (Bratt et al., 2017).

Intimacy versus isolation: Early adulthood (twenties and thirties) and the sick young adult

Erikson's sixth stage of psychosocial development spans the years of the twenties and thirties – the final stage for the focus of this discussion. This stage involves the conflict of intimacy versus isolation (Erikson, 1968). The resolution of this stage is achieved with the establishment of a meaningful and purposeful life, with a sense of connectedness to other people. Erikson (1968) describes this stage as finding oneself, yet also losing oneself in another person. Young adults unable to resolve this conflict are less able to establish close relationships, often fearing rejection and isolating themselves from other people.

During this developmental period, young adults focus predominantly on seeking a career and developing intimate relationships with other people. The major developmental task at this stage is a psychological readiness and a commitment to mutual intimacy. This level of intimacy prepares the young adult for marriage or its alternatives to attain and retain individual identity within joint intimacy. If the young adult finds satisfying friendships, but is also able to achieve intimacy with another, the negative resolution of social isolation will be avoided. A negative resolution results in the young person being unable to establish close relationships, increasing the risk of social problems and relationship difficulties (Erikson, 1968).

For some young people with chronic illness, the ability to have an intimate relationship while remaining largely physically dependent on parents or carers is extremely difficult – and for some it can be impossible. This situation may be a result of delayed emergence of an adulthood identity as a consequence of prolonged poor self-esteem and stalling in efforts for independence and self-regulation.

Young adults with chronic paediatric illness are known to have reduced chances of securing employment, completing education, attaining higher education qualifications, moving out of the family home, marrying and having children (Pinquart, 2014).

REFLECTION POINTS 9.5

- How does psychosocial development influence the way in which children and young people respond to disruptions in health and vice versa?
- Outline the role of the interprofessional team in the care of young people with chronic illness both in the hospital and the community.
- What is the relationship between responsive nursing practice and the psychosocial development of children and young people?
- What role does culture play in influencing the way in which children, young people and their families respond to disruptions in health?

Family considerations

Earlier in this chapter, the centrality of families to the care of children experiencing illness was highlighted and the focus for paediatric care being both the child and family was established. In this section of the chapter, you will be introduced to family considerations when a child or young person experiences illness. In order to care for families effectively, an understanding of contemporary families and their development and strengths is essential. In this section, you will discover the frameworks that can be used to assess families and be invited to consider some of the tensions or challenges experienced by paediatric nurses during care for children and families.

Contemporary families

Families today are diverse in terms of their structure, as well as their membership, functions, beliefs and values. As a consequence, the concept of 'family' is quite challenging to define. It is perhaps useful to think of McCaffery's (1968) reference to pain as being 'whatever the patient says it is' and consider families to be defined by their members; even though members of a family may have no blood relationship, they may consider themselves to be a family.

Contemporary families may be:

- experiencing or adjusting to marital breakdown
- lone-parent households
- blended or step-families
- same-sex parents with children
- migrant and refugee families
- culturally and linguistically diverse
- experiencing domestic violence or coping with disability, injury or illness (AIPC, 2012; Hayes et al., 2010).

The nature of families has an impact on child health and wellbeing, as families are instrumental in ensuring that children's needs are met from birth through to young adulthood and beyond. Families are the social connection between their members and the outside world, and are responsible for role modelling and socialisation. Exposure to a negative or disruptive family environment during early childhood can have a lasting impact on a child's social, cognitive and emotional development and adult opportunities. According to Munns and Shields (2013), these effects may be transferred to the next generation and have real sequalae for the young people.

A variety of models recognise and promote family involvement in a child's care, and this chapter will look at two of these models: the Family Partnership Model and family-centred care.

The Family Partnership Model

The Family Partnership Model was created in the United Kingdom by the Centre for Parent and Child Support (Davis, Day & Bidmead, 2002). The original focus of the model was to support early intervention in child mental health. The model is used primarily within community child health practice, both within Australia and abroad. The principles, however, are relevant to any context where nurses are caring for children and their families. The Family Partnership Model aims to assist parents and children to:

- identify and build upon their strengths
- clarify and manage problems
- develop resilience and the ability to anticipate problems
- enhance/improve child development and wellbeing
- harness social support (Davis et al., 2007).

The model also aims to foster community development, service development and improvement.

The Family Partnership Model also outlines a variety of helper qualities, including respect, genuineness, empathy, humility, quiet enthusiasm, personal strength and integrity, as well as intellectual and emotional attunement (Davis et al., 2007). In addition, helpers use a variety of communication, problem-solving and negotiation skills to establish an effective partnership with parents.

Child health nurses who have trained within the Family Partnership Model and used it in practice have described a shift in their practice so that they are moving away from telling parents what to do to solve a problem towards exploring and facilitating parent needs, thereby enabling them to problem-solve for their family. This involves asking parents what the nurse could do to assist and what parents want from the nurse, which places greater emphasis on parent control during interactions (Fowler et al., 2012). Nurses also develop skills within the foundation of a trusting relationship to challenge negative parent constructions in order to 'develop different, more positive ways of thinking about issues' (Fowler et al., 2012, p. 3310).

Family-centred care

'Family-centred care' is a phrase that has been defined and conceptualised in many ways. It is seen as a paradigm, a philosophy, a model of care and a practice theory (Mikkelsen & Frederiksen, 2011). For the purposes of this chapter, it will be seen as a model of paediatric nursing care, and defined as

> a way of caring for children and their families within health services which ensures that care is planned around the whole family, not just the individual child/person, where all the family members are recognised as care recipients and where family involvement is considered to be central to a child's care. (Shields, Pratt & Hunter, 2006, p. 1318)

Family-centred care is the most frequently used model, with its aim of enhancing the involvement of parents in their child's healthcare. As seen in the above definitions, the whole family is the focus of care (Coyne, 2015). Yet, despite strong agreement among clinicians that this model has benefits for both children and their families (Coyne, 2015; Shields, 2010), there is limited evidence that it impacts their outcomes (Kuo et al., 2012; Shields et al., 2012).

Family-centred care has its challenges, and despite its popularity its definition remains unclear in many settings. The actual application of the model in clinical practice has also been scrutinised (Kuo et al., 2012). This may be because it contrasts with more traditional approaches to care, where responsibility and control rest with healthcare professionals rather than parents (Kuo et al., 2012).

Some of the problems with its application in clinical settings are thought to be due to inadequacies in knowledge and skills. Increasingly, families experience stress when attempting to fulfil their roles, while nurses are challenged to work alongside parents amidst busy workloads and inadequate staffing. Problems emerge with negotiation processes, power struggles between clinicians and parents, and insufficient organisational supports to implement the model effectively (Coyne, 2015). As reported by nurses in the Coyne study, communication with families and the negotiation of care can sometimes be challenging, contributing to challenges with the implementation of family-centred care (Coyne, 2015). Some clinicians may not like to relinquish control of certain aspects of care to parents, and this undermines the notion of partnership that is central to family-centred care (Coyne et al., 2011).

REFLECTION POINTS 9.6

- Families may be quite diverse in terms of their composition and structure. In Australia, contemporary families may be adjusting to marital breakdown, be sole-parent, blended or same-sex parent families, be culturally and linguistically diverse, be experiencing stressors associated with domestic violence, have migration or refugee concerns, or be coping with a family member's disability, injury or illness.
- The Family Partnership Model can be used by nurses to enhance family strengths, problem-solving and resilience in order to optimise child development and well-being. It requires a shift away from the traditional nurse-controlled way of approaching care towards a style of care that explores and facilitates parents' preferences and needs.
- Family-centred care is a model of paediatric nursing care where the child and the whole family are the focus of care. The model is underpinned by family involvement, participation and partnership in the child's care. Nurses caring for children continually negotiate with and empower parents to be involved and lead their child's care.
- Family assessment is integral to planning and providing family-centred care. The model recognises that all families have strengths that will assist them to develop resilience and adapt to stressors.
- What are some examples of ways in which you can promote family-centred care as a paediatric nurse?

Family assessment

In order to provide a high standard of care to children and families, we need to understand both the roles and functions of families, and their strengths and limitations. We need to recognise early stressors and strengthen coping strategies as families grow, despite the presence of chronic illness for their child.

Family assessment is a way to understand each family and to explore how a health problem experienced by one of its members impacts the whole family.

A variety of family assessment models exist and are used by paediatric nurses – for example, the Calgary Family Assessment Model and the Friedman Family Assessment Tool. Most assessment models have a few elements of assessment in common, which usually include:

- a family genogram/ecomap or visual representation of the family structure
- assessment of the developmental stage of the family
- assessment of roles and functions within the family
- assessment of stressors experienced by the family
- assessment of coping strategies used by the family.

We will now discuss these elements of family assessment so you will have a good understanding of these tools in your paediatric nursing practice.

Family genogram/ecomap

The structure of the family is important to understand when considering family assessment. This can often be complex to explain, and **genograms** are a diagrammatic way to map the family structure, specifically each person's relationship within the family unit in relation to the patient over a few generations (Wright & Leahey, 2013).

Figure 9.1 shows a simple genogram of a typical family, with both partners having remarried. The square shapes symbolise males and the circles females. The lines indicate relationships and crosses through lines indicate relationships that have ended (such as by death or divorce or estrangement/separation with a single line). The children are mapped and connected to their parents. The patient who is the focus of the genogram, Milly, is highlighted.

Genogram – A visual representation of a family's structure and relationships in respect to the patient of focus. Some may also include ages, health problems and for some members causes of their deaths.

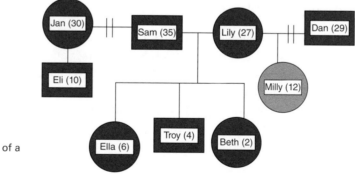

Figure 9.1 An example of a genogram

Further, the nurse can explore the family's interactions within its community and map these external interactions (Holtslander, Solar & Smith, 2013). These diagrams are called **ecomaps**, and can be useful when assisting families to draw on resources to assist them. The family is central in the ecomap, and the support systems are mapped, with the number and boldness of the connecting lines indicating the strength of the relationship and support (Neves, Cabral & da Silveira, 2013). In the ecomap in Figure 9.2, the couple report moderate support from each other, and only one strong source of support from their community. One potential source of support is not linked at all; this could be family members who may be geographically distant.

Ecomap – A visual representation of the identified supports of the family unit.

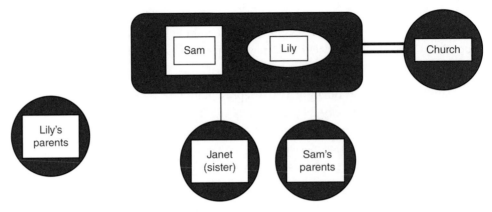

Figure 9.2   An example of an ecomap

More recently, emotion mapping has been used in some studies to represent family member feelings and interpersonal relating within couple and family relationships. This mapping is often set against the background of the couple or family home environment (Gabb & Singh, 2015a, 2015b). Within this approach, emoticon symbols are used to depict the emotions experienced by family members in relation to other members. For example, each family member is given a sticker colour, and emoticons such as laughter, happiness, grumpiness/anger, indifference, upset, sadness and love/ affection are used to depict the feelings experienced by family members in different locations within the family home (Gabb & Singh, 2015a). This strategy can also be used by children to gain an insight into their perceptions regarding their own and family members' feelings.

Family development

Family development can be understood from a variety of standpoints. Family developmental theory and family life-cycle stages (McGoldrick, Carter & Garcia-Preto, 2011) are two ways of thinking about family development. Essentially, it is thought that family roles and tasks are influenced by the stage of the family. For example, a family with teenagers is likely to have different roles and a different focus from a beginning family experiencing the birth of their first child. Understanding the stages of development experienced by families over a lifetime can give paediatric nurses an understanding of significant events, challenges, roles and tasks that may occur during these times.

McGoldrick, Carter and Garcia-Preto's (2011) family life-cycle stages include:

- leaving home: single young adults
- the joining of family through marriage: the new couple
- families with young children
- families with adolescents
- launching children and moving on
- families in later life.

One of the early criticisms of this model was that it was based on understandings of middle-class North American families, so was less equipped to consider the

Table 9.2 Family life-cycle stage tasks and attachments

Family life-cycle stage	Tasks	Attachments
Leaving home: single young adults	Differentiation of self in relation to family of origin Development of intimate peer relationships Establishment of self in relation to work and financial independence	Attachment between young adults and their respective parents Attachment between parents
The joining of family through marriage: the new couple	Establishment of couple identity Realignment of relationships with extended families to include spouse Decisions about parenthood	Attachments between spouses Attachments between each spouse and their respective family of origin Attachments with outside interests
Families with young children	Adjusting the marital system to make space for the child Joining in childrearing, financial and household tasks Realignment of relationships with extended family to include parenting and grandparenting roles	Attachments between parents Attachments between parents and children Attachments between siblings
Families with adolescents	Adjusting parent–child relationships to allow adolescents to move into/out of the family system Mid-life marital and career issues Beginning shift towards joint caring for the older generation	Possible decrease in parental attachment for the young person Adolescent attachment with peer group Attachment between family members
Launching children and moving on	Renegotiation of marital dyad Development of adult-to-adult relationships between parents and grown children Realignment of relationships to include in-laws and grown children Dealing with disabilities and death of grandparents	Attachments between family members Attachments to outside interests
Families in later life	Maintaining own or couple functioning and interest in the face of physiological decline: exploration of new familial and social role options Making room for the wisdom and experience of seniors Dealing with loss of spouse, siblings, peers and preparation for death	Interdependence with the next generation Intergenerational attachments, especially between daughters and parents

Source: Adapted from McGoldrick, Carter & Garcia-Preto (2011); Wright & Leahey (2013).

dynamic and diverse nature of the families that exist in society today. Since it was first developed, a variety of other family life-cycle models have been developed and introduced, including family life-cycles for divorced and remarried, professional and low-income, adoptive, and homosexual, bisexual and transgendered families (Wright & Leahey, 2013). The development of these family life-cycles reflects the limitations of a single model in terms of understanding family development across the lifespan, and acknowledges that families are diverse and constantly changing.

At each stage during the life-cycle, families have particular tasks to fulfil, and attachments between members form and change. Table 9.2 summarises some of the tasks and attachments that may be significant at each stage.

Family roles and functions

Families exist to meet the needs of the individuals within a family, to expand through reproductive functions and to ensure socialisation of new family members. The main functions of the family can be summarised as follows:

- affective function – meeting psychological needs
- social function – meeting social needs and ensuring children become productive within their social group
- reproductive function
- economic function
- healthcare function (Friedman, Bowden & Jones, 2003).

However, over time traditional roles within the family have changed – for example, more families today combine raising children with work commitments as mothers have increased involvement in the workforce compared with previous decades (Cooklin et al., 2016). This change has impacted mother and father roles and expectations within the family. It is important to acknowledge the diverse nature of contemporary families, which may vary in terms of their structure, roles and functioning.

Family strengths

In addition to family development and their associated functions to support family members, it is important to recognise and support the strengths and resilience of families. The family strengths framework acknowledges that families have strengths that develop over time, which promote the resilience of members.

The Australian Family Strengths Nursing Assessment guide was developed in 2000 as part of a family strengths research project. The finding identified that families recognised eight qualities of strong families. Seven qualities were strengths, and the eighth quality – the ability to withstand and bounce back from situations of crisis – was family resilience (Smith & Ford, 2013). The eight qualities form the foundation for the Strengths Assessment Guide (see Table 9.3).

Table 9.3 Australian Family Strengths Nursing Assessment Guide (Version 2)

Family quality	Possible assessment questions
Togetherness The 'invisible glue' that bonds a family together. A sense of belonging and shared values and beliefs is integral to this bond.	In your family, what shared beliefs really matter to you? Do you share beliefs that really matter together, which you would like to follow during this time of healthcare? What are some of the things that cause you to celebrate together? Tell me about some of your family's shared memories.
Sharing activities Planning for and spending time together nurtures the family and its members, and strengthens their sense of togetherness.	When does the family spend time together? What is it you like about when you plan activities together? How often would you play together as a family? Tell me about when you have good times together in your family.
Affection Family members express their concern, care and love for each other regularly, both through words and behaviours.	In your family, when is it most easy to tell others how you feel about them? How best do you show your love for each other? In what ways do you demonstrate consideration for each other? How would others know you care about each other? If I were to ask your best friend about how you care about each other, what would they say? What sort of things do you do for each other?
Support In times of difficulty or need, family members are there for each other and assist, encourage, reassure and look out for one another.	Tell me of times when you as a family 'share the load'. How would an observer seeing your family know that you help each other? Can you think of ways you look out for each other? What does it mean in your family to be 'there for each other'? In what ways do you encourage others to try new things?
Communication Family communication is a strength, especially when it is frequent, positive, open and honest. It is enhanced by complimenting each other, avoiding blame, compromising when there are disagreements, and shared humour.	When do you listen to each other? Tell me about when you talk openly with each other. Tell me about some of the times when you laugh together.

Table 9.3 *(cont.)*

Family quality	Possible assessment questions
Acceptance Family members acknowledge, value and tolerate each other's individuality and uniqueness, and show respect, appreciation and understanding.	In what ways do you accept your individual differences? When are you most likely to give each other space? How do you show the members of your family that you respect each other's point of view? What does forgiveness of each other look like in your family? What different responsibilities does each of you have?
Commitment Dedication and loyalty towards the family is an important strength during challenging times. Commitment is expressed in many ways – to the family as a whole, within the partner relationship, towards children and to extended family or community.	When do you feel safe and secure with each other? How would others know that you trust each other? List some of the things your family does for your community. What rules do you have in your family and how should these be followed during this admission?
Resilience Families and their members have an ability to withstand setbacks and crises, and can adapt, thrive and grow even in the most difficult of circumstances.	In what ways has this admission changed your plans? What helps keep each other hopeful? Can you tell me about when your family pulled together in a crisis? When you have a problem, what helps you discuss your problems? What do other people say they admire in your family?
Spiritual wellbeing The family's and its members' perceived relationship with a higher being, sense of life purpose and satisfaction.	Is spiritual wellbeing an important strength for your family? What do you do as a family to maintain your spiritual wellbeing? Would you like help to maintain any of your spiritual activities during this admission/time of healthcare?

Source: Adapted from Defrain & Asay (2007); Geggie et al. (2000); Marrone et al. (2008); Smith (2008); Smith & Ford (2013).

These qualities include:

- togetherness
- sharing activities
- affection
- support
- communication

- acceptance
- commitment
- resilience (Smith & Ford, 2013).

Following evaluation of the first version of the assessment guide, spiritual wellbeing was added as a family strength (Smith and Ford, 2013).

Stressors

Contemporary families cope with many day-to-day stressors. As already mentioned, a common stressor for modern families is balancing working life with the constant demands of raising children. However, there are more profound stressors that bring about change within a family unit. These can have a significant impact on a child's development and a family's resilience. The family's strength and capacity to cope are important protective factors.

Such stressors can be major life events, such as a death within the family or parental conflict. Other lifetime stressors include a family member affected by a serious chronic disease, low socioeconomic status, environmental events, major life transitions and historic events. High family stress correlates with a lower satisfaction with life for young people (Chappel, Suldo & Ogg, 2014). There is a strong understanding that accumulated stressors and unrelieved stress can intensify the burden of stress. If children and their families do not adapt well to stress that comes with the uncertainty of illness and possible other stressors, the situation can lead to academic, interpersonal and emotional difficulties later in life, and reduce adult opportunities (Valdez, Chavez & Woulfe, 2013). Therefore, it is important for nurses to guide families, recognise stress and work with them towards positive coping strategies and family resilience.

Coping strategies

Each family has its own culture and ways of managing stress, and will thus develop its own coping skills and capacity to problem-solve. When faced with stressors such as the experience of a severely or chronically ill child, family members may react in different ways. Coping is defined by Friedman et al. (2003, p. 466) as 'problem solving efforts by an individual'. These can be positive or negative. Coping was originally conceptualised as being either **emotion-focused coping** or **problem-focused coping**, with the first involving the regulation of negative emotions using strategies such as distancing, seeking emotional support or avoidance. The second type of coping involves a planned approach to addressing the problem using information-seeking and decision-making (Folkman, 2013). More recently, a third type of coping, known as **meaning-focused coping**, has been proposed. This type of coping draws upon inner beliefs and values, revising goals, focusing on the strengths obtained through experience and a reorganising of priorities (Folkman, 2013).

As mentioned earlier in this chapter, families have strengths that will enable them to develop coping skills when faced with stress. The Australian Family Strengths Assessment Guide can be used to identify these strengths to enhance family coping when a child or young person is experiencing illness (Smith & Ford, 2013). Understanding the context of the family and the way each member of the family is situated in that family

Emotion-focused coping – A style of coping where individuals use strategies such as distancing, seeking emotional support or avoidance in order to manage negative emotions.

Problem-focused coping – A style of coping where individuals take a planned approach to addressing problems, using strategies such as information-seeking and decision-making.

Meaning-focused coping – A style of coping often found among individuals encountering life-changing events, such as critical illness or the loss of a family member. Individuals draw upon their inner beliefs and values, revise goals, focus on the strengths gained from the life experience and reorganise their priorities.

group may also assist you to identify and justify the coping strategies employed by that family and provide guidance towards positive coping strategies.

Gender is an important influence when it comes to coping, and mothers and fathers may have quite different coping styles (Brown et al., 2013). For example, in a study of parents with a child diagnosed with developmental delay, mothers tended to engage in emotion-focused coping whereas fathers used a more cognitive and logical style of coping (Barak-Levy & Atzaba-Poria, 2013).

Families cope with stress in many ways. Table 9.4 summarises some of the coping strategies that can be seen in families experiencing stressful situations. You will notice some similarities in relation to family coping with the family strengths discussed earlier.

Table 9.4 Family stress, coping and adaptation

Effective or adaptive coping strategies		Ineffective or maladaptive coping strategies
Developing enhanced relationships within the family: • relying on each other • strengthening cohesion • developing flexible roles	Family social supports: • use of relatives and extended family as support • seeking advice from relatives • practical support from relatives	Denial of family problems and reactive behaviours, such as: • emotional exploitation • blaming (scapegoating) • use of family myths that 'obscure reality and deny real issues' • triangulating of communication – using a third person to choose sides • authoritarianism
Cognitive strategies: • being as 'normal' as possible • passive acceptance • 'reframing' expectations and maintaining a positive outlook • joint problem-solving • being highly informed	Social support of friends: • seeking encouragement and support of friends • sharing concerns with friends • seeking information/advice from friends, particularly those who have experienced similar problems	Family dissolution and addiction: • use of alcohol • use of drugs • use of gambling, leading to family psychosocial issues of loss, abandonment and breakdown
Communication strategies: • honesty and openness • use of humour and laughter	Maintaining links in the community: • self-help groups • spiritual supports, including religious affiliations • more recently, social media networks	Family violence: • partner abuse • child abuse or neglect • sibling abuse or neglect • parent abuse

Source: Adapted from Friedman et al. (2003).

Clearly, families employ both positive and negative coping strategies when faced with stress. The chronic illness of a child may cause families to react with confusion, sadness, anger and anxiety (Johnson & Mendoza, 2018). Families can work through these feelings to develop adaptive mechanisms to cope with the 'new normal'. It is important to identify a family's strengths and their available resources to guide them towards positive coping adaptation (Holtslander, Solar & Smith, 2013). Supported and resourced families working together through the child's illness experience have strengthened resilience and greater ability to cope with stress (Nabors et al., 2018).

CASE STUDY 9.3 AUDREY

You are working in a small hospital in a rural area. Audrey is an 8-year-old girl who has been brought to the hospital by ambulance following a severe asthma attack at her home during the night. This is her fourth admission for asthma in the last six months, and she has missed her last two scheduled outpatients appointments.

Audrey is not accompanied by her mother in the ambulance. Her mother, Conchetta, arrives about an hour and a half later with her three younger children. Conchetta discloses that she could not come in the ambulance as her husband, Trevor, is a fly-in, fly-out mine worker, currently away on a week-long shift.

Conchetta, 28, arrived in Australia six years ago from the Philippines with her daughter, Audrey, and is now married to Trevor, 53. They have since had three more children, now aged 3 years, 2 years and 6 months. The family is renting a house on 2 hectares of land in a rural area about 30 minutes' drive outside a small town. Conchetta states, 'This always happens when Trevor is away. I find it very difficult to cope with all the children when he's away. He is very helpful when he is home. I don't know how I am going to spend time with Audrey this time in the hospital.' Conchetta has no other family in Australia, but reports a close relationship with her church, and says she has a friend 2 kilometres away with whom she is quite friendly, and a sister-in-law who provides occasional help with the children.

Considerations and challenges in conducting family assessments

Performing effective family assessments is vital to plan and provide appropriate nursing care (Wright & Leahy, 2013). Family assessment is often complex, but it is fundamental if we are to provide family-centred care and meet the needs of the child and their family.

However, it is often difficult in the context of nursing practice to perform effective family assessment. There can be many reasons for this. A detailed effective assessment requires the appropriate environment and space to undertake effectively, which can be difficult to achieve in a busy clinical day (Marron & Maginnis, 2009). As with any assessment, interruptions must be minimised and an appropriate confidential environment is used to ensure privacy and comfort for the participants. The presence of the child or other children is often enough of a distractor without the busy clinical environment also impinging on the process. There are self-assessment tools that can be used, such as the McMaster Family Assessment Device. A shortened version of this tool has been found to be effective in a Western Australian study (Boterhoven et al., 2015). The study found that the self-assessment tool was accurate in validating the functioning of families. Using self-assessment tools could prove useful in busy clinical environments where nurses are time-poor.

CASE STUDY 9.4 KYLIE

Kylie is a 21-year-old mother to 6-month-old Skye, who has been admitted to the babies' ward with severe nappy rash. Kylie is a patient in a methadone program as she struggles to overcome her drug addictions. Her partner, Steve, is a recovering alcoholic and has sole custody of his 3-year-old son, Lucas. At 1 month of age, Skye was seen on a previous admission by the Suspected Child Abuse and Neglect (SCAN) team for failure to thrive. Kylie and Steve live in a caravan park an hour's drive from the hospital. In the few days since Skye's admission, you have heard other nurses making very critical and judgemental comments about Kylie and her parenting ability. You have noticed that Kylie hasn't been visiting as much during the day and did not stay overnight last night. When you ask Kylie how she's going, she bursts into tears and says, 'All you nurses are such bitches – you make out like I'm a bad mother and I don't need this crap. I'm taking Skye home right now. I don't care if it's against orders!'

When doing family assessments, it is necessary to form a therapeutic relationship with the family to encourage disclosure (Holtslander, Solar & Smith, 2013). Many nurses report discomfort with approaching more difficult topics such as child abuse or domestic violence, which may make the parent feel uncomfortable or challenged (Marron & Maginnis, 2009). This can be difficult for the family member to discuss, and such a conversation may not be possible when the child or other family members are present. There can also be an emotional impact for you as the nurse, based on your own family experiences (Lee, Leung & Mak, 2012). You therefore need to be aware of your own feelings and prejudices when you are working with families, and alert for judgemental thinking and conversations. You need to avoid preconceived ideas about what families should be or how they should behave. Tweedlie and Vincent (2019) studied student nurses exposed to child abuse cases and found that acknowledgement of preconceived ideas about family, critical reflection on the experience and appropriate support to manage negative emotions were important.

When caring for children and families where domestic violence, substance abuse or child protection issues are present, it may be helpful to consider that such parents are experiencing their own multifaceted health problems, which are often the result of their own adverse life experiences. Many parents who are engaged with child-protection services have themselves been subjected to abuse or rejection as children, and are often marginalised as adults, and this behaviour can repeat over generations (Pasalich et al., 2019). While many parents with a history of child abuse do not abuse their own children, they can struggle with forming attachments and appropriate responses to the needs of their children (Pasalich et al., 2019).

Parents who have experienced abuse or neglect themselves may be at higher risk of perpetuating child abuse, and often have a negative response to support offered (Pasalich et al., 2019). In addition, mothers who are struggling with substance abuse have often been subjected to previous trauma in their lives, or may have mental health problems such as anxiety or depression (Cleveland & Gill, 2013). If they are met with poorer quality care or judgemental attitudes by healthcare professionals, this can worsen their vulnerability and sense of isolation and rejection, and lead to avoidance of services. Sadly, healthcare professionals working with these families have been found to be judgemental and perceived to be uncaring (Fraser et al., 2007; Maguire, 2014). The imperative for nurses to partner with these families cannot be understated in order to build parenting skills and to protect their children. This partnership requires a respectful and supportive relationship, working with the strengths of the family (Caneira & Myrick, 2015). The current approach to child abuse is to take a preventative role, by identifying and resourcing at-risk families (Caneira & Myrick, 2015).

The relationship between nurses and mothers can have a powerful effect on the mother–child relationship and engender greater confidence and assertiveness in the mothering role (Cleveland & Gill, 2013). Nurses who express caring attitudes towards both mother and baby, and who engage mothers in the care of their infant, are valued by mothers who are struggling with drug addiction. Conversely, non-verbal behaviours such as eye-rolling, obvious surveillance and judgemental conversations among staff are a heavy burden for mothers. These mothers perceive that nurses fail to see the person behind the drug addiction and don't notice their efforts to be a good mother (Cleveland & Gill, 2013).

Nurses can empower mothers by ensuring that they collaborating with them, rather than treating them as if they are inferior. Reducing real or perceived power differentials is essential for an effective helping relationship (Caneira & Myrick, 2015). Working with drug-dependent parents can be very challenging, and healthcare professionals can find it difficult to support these families professionally. Given the stigma and the association of issues such as domestic violence, poverty and mental health problems with illicit drug dependence, acceptance is challenging for some healthcare professionals (Whittaker et al., 2016). Nurses can speak out against unprofessional care and encourage mothers to make formal complaints if they receive such care. Nurses can role-model their regard and respect for the dignity of mothers like Kylie in Case study 9.4. Nurses should also be encouraged to connect mothers like Kylie with supports who can continue to help them with their recovery from drug addiction alongside clinicians helping with parenting skills. Small gestures from the nurse, such as giving a mother praise for positive interactions and good parenting of their child, can also have a positive impact. Parents appreciate healthcare professionals who are respectful and supportive (Caneira & Myrick, 2015). Further, it is recognised that parenting can be an opportunity for positive change with the appropriate supports (Whittaker et al., 2016).

Nurses should not make assumptions about families based on gender, culture, ethnic, political, socioeconomic or religious background. These groups are not homogeneous, but instead enjoy great diversity (Manchester, 2013). However, these considerations can be incorporated into your family assessment. Culture is not necessarily linked to ethnicity, although this is a common belief (Manchester, 2013). We are all members of many cultures, and this will change as we move through life stages, and our interactions with others and needs alter (Friedman, Bowden & Jones, 2003). For example, as a nursing student you are part of the university culture and way of life, and you will move into the workplace culture when you graduate. You will move through many different cultures and experience many people in your personal and professional life.

Developing an understanding of the individual family's cultural, ethnic and spiritual perspective will assist you to understand the family and their needs, and the ways these factors contribute to care planning. Asking open-ended questions can lead to deeper exploration of these topics and a greater respect for diversity. This will help you to understand the family's needs and how members make decisions to provide culturally safe, sensitive and individualised care.

As a paediatric nurse, you need to identify those children and families requiring detailed family assessment. This may involve collaborating with or referral to other health professionals – particularly social workers, who are experts in interviewing and family assessment.

SUMMARY

- When a child is hospitalised, they not only need to adapt to stressors and pain associated with their injury, illness and course of treatment; they also experience separation from their family and a loss of control, and they encounter health professionals who are, in the main, strangers to them.
- Psychosocial responses to stress will depend on the child's growth, stage of development, maturity, family factors and the repertoire of previous similar experiences.
- In this chapter, we have used a framework of psychosocial development to present responses to illness experiences for children and young people. Using respectful and therapeutic strategies to ameliorate the negative impacts of illness and hospitalisation for the child and family is a key responsibility of paediatric nurses.
- The Family Partnership Model and family-centred care are two models that recognise the centrality of families in paediatric nursing. The approaches encourage nurses to work in partnership with families to ensure optimal health outcomes for the child and their family.
- Family assessment is integral to the effective psychosocial care of children and families. The principles of family assessment incorporate consideration of family composition, structure, functioning, family development/life-cycle stage, family strengths and resilience, member roles and life experiences, stressors and coping strategies.

LEARNING ACTIVITIES

9.1 Describe the major stress-related factors for a hospitalised child. What responses to separation are expected? Discuss in relation to the developmental stage of the child.

9.2 Explain the potential reactions you will encounter in response to injury and pain:
- for an infant
- for a toddler
- for a school-aged child
- for a child older than 12.

9.3 What reactions might parents or caregivers and siblings have to the hospitalisation of their child or sibling?

9.4 What strategies can the paediatric nurse implement to ameliorate the effect of hospitalisation on the child and family? Consider siblings in your answer.

9.5 Re-read Case study 9.3.
- Draw a genogram of this family's structure. Try drawing an ecomap of Conchetta's support system.
- Based on your reading so far, what family life-cycle stage is this family in?
- What are the stressors for both Audrey and Conchetta? Write these down and consider how understanding these stressors may be useful when planning care for Audrey and her family.

FURTHER READING

The companion paediatric skills text has a whole chapter dedicated to caring for adolescents, and is worthwhile reading to further your understanding of the needs of young people experience illness. In addition, there are web resources including a case study of a young person with cystic fibrosis.

Hutchinson, L & Fraser, J 2018, Adolescent nursing skills, in E Forster & JA Fraser (eds), *Paediatric nursing skills for Australian nurses*, Cambridge University Press, Melbourne.

Caring for infants when parents are experiencing or recovering from drug addiction can be challenging for paediatric nurses. For further insights into the pathophysiology of drug addiction and the need to respond compassionately to families see the following article:

Maguire, D 2014, Drug addiction in pregnancy: Disease not moral failure, *Neonatal Network*, 33(1), pp. 11–18.

REFERENCES

Ainsworth, MDS, Blehar, MC, Waters, E & Wall, S 1978, *Patterns of attachment: A psychological study of the strange situation*, Lawrence Erlbaum, Hillsdale, NJ.

Aldiss, S, Cass, H, Ellis, J & Gibson, F 2016, 'We sometimes hold on to ours': Professionals' views on factors that both delay and facilitate transition to adult care, *Frontiers in Pediatrics*, 4, pp. 125–37.

Anderson, K. Anderson, L. & Glanz, W. 1998, *Mosby 's medical, nursing, and allied health dictionary*, Elsevier, St Louis, MI.

Australian Institute of Professional Counsellors (AIPC) 2012, *Trends and statistics of the contemporary family,* viewed 24 March 2014, www.aipc.net.au/articles/trends-and-statistics-of-the-contemporary-family.

Barak-Levy, Y & Atzaba-Poria, N 2013, Paternal versus maternal coping styles with child diagnosis of developmental delay, *Research in Developmental Disabilities,* 34(6), pp. 2040–6.

Barnett, MA, Neppl, TK, Scaramella, LV, Ontai, LL & Conger, RD 2010, Grandmother involvement as a protective factor for early childhood social adjustment, *Journal of Family Psychology,* 24(5), pp. 635–45.

Beardon, DJ, Feinstein, A & Cohen, L 2012, The influence of parent preprocedural anxiety on child procedural pain: Mediation by child procedural anxiety, *Journal of Pediatric Psychology,* 37(6), pp. 680–6.

Bell, MF, Bayliss, DM, Glauert, R, Harrison, A & Ohan JL 2016, Chronic illness and developmental vulnerability at school entry, *Pediatrics,* 137(5), p. e20152475.

Bellis, MA, Hughes, K, Leckenby, N, Perkins, C & Lowey, H 2014, Measuring mortality and the burden of adult disease associated with adverse childhood experiences in England: a national survey, *Journal of Public Health,* 37(3), pp. 445–54.

Boterhoven de Hann, KL, Hafekost, J, Lawrence, D, Sawyer, MG & Zubrick, SR 2015, Reliability and validity of a short version of the general functioning subscale of the McMaster Family Assessment Device, *Family Process,* 54(1), pp. 116–23.

Bowlby, J 1951, *Maternal care and mental health,* World Health Organization, Geneva.

——1969, *Attachment and loss. Volume 1: Attachment,* Basic Books, New York.

——1988, *A secure base: Clinical applications of attachment theory,* Routledge, London.

Bratt, EL, Burström, A, Hanseus, K, Rydberg, A & Berghammer, M 2017, Do not forget the parents: Parents' concerns during transition to adult care for adolescents with congenital heart disease, *Child: Care, Health and Development,* 44(2) pp. 278–84.

Bretherton, I 1992, The origins of attachment theory: John Bowlby and Mary Ainsworth, *Developmental Psychology,* 28, 759–75.

Brown, F, Whittingham, K, Boyd R & Sofronoff, K 2013, Parenting a child with traumatic brain injury: Experiences of parents and health professionals, *Brain Injury,* 27(13–14), pp. 1570–82.

Burns-Nadar, S, Hernadez-Reif, M & Porter, M 2014, The relationship between mothers' coping patterns and children's anxiety about their hospitalization as reflected in drawings, *Journal of Child Health Care,* 18(1), pp. 6–18.

Caneira, L & Myrick, K 2015, Diagnosing child abuse: The role of the nurse practitioner, *The Journal for Nurse Practitioners,* 11(6), pp. 640–6.

Chappel, AM, Suldo, S & Ogg, JA 2014, Association between adolescents' family stressors and life satisfaction, *Journal of Child & Family Studies,* 23, pp.76–84.

Children's Hospital Foundation, 2021, Juiced TV: The TV show made by the kids in hospital, for the kids in hospital, viewed 20 February 2021, www.childrens.org.au/what-we-do/patient-and-family-support/juiced-tv/?cli_action=1616632739.232#tabs-2

Cleveland, L & Gill, S 2013, Try not to judge: Mothers of substance-exposed infants, *American Journal of Maternal Child Nursing,* 38(4), pp. 200–5.

Cooklin, AR, Westrupp, EM, Strazdins, L, Giallo, R, Martin, A & Nicholson, M 2016, Fathers at work: Work–family conflict, work–family enrichment and parenting in an Australian cohort, *Journal of Family Issues,* 37(11), pp. 1611–35.

Coyne, I 2015, Families and health-care professionals' perspectives and expectations of family-centred care: Hidden expectations and unclear roles, *Health Expectations*, 18(5), pp. 796–808.

Coyne, I, O'Neill, C, Murphy, M, Costello, T & O'Shea, R 2011, What does family-centred care mean to nurses and how do they think it could be enhanced in practice?, *Journal of Advanced Nursing*, 67(12), pp. 2561–73.

Davis, H, Day, C & Bidmead, C 2002, *Working in partnership with parents: The parent advisor model*, Psychological Corporation, London.

Davis, H, Day, C, Bidmead, C, MacGrath, M & Ellis, M 2007, *Current family partnership model,* Centre for Parent and Child Support, London.

DeFrain, A & Asay, S 2007, *Strong families around the world: Strengths-based research and perspectives*, Haworth Press, New York.

Ernst, M, Brähler, E, Klein, EM, Jünger, C, Wild, PS, Faber, J, Schneider, A & Beutel, ME 2019, Parenting in the face of serious illness: Childhood cancer survivors remember different rearing behavior than the general population, *Psycho-oncology*, 28(8), pp. 1663–70.

Erikson, EH 1968, *Identity youth and crisis*, WW Norton, New York.

Falvo, D 2013, *Medical and psychosocial aspects of chronic illness and disability* (4th ed.), Jones & Bartlett Learning, Boston.

Flynn, KE, Kliems, H, Saoji, N, Svenson, J & Cox, ED 2018, Content validity of the PROMIS [R] pediatric family relationships measure for children with chronic illness, *Health and Quality of Life Outcomes,* 16(1) pp. 203–11.

Flynn, S & McGregor, C 2017, Disabled children and child protection: Learning from literature through a non-tragedy lens, *Child Care in Practice : Northern Ireland Journal of Multi-disciplinary Child Care Practice*, 23(3), p. 258.

Folkman, S 2013, Stress, coping and hope, in BI Carr & J Steel (eds), *Psychological aspects of cancer*, Springer, New York, pp. 119–27.

Fowler, C, Rossiter, C, Bigsby, M & Dunston, R 2012, Working in partnership with parents: The experience and challenge of practice innovation in child and family health nursing, *Journal of Clinical Nursing*, 21, pp. 3306–14.

Fraser, JA, Barnes, M Biggs, HC & Kain, VJ 2007, Caring, chaos and the vulnerable family: Experiences in caring for newborns of drug-dependent parents, *International Journal of Nursing Studies*, 44(8), pp. 1363–70.

Frederick, J, Devaney, J & Alisic, E 2019, Homicides and maltreatment-related deaths of disabled children: A systematic review, *Child Abuse Review*, 28, pp. 321–38.

Friedman, MM, Bowden, VR & Jones, EG 2003, Family stress, coping and adaptation, in MM Friedman, VR Bowden & EG Jones, *Family nursing: Research, theory and practice*, Pearson Education, Englewood Cliffs, NJ, pp. 463–510.

Gabb, J & Singh, R 2015a, The uses of emotion maps in research and clinical practice with families and couples: Methodological innovation and critical inquiry, *Family Process*, 54(1), pp. 185–97.

—— 2015b, Reflections on the challenges of understanding racial, cultural and sexual differences in couple relationship research, *Journal of Family Therapy*, 37, pp. 210–27.

Geggie, J, DeFrain, J, Hitchcock, S & Silberberg S 2000, *The family strengths research report,* Family Action Centre, University of Newcastle.

Guite, JW, Russell, BS, Homan, KJ, Tepe, RM & Williams, SE 2018, Parenting in the context of children's chronic pain: Balancing care and burden, *Children (Basel)*, 5(12), p. 161.

Hayes, A, Weston, R, Qu, L & Gray, M 2010, *Families then and now 1980–2010*, AIFS, Melbourne.

Helgeson,VS, Honcharuk, E, Becker, D, Escobar, O & Siminerio, L 2011, A focus on blood glucose monitoring: Relation to glycemic control and determinants of frequency, *Pediatric Diabetes*, 12, pp. 25–30.

Holtslander, L, Solar, J & Smith, NR 2013, The 15-minute interview as a learning strategy for senior undergraduate nursing students, *Journal of Family Nursing*, 19(2), pp. 230–48.

Johnson, EJ, & Mendoza, SO 2018, Care-giving coping strategies among mothers with chronically ill children, *Journal of Social Service Research*, 44(3), pp. 400–13.

Kuo, DZ, Houtrow, AJ, Arango, P, Kuhlthau, KA, Simmons, JM & Neff, JM 2012, Family-centred care: Current applications and future directions in pediatric health care, *Maternal Child Health Journal*, 16, pp. 297–305.

Lambert, V, Coad, J, Hicks, P & Glacken, M 2013, Social spaces for young children in hospital, *Child: Care, Health and Development*, 40(2), pp. 195–204.

Lee, ACK, Leung, SSK & Mak, YW 2012, The application of family-nursing assessment skills: From classroom to hospital ward among final-year nursing undergraduates in Hong Kong, *Nurse Education Today*, 32, pp. 78–84.

Lerwick, JL 2013, Psychosocial implications of pediatric surgical hospitalization, *Seminars in Pediatric Surgery*, 22(3), pp. 129–33.

Lulgjuraj, D & Maneval, RE 2021, Unaccompanied hospitalized children: An integrative review, *Journal of Pediatric Nursing*, 56, pp. 38–46.

Lum, A, Wakefield, CE, Donnan, B, Burns, MA, Fardell, JE & Marshall GM 2017, Understanding the school experiences of children and adolescents with serious chronic illness: A systematic meta-review, *Child: Care, Health & Development*, 43 (5), pp. 645–62.

Maguire, D 2014, Drug addiction in pregnancy: Disease not moral failure, *Neonatal Network*, 33(1), pp. 11–18.

Manchester, A 2013, Cultural safety should be reviewed, *Kai Tiaki Nursing New Zealand*, 19(9), p. 14.

Marron, CA & Maginnis, C 2009, Implementing family health assessment: Experiences of child health nurses, *Neonatal, Paediatric and Child Health Nursing*, 12(1), pp. 3–8.

Marrone, C, Lane, T, Deal, R, Silberberg, S & University of Newcastle (NSW) Family Action Centre 2008, *Our scrapbook of strengths: strong families, strong communities* (2nd ed.), St Luke's Innovative Resources, Bendigo, Vic, pp. 12–15.

McCaffery, M 1968, *Nursing practice theories related to cognition, bodily pain and man–environment interactions*, UCLA Students Store, Los Angeles.

McGoldrick, M, Carter, B & Garcia-Preto, NA 2011, *The expanded family life cycle: Individual, family, and social perspectives* (4th ed.), Allyn and Bacon, Boston.

Mikkelsen, G & Frederiksen, K 2011, Family-centred care of children in hospital: A concept analysis, *Journal of Advanced Nursing*, 67(5), pp. 1152–62.

Morawska, A, Calam, R & Fraser, J 2014, Parenting interventions for childhood chronic illness: A review and recommendations for intervention design and delivery, *Journal of Child Health Care*, 19(1), pp. 5–17.

Munns, A & Shields, L 2013, Indigenous families' use of a tertiary paediatric hospital in Australia, *Nursing Children and Young People*, 25(7), pp. 16–23.

Nabors, L, Cunningham, JF, Lang, M, Wood, K, Southwich, S & Stough, CO 2018, Family coping during hospitalization of children with chronic illnesses, *Journal of Child and Family Studies*, 27, pp. 1482–91.

National Child Traumatic Stress Network 2016, *Health care tool box: Guide to helping children and families with illness and injury*, Children's Hospital of Philadelphia, Philadelphia, PA.

Neves, ET, Cabral, IE & da Silveira, A 2013, Family network of children with special needs: Implications for nursing, *Review Latino-Am Emfermagem*, 21(2), pp. 562–70.

Newman, BM & Newman, PR 2011, Is there a sensitive period for attachment?, in BM Newman & PR Newman, *Development through life: A psychosocial approach*, Wadsworth/Cengage, Belmont, CA, pp. 166–238.

Pao, M & Bosk, A 2011, Anxiety in medically ill children/adolescents, *Depression and Anxiety*, 28(1), pp. 40–9.

Park, H & Walton-Moss, B 2012, Parenting style, parenting stress, and children's health-related behaviours, *Journal of Developmental and Behavioral Pediatrics*, 33(6), pp. 495–503.

Pasalich, DS, Fleming, CB, Spieker, SJ, Lohr, MJ & Oxford, ML 2019, Does parents' own history of child abuse moderate the effectiveness of the Promoting First Relationships® intervention in child welfare?, *Child Maltreatment*, 24(1) pp. 56–65.

Pinquart, M 2013, Do the parent–child relationship and parenting behaviors differ between families with a child with and without chronic illness? A meta-analysis, *Journal of Pediatric Psychology*, 38(7), pp. 708–21.

—— 2014, Achievement of developmental milestones in emerging and young adults with and without pediatric chronic illness: A meta-analysis, *Journal of Pediatric Psychology*, 36(6), pp. 577–87.

Pinquart, M & Shen, Y 2011, Behavior problems in children and adolescents with chronic physical illness, *Journal of Paediatric Psychology*, 36(9), pp. 1003–16.

Pinquart, M & Teubert, D 2012, Academic, physical, and social functioning of children and adolescents with chronic physical illness: A meta-analysis, *Journal of Pediatric Psychology*, 37(4), pp. 376–89.

Shave, K, Ali, S, Scott, SD & Hartling, L 2018, Procedural pain in children: A qualitative study of caregiver experiences and information needs, *BMC Pediatrics*, 18(1), pp. 324–34.

Shields, L 2010, Questioning family centred care, *Journal of Clinical Nursing*, 7(18), pp. 2629–38.

Shields, L, Pratt, J & Hunter, J 2006, Family centred care: A review of qualitative studies, *Journal of Clinical Nursing*, 15(10), pp. 1317–23.

Shields, L, Zhou, H, Pratt, J, Taylor, M, Hunter, J & Pascoe, E 2012, Family-centred care for hospitalised children aged 0–12 years, *Cochrane Database of Systematic Reviews*, 10, CD004811.

Smith, BA & Kaye, DL 2012, Treating parents of children with chronic health conditions: The role of the general psychiatrist, *Focus*, 10, doi:10.1176/appi.focus.10.3.255

Smith, L 2008, Family assessment and the Australian Family Strengths Nursing Assessment Guide, in M Barnes & J Rowe (eds), *Child, youth and family health: Strengthening communities*, Churchill Livingstone, Sydney, pp. 11–14.

Smith, L & Ford, KM 2013, Family strengths and the Australian Family Strengths Nursing Assessment Guide (version 20, in M Barnes & J Rowe (eds), *Child, youth and family health: Strengthening communities* (2nd ed.), Elsevier, Sydney, pp. 11–18.

Svensson, B, Bornehag, CG & Janson, S 2011, Chronic conditions in children increase the risk for physical abuse – but vary with socio-economic circumstances, *Acta Paediatrica*, 100(3), pp. 407–12.

Tennant, M, McGillivray, J, Youssef, GJ, McCarthy, MC & Clark, T-J 2020, Feasibility, acceptability, and clinical implementation of an immersive virtual reality intervention to address psychological well-being in children and adolescents with cancer, *Journal of Pediatric Oncology Nursing*, 37(4), pp. 265–77.

Thabrew, H, Ruppeldt, P & Sollers, JJ 2018, Systematic review of biofeedback interventions for addressing anxiety and depression in children and adolescents with long-term physical conditions, *Applied Psychophysiology Biofeedback*, 43, pp. 179–219.

Tweedlie, J & Vincent, S 2019, Adult student nurses' experiences of encountering perceived child abuse or neglect during their community placement: Implications for nurse education, *Nurse Education Today*, 73, pp 60–4.

Valdez, CR, Chavez, T & Woulfe, J 2013, Emerging adults' lived experience of formative family stress: The family's lasting influence, *Qualitative Health Research*, 23(8), pp. 1089–1102.

White, K, Issac, MS, Kamoun, C, Leygues, J & Cohn, S 2018, The THRIVE model: A framework and review of internal and external predictors of coping with chronic illness, *Health Psychology Open*, 5(2), doi:10.1177/2055102918793552

Whittaker, A, Williams, N, Chandler, A, Cunningham-Burley, S, McGorm, K & Mathews, G 2016, The burden of care: a focus group study of healthcare practitioners in Scotland talking about parental drug misuse, *Health and Social Care in the Community*, 24(5), e72–e80.

Wright, LM & Leahey, M 2013, *Nurses and families: A guide to family assessment and intervention* (6th ed.), FA Davis, Philadelphia, PA.

The acutely ill or injured child and adolescent: Nursing assessment and interventions

10

Elizabeth Forster and Lee O'Malley

With acknowledgement to Nicola Brown,
Nerralie Shaw and Robyn Galway
for the second edition

LEARNING OBJECTIVES

In this chapter you will:

- Develop your understanding of the evidence-based nursing assessments and interventions used in the care of acutely ill infants, young children and adolescents
- Develop your understanding of the aetiology, signs and symptoms of key acute illnesses experienced by infants, young children and adolescents
- Consider the developmental needs of infants, young children and adolescents in the planning and implementation of nursing care
- Explore the impact of illness, injury and hospitalisation on infants and young children
- Gain an understanding of the nursing skills required for paediatric perioperative care

Introduction

Children contract infections regularly during early childhood, and thus can experience episodes of acute illness. They are also at greater risk of injury. For the most part, these episodes are of short duration and resolve with the care of parents at home, sometimes with support from community healthcare professionals such as a general practitioner. However, in some instances the illness can reach a level of severity that requires nursing care and medical treatment in a hospital setting. Children aged 0–4 years are the most common age group presenting to an emergency department (AIHW, 2018). Infants and children are still developing, so they have physiological and anatomical differences from adults that require specialist skills and knowledge. Hospital environments can be challenging for both the young child and their family. For many families, visiting the emergency department with their sick child or adolescent may be the first time they have ever had to seek acute care from a hospital. Adolescence is a complex and critical period of development, with significant social, emotional and physical changes. Similar to childhood, adolescent development and maturation is complex, and differs between individuals. It is most commonly considered the period between the onset of puberty and the time an individual is legally recognised as an adult – anywhere from 10 to 18 years. However, it is not one discrete period of development; there is considerable individual variation in development, and evidence that final brain development is not complete until the mid-twenties.

It is important that nurses understand this, and that we ensure the child's or adolescent's care is delivered in a way that is supportive and respectful of the individual and their family.

In Chapter 11, you will be introduced to primary assessment of infants and children, and recognition of the sick or deteriorating child. In this chapter, some key nursing considerations and interventions for the acutely unwell and injured child and adolescent will be discussed. Following this, you will explore some of the illnesses and injuries that children and adolescents can acquire, which may require hospital care. You will be asked to reflect on the nursing management of some of these conditions through review of case studies and reflective questions.

Key nursing considerations for the acutely unwell child and adolescent

The five most common illnesses with which paediatric patients present to emergency departments in Australia are: respiratory illnesses; infections and parasitic diseases; skin and subcutaneous tissue injuries; illnesses of the digestive system; and diseases of the musculoskeletal system and connective tissue (AIHW, 2018). The most common group of illnesses diagnosed in paediatric patients presenting to emergency departments is respiratory illnesses, with 195 566 (0–4 years) and 66 828 (5–14 years) presenting during 2017–18 (AIWH, 2018). In further review of this diagnostic group, the most common respiratory illnesses are upper respiratory tract infections (URTIs), croup, acute bronchiolitis and acute asthma.

In New Zealand, the reasons for paediatric presentations are similar, with asthma and wheeze, dental, acute URTIs (excluding croup), gastroenteritis and skin infections being the most common reasons for emergency department among 0–4-year-old Māori and non-Māori and non-Pacific children (Simpson et al., 2017). Rates of hospital presentation for Māori children aged 0–4 years are significantly higher than for non-Māori and non-Pacific children (Simpson et al., 2017). For Māori children aged 0–14 years, the most common health illness that is identified for hospital presentations is injury or poisoning, followed by respiratory illnesses such as bronchiolitis and asthma (Simpson et al., 2017). Dental and skin conditions also feature strongly among hospitalisations for 5–12-year-old children in New Zealand, and these rates are influenced by ethnicity, with rates being higher among Māori and Pacific children compared with non-Māori and non-Pacific children. There are also differences related to rural or urban location (Hobbs, Tomintz & Kingham, 2019).

The second most common group of diagnoses of paediatric patients presenting to emergency departments comprises those with infections and parasitic diseases, which can be bacterial or viral. The most common causative pathogen in the viruses group is the Respiratory Syncytial Virus (RSV) within the respiratory illnesses group and Rotavirus as the most common pathogen in the digestive system causing gastroenteritis (Kesson, Benwell & Elliott, 2010; AIWH, 2018; RCHM, 2019). These viruses manifest in various symptoms experienced by children through signs of fever and dehydration, and more specifically for respiratory illnesses, the need for oxygenation support. For these illnesses, symptoms can include pain, nausea and difficulty/challenges in breathing.

In New Zealand, the most common cause of ambulatory sensitive hospitalisation, including via the emergency department, among 0–4-year-olds is asthma and wheeze, with dental conditions the second most common cause (Simpson et al., 2017). This is followed by acute upper respiratory tract infections (excluding croup) (Simpson et al., 2017). Communicable diseases are still one of the most common causes for hospitalisations in New Zealand up to 15 years of age, with respiratory infections 'among the top 10 leading conditions in this age group, especially in infants' (Ministry of Health, 2020, p. 46).

The most commonly diagnosed illnesses in children and their causative pathogens include *Escherichia coli* in urinary tract infections and *Staphylococcus aureas* in respiratory infections and skin conditions such as eczema and impetigo (Desai, Gilbert & McBride, 2016; RCHM, 2018). Again, with this diagnostic group of illnesses, the most commonly experienced signs and symptoms identified in paediatric patients include fever, dehydration, and pain and discomfort. It is these categories that will now be discussed further relative to the different illnesses introduced here.

Fever

Fever is a common and normal response to infection; however, the mechanisms by which fever occurs are still not fully understood (Meremikwu & Oyo-Ita, 2009a). What is known is that infection by organisms such as viruses or bacteria can stimulate the release of pyrogenic cytokines, which stimulate the pre-optic area of the hypothalamus via humeral and neural pathways to raise body temperature to a higher level than normal (Ogoina, 2011). At a higher body temperature, it seems that the environment for replication of bacteria and viruses can become unfavourable and that immunological factors in the blood, such as white blood cells, may be enhanced (Ogoina, 2011). The fact that fever may be a normal and potentially beneficial response to invasion by pathogens has influenced current practice in the care of children with fever.

In most cases, measurements around 38°C (centrally measured) and higher are regarded as a fever. Key issues in the monitoring and management of fever in children include definitions of normal body temperature and fever. It is generally accepted that the mean range of normal body temperature is 36.5–37.5°C (Forbes, 2013); however, there is some variation in temperature between individuals and the site of measurement. For example, temperature measurements via the axilla site will be cooler than temperature measurements made via more central sites such as the frontal lobe or tympanic membrane. The variations in range between sites can present an issue when monitoring a trend in temperature over time. It is essential that the site of measurement and the thermometry equipment used are consistent in order to ensure accurate monitoring of temperature.

The management of fever has not always been based on the best available evidence. The decision to tolerate or treat fever in children traditionally has been controversial. Fever can contribute to the discomfort of illness for children, and can cause anxiety for parents (Walsh, Edwards & Fraser, 2008); as a result, healthcare professionals and parents can feel the need to intervene. However, traditional methods of intervening to reduce fever, such as non-pharmacological methods of tepid sponging and fans, may not be appropriate and are not recommended (Meremikwu & Oyo-Ita, 2009b; Watts & Robertson, 2012). If intervention is warranted – for example, pain relief for discomfort for a sore throat – then anti-pyretic medication may be required. It is more important to maintain the child's level of comfort with supportive rest, keeping them covered in light clothing and wiping perspiration away from the face with a slightly warm cloth, not a cool or cold cloth (RCHM, 2020). Attempts to reduce a child's fever won't help in treating the underlying illness; instead, the fever helps the body's immune system to fight the infection (RCHM, 2020).

Fever also causes metabolic effects, such as increased heart and respiratory rates, so a greater need for oxygen and fever can also result in the use of proteins rather than glucose for energy. This can lead to protein and fat breakdown (Balli & Sharan, 2020). These effects of fever may not be desirable in ill paediatric patients who are, for example, in respiratory distress with an increased need for maintaining adequate oxygenation or who are ill and therefore have increased caloric requirements.

Anti-pyretic medications –
These include paracetamol and non-steroidal anti-inflammatory medications such as ibuprofen; they are used to reduce fever.

Anti-pyretic medications are generally considered 'safe' medications and are widely available without prescription. Yet the use of anti-pyretic medications such as paracetamol or ibuprofen to reduce fever (Crook, 2010) is not entirely without risk (Meremikwu & Oyo-Ita, 2009b; van den Anker, 2013), particularly when the dosage recommendation is exceeded. For example, over-dosing on paracetamol can cause liver damage and over-dosing on ibuprofen can lead to renal dysfunction. The action of anti-pyretic medications is not fully understood, but it is postulated that these medications work by reducing the 'set point' of the hypothalamic control of body temperature (Rang, Dale & Ritter, 2011). Generally, aspirin should not be used in children due to concerns about the relationship between the use of aspirin and either influenza or varicella, and the development of Reye's Syndrome – a life-threatening illness (Butters, Curtis & Burgner, 2020). However, aspirin has been prescribed for children with Kawasaki disease, which causes vasculitis of small and medium-sized blood vessels and can lead to coronary artery aneurysms (Butters, Curtis & Burgner, 2020).

Dehydration

Dehydration is a common reason for presenting to hospital or community healthcare, and the most common condition causing dehydration is acute gastroenteritis.

Dehydration from acute gastroenteritis is a leading cause of mortality for children in developing countries (WHO & UNICEF, 2013). Viral gastroenteritis causes injury to the small bowel, resulting in low-grade fever and increased fluid losses through vomiting and diarrhoea (Prisco et al., 2020). Children can also develop bacterial gastroenteritis, primarily through food poisoning. There is an additional risk that bacterial gastroenteritis can progress to become a more systemic infection, resulting in sepsis and shock (Dalby-Payne & Elliott, 2011).

Additional clinical conditions that may also result in dehydration in paediatric patients include diabetic ketoacidosis, cardiac, renal and liver disease, and it is also important to assess for dehydration in children undergoing surgery (Prisco et al., 2020). Additionally, although the focus of our discussion is dehydration, paediatric nurses need to be vigilant for over-hydration. This may be due, for example, to fluid overload due to intravenous fluid therapy in the paediatric patient. Meticulous daily fluid intake and output monitoring and recording are therefore needed, along with clinical assessment of the child (Forster & Scaini-Clarke, 2017).

Assessment of dehydration

Under-estimating the degree of dehydration and not replacing lost fluids and electrolytes can result in acidosis, electrolyte imbalance, renal damage or death. Consistent assessment of dehydration is a crucial step in determining required treatment and need for hospitalisation.

Several scales and algorithms have been developed to assess and treat dehydration. Commonly used assessment scales include the World Health Organization's (WHO) Scale, the Gorelick Scale and the Clinical Dehydration Scale (CDS) (Pringle et al., 2011). Each scale predicts the percentage of estimated weight loss due to fluid loss for different age groups. For example, the WHO and Gorelick Scales are used in children aged from 1 month to 5 years, and the CDS is used in children aged from 1 month to 3 years. Each scale assesses a range of clinical signs associated with dehydration. In Australia, some modifications of these scales have been developed by expert groups (see Table 10.1).

Essentially, the differences between mild, moderate and severe dehydration are based on changes in the signs of circulation – especially colour, heart rate, activity level, peripheral perfusion, urine output and blood pressure. Early signs of mild dehydration, such as pallor, dry mucous membranes and diminished urine output, are the result of compensatory mechanisms in response to decreased fluid volume. As dehydration becomes moderate and then severe, signs that the circulation is compromised become more apparent. Signs of moderate to severe dehydration include worsening colour, deterioration in level of consciousness, increasing tachycardia, decreased capillary refill, deterioration in skin turgor and lastly hypotension. Hypotension in infants and children is considered an ominous sign of severe dehydration, indicative of hypovolaemic shock.

Table 10.1 Commonly used scales for assessment of dehydration

	WHO	CDS	Gorelick	NSW Health
Age group	**1 month–5 years**	**1 month–3 year**	**1 month–5 years**	**Not stated**
Signs	Condition/level of consciousness	General appearance	General appearance	Lethargy
	Eyes (normal or sunken)	Eyes	Capillary refill	Capillary refill
	Thirst	Mucous membranes	Tears	Mucous membranes
	Skin pinch	Tears	Mucous membranes	Eyes
			Eyes	Breathing
			Breathing	Quality of pulses
			Quality of pulses	Skin turgor
			Skin elasticity	Heart rate
			Heart rate	Urine output
			Urine output	

Hydration and diet for children with acute gastroenteritis

Oral rehydration therapy (ORT) using commercially developed modified glucose and sodium solutions is one of the safest and most effective methods of treating mild to moderate dehydration caused by diarrhoea and vomiting (Dalby-Payne & Elliott, 2011). In most instances, ORT is used orally; it is given in small frequent amounts over several hours as a 'trial of oral fluids' to see whether increased fluid and electrolyte intake via the oral route can result in rehydration without the need for intravenous cannulation and fluid therapy (Santillanes & Rose, 2018). If vomiting persists or a child refuses to drink ORT, consideration may be given to administering ORT via a nasogastric tube. Prescription of oral ondansetron has also been shown to be effective in paediatric patients for managing nausea and vomiting (Santillanes & Rose, 2018).

For children with moderate to severe dehydration, intravenous fluids may be required. Children with clinical signs of severe dehydration, including hypotension, may require fluid resuscitation with fluid boluses to ensure adequate circulation and there are a number of algorithms governing intravenous fluid therapy for children and young people in hospital (NICE, 2009, 2020).

An early return to normal diet and the reintroduction of milk are now encouraged for infants and children with acute gastroenteritis once vomiting has subsided. Breastfeeding can continue through the illness period. Evidence suggests that early resumption of diet is associated with a reduction in number of bowel motions, reduced duration of illness and lower weight loss (NICE, 2009). There is growing interest in the use of probiotics in managing paediatric acute gastroenteritis, and evidence to date indicates some weak evidence for some strains of probiotics and some recommendations against the use of other strains (Szajewska et al., 2020). More research is needed in this area to determine the safety and effectiveness of probiotics in paediatric acute gastroenteritis (Szajewska et al., 2020).

Intravenous therapy

Restoration or maintenance of normal fluid and electrolyte balance is an essential component of care of the sick infant or child. For many reasons, infants or children may be unable to maintain a normal intake of fluids because they are sick, or because they are being kept nil by mouth. Children with acute illness frequently require intravenous access for a range of reasons, including the administration of fluids, medication, blood products and/or blood sampling. Most often, intravenous access for short-term use is obtained via peripheral venous cannulation. Obtaining and maintaining intravenous access in infants and children can be challenging for many reasons, including the smaller relative size of children's blood vessels and the fear, anxiety and pain caused by the procedure.

Generally, the site of intravenous cannulation is determined on the basis of the child's history and the type of medication or fluid that is to be administered (Rathnayake, 2012). In most instances, the first site of choice will be the dorsal aspect of the child's non-dominant hand. Other sites that may be considered are the wrist, leg, foot and scalp.

Topical anaesthetics (such as EMLA or amethiocaine) can be applied prior to cannulation to the site(s) of choice to reduce the pain associated with venipuncture, but these generally need to be applied 45 minutes to one hour before cannulation is attempted. Although there is good evidence that topical anaesthesia reduces the pain associated with venipuncture and cannulation (Rathnayake, 2012), some clinicians may elect not to use it as it may cause transient vasoconstriction of superficial vessels. However, results from the first prospective study to compare the success rate of cannulation with or without EMLA found no significant difference in success rate (Schreiber et al., 2013). While these results suggest that EMLA may not reduce the success of cannulation, further studies are required to confirm these findings and reduce clinicians' concerns.

Preparing the child and family for intravenous cannulation

Depending on the age of the child, their capacity to cooperate during cannulation may be limited by their development, and their feelings of fear and anxiety. It is important that these factors are taken into consideration when preparing the child and family. In the first instance, parental consent will need to be obtained for the procedure, and details of the approach to the procedure discussed initially with the parent, and then with the child using developmentally appropriate language. It may be necessary to hold the child or their limb during the procedure, and parents should be given a choice about their role in this. At a minimum, children will need their parent close by to provide comfort after the procedure. Partial wrapping of the child's body, leaving the limb intended for cannulation free, can help the parent to hold the child more easily during the procedure.

In addition to topical anaesthetics to reduce the pain of cannulation mentioned earlier, we should consider the use of distraction and other methods to reduce pain. For infants, parent presence, physical comfort and non-nutritive sucking with sucrose or a dummy are simple interventions that may provide comfort during the pain of cannulation. For children, looking at books, blowing bubbles, watching a movie or listening to music are some techniques that can be used.

Monitoring the intravenous site and infusion

Intravenous cannulation is painful and distressing for children, and may be technically difficult for clinicians, so protection of a patent cannula is essential. It is important that the child's developmental stage, the condition of their skin, the location of the site and the child's mobility are taken into consideration. The cannula is normally secured at the insertion site with sterile opaque dressing or tape, so the site can be visualised and monitored for inflammation, leaking and infiltration. Depending on the position of the site and the mobility of the limb, it may be necessary to splint the limb to ensure patency of the cannula. Accessing the intravenous line should be performed using an aseptic non-touch technique (NHMRC, 2010). The site should be checked frequently – up to hourly as required. An intravenous infusion pump is used to ensure the accurate rate of fluids is infused. Administration of intravenous fluids should be recorded accurately in the fluid balance chart, in addition to other fluid intake and output.

Extravasation occurs when fluids leak unintentionally from the cannulated blood vessel into surrounding tissues. This may occur due to dislodgment of the cannula from the vessel, or occlusion. The incidence of extravasation may be higher in children due to factors such as smaller, fragile vessels and the risk of child interference with the cannula. Even though the flow rates of fluid may be comparatively smaller in children, their smaller body mass means that the swelling associated with extravasation may cause a significant injury to the tissues if not recognised early. It is essential that when extravasation is suspected, the infusion should be stopped and the site of extravasation assessed to determine the severity of the injury. Awareness of the risk and management of extravasation is an important part of the skill of caring for a patient with an intravenous infusion.

Intravenous fluids: Types and volumes

Infants have higher total body water than older children and adults, and turn their body water over more frequently. In addition, infants have a higher body surface area: mass ratio and are therefore more susceptible to insensible fluid losses. As a result, accurate and careful calculation of fluid volumes is required. Infants and children are generally prescribed fluids based on body weight. Sometimes their fluids may be calculated based on body surface area. There are different methods for calculating fluid requirements, based either on total daily amounts or hourly amounts.

In addition to different fluid volumes, the types of intravenous fluids used in children are slightly different from those used for adults. Intravenous fluids used for maintaining hydration generally contain a mixture of sodium chloride and glucose. Younger infants have higher energy needs, so they may be prescribed a higher concentration of glucose than older infants and children. For intravenous rehydration fluids, generally 0.9 per cent sodium chloride with 5 per cent glucose is the fluid of choice (New South Wales Health, 2015).

Body surface area (BSA) – A calculation of the surface area of the human body, expressed in square metres. BSA may be calculated using software or a nomogram. In order to calculate BSA, an accurate weight and height/length of the patient are required.

Administering oral medications

For infants and children, the dose of medication prescribed is usually calculated based on weight. In some instances, **body surface area (BSA)** may be used to calculate medications.

In addition to the usual precautions taken in administering medications to anyone (right medication, right dose, right route, right time, right person), consideration needs to be given to the age and the development of the child. For example, infants are not able to swallow tablets, so wherever possible a liquid preparation of the oral medication would be preferred. The smaller size of children and the variation in size across age groups means that health professionals need to calculate doses and check prescribed doses of medication carefully. Other challenges in administering medication to children include identifying children who are pre-verbal. It is important that the identity of the child is confirmed, either by the parent or medical identification bracelet, prior to the administration of medications.

Not all oral medications may be available in liquid form. For advice on preparing solid oral medications for administration to infants or younger children, seek advice from a reputable medication information source such as the Children's Dosing Companion from the *Australian Medicines Handbook* (2017) or a pharmacist.

Administering oral medications to children can be challenging, especially if the child does not want to take the medication or the taste is unpleasant. Some children may be better with a medication spoon, but you may be more comfortable using a syringe – particularly when the child is younger or less cooperative. Wherever possible, nurses should try to make the experience positive.

For practical and comfort reasons, it is wise to sit the child in your lap for administration. It can help to tuck their arm closest to you behind your back and hold the other arm still. Gently administer the oral medication liquid into the mouth, along the inside of the cheek. Administer small amounts, allowing the child to swallow. If you try to administer too much at once, the child may spit it out. Encourage the child to swallow the medication and give a lot of positive feedback once the process is complete – even if it was a struggle!

REFLECTION POINTS 10.1

If a parent or carer is present, consider asking them to assist in administration of a medication as the child will be more likely to take the medication when it is given to them by someone they know. Inclusion of parent or carer supports family-centred care and assists in maintaining a therapeutic relationship between the nurse and the patient, particularly if the child is a toddler.

What could you do to provide that positive support and feedback to the child while the parent or carer is administering a medication?

- Even mild episodes of acute illness and fever can make us feel discomfort from pain such as headaches or myalgia.
- In some cases, where children are miserable but without a fever, or with only a mild fever, it can be more appropriate to give a medication such as paracetamol for its analgesic properties and the relief of pain and discomfort than to use it as an anti-pyretic.
- Consider any alternatives that can be used prior to administrating the medication, and what these may include. Who would you ask for further information to assist you?

For further information on the administration of medications and management of intravenous therapy in paediatric patients, see Forster, Maher and Patane (2018) and Brown and Green (2018) in the Further reading section.

Pain assessment and management

Pain is a common symptom of many childhood illnesses, so assessment of pain is a nursing priority. Assessment of pain in children can be challenging, and can only be truly expressed by the person experiencing it. Self-reporting is therefore the most accurate assessment. When caring for children, however, self-report may not be possible due to factors including the developmental age and a child who is not verbally communicating, language levels, previous experiences and cognitive development. Nurses can detect for changes in the child's facial expressions and behaviours, as well as physiological parameters, such as a rise in heart rate or changes in respiratory rates and patterns. However, these are not always reliable (Brummelte, Oberlander & Craig, 2014), as they may also be signs of the underlying illness. Therefore, inclusion of the parent/carer's interpretation of the non-verbal assessments of the non-verbal child as an indicator of pain is important, either from their previous identifications or from observed difference to the child's normal behaviour. Some children may deny pain if they have concerns that intervention by healthcare professionals may worsen pain or lead to procedures (such as cannulation) that may result in further pain. The three main approaches to the assessment of pain in children include self-reporting of pain by children or their parent/s, observation of behaviours and physiological signs that are known to reflect pain (APAGBI, 2012). No single pain-assessment tool can be recommended for use in all children. Recent evidence-based practice guidelines for pain management have made recommendations for the use of behavioural and self-report tools in the assessment of pain in children (see Table 10.2).

Table 10.2 Recommended measures for the procedural and postoperative pain assessment based on chronological age with no cognitive impairment

Child's age	Measure
Newborn–3 years	COMFORT or Revised Face Legs Arms Cry Consolability (FLACC) Scale
4 years	Revised Faces Pain Scale + COMFORT or FLACC
5–7 years	Revised Faces Pain Scale
7 years	Numerical rating scale, visual analogue scale or revised Faces Pain Scale
>7 years	Visual analogue scale

Note: The Revised FLACC Pain Scale has been validated for children with cognitive impairment (Beltramini et al., 2017).
Source: Adapted from APAGBI (2012).

Observational and behavioural pain-assessment tools

The signs and symptoms of pain can be similar to fear or distress, and at times it can be difficult for the practitioner to determine which of these they are observing. This can be particularly challenging in infants and younger, pre-verbal children. For these groups of children, observational and behavioural tools are used for pain assessment. Currently, the COMFORT and Face Legs Arms Cry Consolability (FLACC) scales are most commonly recommended for use as observational and behavioural pain-assessment tools.

The COMFORT behaviour scale was initially developed to assess distress in infants in the paediatric intensive-care setting (Ambuel et al., 1992), but has since been validated for the assessment of pain intensity and distress in other age groups, including ventilated adults in intensive care settings (Ashkenazy & DeKeyser-Ganz, 2011) and older infants and toddlers (van Dijk et al., 2000). The scale is based on behavioural and physiological signs. Scores are given for alertness, calmness, respiratory distress, crying, physical movement, muscle tone, facial tension, mean arterial pressure and heart rate.

The FLACC scale is used to quantify pain behaviours in children. It was first developed for assessing post-operative pain in infants and children aged under 7 years (Merkel et al., 1997), and it has since been validated in other studies with similar-aged children (Manworren & Hynan, 2003; Willis et al., 2003), older children and adolescents (Nilsson, Finnstrom & Kokinsky, 2008), children with cognitive impairment (Malviya et al., 2006) and in one study of non-Western children (Bai et al., 2012). The FLACC scale requires the healthcare practitioner to assess the degree of tension evident in the face and legs, the level of activity, the extent of crying and how easily the infant or child can be consoled.

To assist in the pain assessment of children with cognitive impairment, the revised FLACC scale (r-FLACC) can be utilised and has been validated (Beltramini, Milojevic & Pateron, 2017).

Self-report tools

Self-report tools are commonly used in children over the age of 5 years, who are able to provide a verbal self-report of pain. While many self-report tools have been developed as a way to measure children's self-reporting of pain, not all are used effectively or consistently, or they lack repeated evaluation data. The self-report tools most commonly evaluated, used and recommended are the Faces Pain Scale – Revised (FPS–R), visual analogue scale (VAS) and numerical rating scores (NRS). For children older than 7 years, the visual analogue scale is considered the gold standard in pain assessment scales in children and is the most validated self-reporting pain tool recommended (Beltramini, Milojevic & Pateron, 2017).

Pain management

There are many different reasons why a child may experience pain. The pain may be acute, chronic or related to a procedure. Whatever the source of the pain, it is vital that pain is managed adequately so ongoing negative physiological and psychological impacts are minimised. Examples of these negative outcomes are changes in vital signs, fear, anxiety and developmental regression (Koller & Goldman, 2012;

Woragidpoonpol et al., 2013). Pain management, like pain assessment, will be individualised. The type and source of the pain will assist in determining the management and can be a mix of non-pharmacological and pharmacological methods.

Non-pharmacological pain management has been comprehensively researched, and can be used as an effective standalone measure or as an adjunct to pharmacological treatment (Woragidpoonpol et al., 2013; Wente, 2012; Koller & Goldman, 2012; Pillai Riddell et al., 2015; Srouji, Ratnaplan & Schneeweiss, 2010). Nurses are able to institute many common non-pharmacological measures, which can be a simple as swaddling, administration of sucrose prior to procedures, singing, holding and simple distraction with toys, games or books. Other more complex measures, such as guided imagery, breathing exercises, positive reinforcement and comfort positioning, can be implemented with the assistance of colleagues trained in these procedures.

Simple analgesics such as paracetamol and ibuprofen are frequently used as first-line pharmacological pain management for mild to moderate pain such as earache (otalgia) through to acute post-operative pain (Penrose, Palozzi & Dowden, 2013). These medications may be used under medical supervision in combination with each other or with opioids when pain is more severe (Bearde & Greco, 2011). Opioids such as morphine are recognised as safe and effective analgesics, and are available in many different preparations to enable effective delivery. Whether they are administered orally, rectally, via inhalation or intravenously, all children require close monitoring for side-effects such as sedation, respiratory depression, urinary retention, pruritus, and nausea and vomiting (Penrose, Palozzi & Dowden, 2013).

REFLECTION POINTS 10.2

- There are many validated pain-assessment tools available in various texts and clinical guidelines. Take time now to find a few, such as FLACC, FPS-R or VAS, and think about how they might be used when caring for a child with acute pain. For example, the FLACC scale is available on the companion website.
- Topical analgesia has been discussed in this chapter as an example of assisting in a painful procedure: cannulation. Take time to review this section again and reflect upon other combinations of pharmacological and non-pharmacological methods that you might use when caring for a child with pain.
- One of the more challenging aspects of caring for children can be communicating our intentions to perform procedures that may cause fear, anxiety or pain. When we plan to talk to children about a procedure such as intravenous cannulation, there are a number of issues to take into consideration:
  - their stage of cognitive development
  - their understanding of language – for example, whether their primary language is the same as ours
  - the presence of parents
  - the timing of the information
  - prior experiences of painful or distressing procedures.

Discuss the implications of each of these when undertaking a procedure on a child.

Regional anaesthesia, which is the administration of local anaesthetic, is also an effective method to address acute pain. This method is often used post-surgery, either into the epidural space for pain relief below the waist or peripherally into a nerve plexus. It provides complete blockage of pain transmission.

All methods of pain management have protocols to ensure safe and effective care. Healthcare facilities will specify nursing guidelines to adhere to. Before providing nursing care to children with complex pain management in place, it is the responsibility of each nurse to familiarise themselves with the pharmacokinetics and side-effects of all analgesic medications.

For further information regarding pain assessment and management for paediatric patients see Forster and Kotzur (2018) in the Further reading section.

Common acute illnesses in childhood and adolescence

Most children will experience short-term acute illnesses during childhood that resolve without the need for admission to hospital. However, for some the extent of the illness may be of sufficient severity to require admission to hospital. While it is beyond the scope of this chapter to cover all the illnesses that may require acute nursing and medical care in hospital, we will briefly explore some common conditions, including their likely causes, signs and symptoms. In consideration of why adolescents require admission to hospital, it is believed it is for reasons more likely related to an injury or chronic condition. While most injuries are mild and can be managed at home by parents, there are times when care and treatment for injury or illness results in the admission of the young person to hospital.

In the previous section, we discussed key interventions for children with acute illness, including management of fever, dehydration and pain management. This section presents case studies of children with common illnesses. Take some time to consider how the assessments and interventions we have explored previously may be used for children with the illnesses outlined below.

Febrile seizures

CASE STUDY 10.1 YING

Ying is an 18-month-old girl brought to the emergency department by her mother and father. Ying's mother explains that Ying has been vomiting sporadically for 12 hours and experienced a brief seizure at home. She is not sure how long the seizure lasted, but thinks it was less than a minute. Ying's father explains that during the seizure, Ying was staring, had rhythmic clenching of both fists and her body and limbs were rigid.

Ying is pale, sleepy and lethargic. She feels peripherally warm to touch. Her heart rate is 165/min, respiratory rate is 35/min, blood pressure 95/60 and temperature 39.0°C. Her mouth and lips are dry. Her parents report that she has not kept down any fluids for 12 hours. Each time Ying drinks fluids, she vomits, and she has only passed urine once since the vomiting began.

Approximately 2–5 per cent of children will experience a single, brief febrile seizure before the age of 5 years and it is the most common type of seizure experienced in this age group (Cullen, 2021). Typically, it will be a generalised tonic-clonic seizure, lasting only a minute or two. In most instances, the seizure is caused by a sudden rise in core body temperature. In infancy and early childhood, children are more susceptible to such seizure triggers, as the cerebral cortex is quite excitable, and consequently the threshold for a seizure is lower (Lux, 2010). However, in a few cases, repeated or longer seizures may indicate a more serious condition, such as meningitis or epilepsy (Lux, 2010). If an infant or child has a seizure, it is considered a medical emergency in the first instance.

Studies into the use of prophylactic treatment of febrile seizures do not support the use of anti-epileptic medications or anti-pyretic medications in simple febrile seizures (Cullen, 2021), particularly as some of the anti-epileptic medications have undesirable side-effects. More importantly, parents should be advised on the first aid response to a seizure, the risk of recurrence and when to seek medical advice. For most parents, their child's febrile seizure is their first experience ever of a seizure and can be a frightening experience. It is important that health professionals are sensitive to the distress that parents have experienced, even though the relative risk associated with a simple febrile seizure may be mild.

Acute respiratory illness

Acute respiratory illnesses that are characterised by some degree of upper or lower airway obstruction require nursing care and hospitalisation. The extent to which infants and children become unwell with respiratory illness can vary considerably between individuals and, depending on the cause and site of the obstruction, sick infants and children can further deteriorate in a relatively short timeframe, as outlined in Chapter 11.

Respiratory tract infections

As stated in the introduction to this chapter, respiratory tract illnesses and infections caused by viruses are a very common in children, particularly a child less than 4 years of age. In most instances, children have a mild illness that resolves within a few days, and some children will develop a severe infection that requires admission to hospital. Symptoms vary, depending on the site and cause of the infection, but in general children are more likely than adults to have symptoms of fever, discomfort and decreased fluid intake.

Croup

Croup (laryngotracheo-bronchitis) is the most common obstructive disorder of the upper airway, usually caused by viruses such as Para influenza types 1 and 2 (Schomacker et al., 2012; Woods, 2015). The signs of croup are characteristic – an inspiratory stridor, barking cough and onset in the evening and at night. In mild cases, these symptoms resolve within a few days. Nonetheless, the symptoms of croup can be frightening for the child and parent.

Croup is usually mild in children, and can be cared for at home, usually after review by a general practitioner. Children with moderate or severe croup require review and close monitoring by health professionals in an emergency department and may require admission. However, the early use of oral corticosteroids, which can quickly reduce the inflammation in the upper airways (usually by two hours post administration) and thus reduce obstruction, have significantly reduced the duration of hospital stay as well as re-presentations (Gates et al., 2018).

Any child with stridor requires close and careful monitoring and assessment, as it can worsen and lead to severe airway obstruction. Furthermore, stridor with drooling and without coughing may indicate the presence of epiglottitis or bacterial tracheitis (El Hitti, 2020; Tibballs & Watson, 2011), conditions associated with acute airway obstruction. Epiglottis is a medical emergency that requires immediate medical management for safe airway maintenance, preferably by an experienced paediatric medical team, and supplemental oxygen for hypoxia if tolerated by the child (El Hitti, 2020). It is vital to avoid upsetting the child, as anxiety can worsen respiratory distress (El Hitti, 2020).

It is essential to establish the extent of airway obstruction, as this is the main criterion for determining the degree of severity of illness in a child with croup; for this reason, very careful respiratory assessment is required (see Chapter 11). Children with croup are generally considered to have mild croup when they are interacting normally with parents and their environment. These children may have an audible inspiratory stridor when they are active, but the stridor is absent at rest. When stridor is present even at rest, then children are considered to have moderate croup. More severe croup is characterised by worsening airway obstruction, causing anxiety, sleepiness, marked tachycardia and pallor. Severe airway obstruction is an emergency, and intubation may need to be considered (Woods, 2015; Zoorob, Sidani & Murray, 2011).

Children with mild croup require close parental supervision and care at home. Historically, parents have often been advised to reduce stridor by exposing their child to a warm, humidified environment, such as a bathroom with a warm shower running, or steam inhalations. However, there is little evidence that this is effective, and there are also concerns that the use of steam inhalations increases the risk of burns and scalds (Fitzgerald & Kilham, 2003; Zoorob, Sidani & Murray, 2011). It is more important to ensure that parents are aware of, and watching for, the signs of increasing airway obstruction.

Medications are the mainstay of treatment for children with moderate and severe croup. The use of corticosteroids such as oral dexamethasone or nebulised budenoside in the management of croup has significantly reduced the length of time required in hospital for children with croup (New South Wales Health, 2010). Children with moderate and severe croup will generally be prescribed oral or nebulised corticosteroids (Mazza et al., 2008). Some children with mild croup may also be prescribed a single dose of oral corticosteroid (Russell et al., 2011). Nebulised adrenaline may be required to reduce bronchial and tracheal oedema in children with severe croup, and can rapidly reduce the symptoms of croup in 30 minutes (Bjornson et al., 2011). Further doses may be required after two hours.

Discharge from hospital can occur when no stridor is present. At the time of discharge, the parents should be provided with education or a fact sheet and have organised follow-up with a general practitioner (New South Wales Health, 2010).

Bronchiolitis

Bronchiolitis, a common respiratory illness in children less than 12 months, is a viral infection of the lower airways and can cause wheezing-like symptoms. Causation can be related to several viruses, including RSV, adenovirus, rhinovirus and influenza. Signs and symptoms of bronchiolitis include wheezing, difficult feeding, pallor and respiratory distress. For those who do experience respiratory distress, hypoxia, lethargy or inability to maintain adequate fluid intake due to poor feeding, admission to hospital will be required. Treatment is essentially supportive, and may include oxygen administration using various delivery devices to prevent hypoxia, intravenous fluids to maintain hydration or nasogastric feeding (Piedra & Stark, 2016). The Australasian Bronchiolitis Guidelines (PREDIC, 2016) outline the current recommendations for management of bronchiolitis. Case study 11.1 in Chapter 11 discusses the case of Maggie, an infant with bronchiolitis, and outlines the nursing management required.

CASE STUDY 10.2 LEILA

Leila is a 7-year-old girl brought into the emergency department by her parents one evening, complaining of a persistent dry cough and some difficulty with breathing. On assessment, it is identified that Leila looks tired in appearance, speaks in short phrases of no more than five words and has an audible expiratory wheeze when answering questions. She is sitting on the edge of the bed, leaning forward, and this position is the most comfortable for her to breathe.

On observation, she has clear nasal discharge and her mother states that she has had a runny nose the past two days and hasn't been sleeping due to her tight, dry cough. She has increased work of breathing with obvious nasal flaring, tracheal tug and intercostal recession. She is tachypnoeic and tachycardic, and oxygen saturations are measured at <92 per cent.

It is decided that Leila will be admitted into the short stay unit in the emergency department for further monitoring and treatment.

Asthma

Asthma is an inflammatory disorder of the airways, and is one of the most common paediatric emergency presentations in Australia and New Zealand. It can be an acute illness; however, with repeated acute episodes from exposure to triggers, asthma can become a chronic illness requiring long-term management (CHQ, 2019). It is a reversible airway obstruction that is characterised by airway inflammation, thickened mucous production and bronchospasm, leading to a narrowing of the airways that contributes to air trapping and reduced airflow (RCHM, 2018). Children who present to hospital with acute asthma experience symptoms such as a cough, audible wheeze and difficulty breathing or a feeling of tightness in the chest (National Asthma Council Australia, 2020). Signs of acute asthma in children include nasal flaring, tracheal tug and intercostal recession, with associated tachypnea and tachycardia. If untreated, the bronchospasm and bronchoconstriction contribute to reduced oxygenation levels, requiring supplemental oxygen support.

For children older than 5 years, asthma is treated with similar clinical practice guidelines recommending a combined approach of the inhaled bronchodilators salbutamol and ipratropium bromide (Atrovent), a useful anticholinergic adjunct that acts directly on the smooth muscle of the airways. Corticosteroids such as prednisolone and hydrocortisone are also included for systemic support (CHQ, 2019; Plotnick & Ducharme, 2000; RCHM, 2018; Sydney Children's Hospital, 2019). For children between 1 and 5 years of age, asthma treatment is not inclusive of steroids and instead a pathway of pre-school wheeze management is recommended in Australia, with an emphasis on salbutamol to treat wheeze.

Children presenting to hospital emergency departments with an acute episode of asthma are promptly treated following the national guidelines to prevent further deterioration and ideally an admission from the short-stay unit in the emergency department to the ward. Treatment approaches such as 'burst therapy', or three doses of salbutamol inhalers at 20-minute intervals (CHQ, 2019), are used.

Pneumonia

Pneumonia is a lower respiratory tract infection with presenting signs of cough (although cough may not always be present early in pneumonia), increased secretions, pain in the chest (or commonly the abdomen in children), fever and respiratory distress (Haq et al., 2017). Pneumonia is a common illness in young children, and is the largest cause of morbidity and mortality among infants and children aged from 1 month to 5 years internationally (de Benedictis et al., 2020). This illness is more prevalent in lower socioeconomic groups due to overcrowding, and thus ease of transmission of the infective agents. Children who have underlying cardiopulmonary conditions such as asthma, congenital heart disease and immunity disorders have a higher risk of contracting pneumonia.

Treatment of pneumonia is supportive and similar to bronchiolitis, with the addition of intravenous antibiotics. Pneumonia is predominantly bacterial in origin, with streptococcus pneumonia the most common bacterial cause in children (Haq et al., 2017). However, viral infection is also common due to respiratory syncytial virus and parainfluenza and influenza viruses (Haq et al., 2017). Pneumonia can be prevented by immunisation with the *Haemophilus influenzae* type B (HIB) and pneumococcal conjugate vaccines (Barson, 2015), so opportunistic parental education and immunisation is another important nursing consideration.

Acute otitis media

Acute otitis media (AOM) refers to an infection or inflammation of the middle ear, characterised by fluid collection in the middle ear and a bulging tympanic membrane. Up to 60 per cent of children aged under 3 years will have at least one episode of otitis media during early childhood (Klein & Pelton, 2015; Wood & Vijayasekaran, 2014), and the incidence is higher still in Aboriginal and Torres Strait Islander children (AIHW, 2018). Children of this age are more likely to develop ear infections as they have short, horizontal Eustachian tubes that are less likely to drain fluid produced during an upper airway infection. AOM is more likely to occur in households with smokers, where there has been a lack of breastfeeding, in infancy and toddlerhood, in children exposed to more frequent URTIs through childcare attendance and in lower socioeconomic groups (Klein & Pelton, 2015).

CASE STUDY 10.3 LUCAS

Lucas is a 7-month-old infant brought to the after-hours general practice clinic. Lucas's parents report that he has cried inconsolably for six hours and has little interest in breastfeeding or solids. Lucas appears pale and is peripherally warm. He is noticeably irritable and crying, despite being held by his mother. He has profuse nasal secretions and a dry mouth. His parents are concerned that he has not had a wet nappy for six hours. The general practitioner inspects his ears and notes bilateral inflamed tympanic membranes, with a bulging right tympanic membrane. Lucas has a heart rate of 172/minute, a respiratory rate of 44/minute and his axilla temperature is 39.7°C.

The signs of AOM are usually fairly rapid in onset. Most children will present initially with vague or non-specific complaints such as being irritable and difficult to settle, and may have a loss of appetite and little interest in drinking their usual fluids. More definitive signs include fever, earache (or rubbing of the ear in pre-verbal children) and sometimes discharge from the ear if the tympanic membrane ruptures. Many children will have had a recent history of an URTI, including a sore throat and rhinitis. A diagnosis of AOM is made based on these clinical signs with confirmation of a bulging and reddened tympanic membrane. The tympanic membrane is visualised using an otoscope. Normally, a tympanic membrane is a pale pearl-pink colour. In AOM, the membrane is redder and may bulge from the build-up of fluid in the middle ear.

REFLECTION POINT 10.3

An earache can be very painful and distressing for an infant or child. Take some time to review the methods of pain assessment provided at the beginning of the chapter and consider which tools would be useful for assessing pain in children younger than 3 years of age.

Management of pain associated with AOM is an important intervention. Relief from pain can help the child to settle to sleep and may improve their intake of oral fluids. In most cases, oral analgesics such as paracetamol or ibuprofen can be used to reduce the pain. Although the main purpose of using either paracetamol or ibuprofen is to reduce pain in this circumstance, these medications can also reduce any fever that is present.

Pain and fluid management are the primary considerations for managing AOM, with most incidences resolving over a period ranging from two days to two weeks. Concerns about the over-use of oral antibiotics in the community have led to the development of evidence-based guidelines to encourage more judicious use of antibiotic therapy in the treatment of AOM. To date, evidence suggests that antibiotics are appropriate for the treatment of children under 2 years of age with bilateral AOM or for children with both bilateral AOM and a discharge from the ear (otorrhoea) (Venekamp et al., 2015; Wood & Vijayasekaran, 2014). If pain persists for longer than 48 hours, the child should be reviewed and antibiotic therapy may be considered. An important consideration with recurrent or undiagnosed episodes of AOM is that this may lead to a chronic collection of fluid. Chronic otitis media may lead to conductive hearing loss, with subsequent delays in cognitive, speech and language development (Monasta et al., 2012; Wood & Vijayasekaran, 2014).

Abdominal pain

CASE STUDY 10.4 BO

Bo is a 15-year-old girl who presents to the general medical practice accompanied by her mother and older sister. Bo has had abdominal pain for several days, but it has increased in severity over the past 12 hours. During examination, it becomes apparent that the pain is difficult to localise, although it increases when Bo moves. Bo has not eaten or had a drink since yesterday. Her mother reports that she has been 'off her food' for a day or two. Her bowel movements have not changed recently. Bo has a low-grade fever (37.8°C), a heart rate of 110/minute and blood pressure of 95/55 mmHg. The medical officer is not certain of the cause of the pain, but considers that it may be early appendicitis and refers Bo to the emergency department of her local hospital. The team at the hospital decides that there are reasonable grounds to suspect appendicitis. Bo is prepared for transfer to theatre for an emergency laparoscopy and possible laparoscopic appendicectomy.

Children and young people with abdominal pain are a common group seeking care in emergency departments and general practice. It can be difficult to determine the cause of such pain, as there are many potential causes, and the child or young person may find it difficult to pinpoint the exact location of the pain and describe it clearly. Symptoms of abdominal pain in younger children are less specific and more difficult to localise, whereas a young person should be able to localise and describe the pain in more detail. However, the nature of abdominal pain seems to vary considerably between individuals and conditions. Abdominal pain may indicate a range of conditions from mild issues such as constipation to more serious problems that are the result of acute conditions, such as appendicitis or trauma.

Assessment and management

Assessment of the child or young person with abdominal pain is essential, especially when the cause is not clear. While in many cases abdominal pain may resolve or be related to relatively non-urgent conditions, there is a possibility that the symptom of pain indicates a more serious and urgent problem.

Chapter 11 outlines the principles for recognising and responding to signs of deterioration. These principles are the framework that we would use in practice for Bo – monitoring cardiovascular stability through the measurement of vital signs such as pulse and blood pressure, and the assessment of other clinical signs including colour, behaviour, peripheral circulation and pain.

In the past, clinicians were reluctant to give analgesia to relieve abdominal pain until a diagnosis of the cause of the pain was made. Contemporary clinical guidelines indicate that there is no evidence to support the withholding of analgesia in children or young people with acute abdominal pain, nor does the use of analgesia impede diagnosis or treatment (National Institute of Clinical Studies, 2011; New South Wales Health, 2013).

Appendicitis

Acute appendicitis is the most common surgical emergency in children and young people, although in some cases appendicitis may be treated conservatively. Approximately 16 per cent of people in developed countries will have an appendicectomy during their lifetime, with the peak incidence between the age of 8 and 14 years (Bradbury, Forsythe & Parkes, 2012). Although it is relatively common compared with other abdominal conditions, the causes of acute appendicitis are not fully understood. It may be related to some degree of obstruction of the appendix that triggers an inflammatory response in the mucosa of the appendix (Agency for Healthcare Research & Quality, 2015). The inflammation may cause venous congestion and diminish arterial blood supply, leading to ischaemia and infarction (Bradbury, Forsythe & Parkes, 2012). If this does not resolve, appendicitis can result in perforation and sepsis.

There is no definitive test to diagnose appendicitis, apart from direct visualisation via laparoscopy. Thus clinicians rely on clinical signs and symptoms, and blood test results such as white blood count, in deciding whether to proceed to laparoscopy and, if required, appendicectomy, or to wait, watch and observe to see whether the pain decreases or increases, and whether other symptoms develop (Agency for Healthcare Research & Quality, 2015). In addition to abdominal pain, individuals with appendicitis may have nausea, vomiting, diarrhoea, fever, pallor or abdominal distension (Howell et al., 2010). None of these signs or symptoms is conclusively indicative of appendicitis – they can indicate other conditions such as inflammatory bowel diseases, mesenteric adenitis or gynaecological conditions such as pelvic inflammatory disease or ectopic pregnancy, to name just a few.

For the young person, it is important to establish whether they have commenced menstruation and whether they are sexually active in order to exclude pregnancy.

Discussions about puberty, sexual activity and any related tests need to be handled with great tact and diplomacy. Please recognise that the young person may not be willing to disclose their sexual history in front of parents, friends or family. Furthermore, young people may deny that they are sexually active even when they are.

For further information on assessing and communicating with adolescents, see Hutchinson & Fraser (2018) in the Further reading section.

REFLECTION POINTS 10.4

Imagine that you are required to ask Bo to provide a urine sample for a pregnancy test. Think about who might be present, the environment you may be in and the words you might use.

- What will you say to Bo?
- What will you do to maintain her privacy?
- What right does Bo have to consent to or refuse this urine sample?
- What right does Bo have to confidentiality of the results of such a test?

Injuries in children and adolescents

Injury is a leading cause of hospitalisation and death for children and young people in Australia (Mitchell, Curtis & Foster, 2018). In children aged 10–14 years, approximately 16 per cent of all admissions to hospital are related to injury (Pointer, 2014). The most common causes of injuries for childhood injury are falls, injuries due to striking or being struck by objects, and road transport-related injuries (Mitchell, Curtis & Foster, 2018). Rates of injury are also higher in rural and remote areas and for Aboriginal and Torres Strait Islander children and young adults (Harrison, Berry & Jamieson, 2012; Pointer, 2016). Young people who live in a remote area are twice as likely to sustain an injury that requires hospitalisation compared with young people living in major cities (Harrison, Berry & Jamieson, 2012). In New Zealand, the most common reason for hospital presentations of children aged 5–9 years is falls, with 48 per cent of children identified as being injured from increasing exposure to mechanical forces and activities involving playground equipment (Ministry of Health, 2020; Safekids Aotearoa, 2015).

When it comes to young people aged 15–17 years, self-harm is one of the primary reasons for admission to hospital. Girls of this age group are also more likely to be injured as a result of intentional self-harm compared with other children (Griffin et al., 2014). This is also reflected in the hospital admission rates for self-harm, with young girls accounting for 35 per cent of admissions to hospital while boys only account for 4 per cent (Pointer, 2014). It is important to highlight that self-harm is often associated with other psychological factors and negative life events – for example, depression and suicide attempts by a family member (Doyle, Treacy & Sheridan, 2015).

Hospitalisation for a physical injury may be an opportune time to intervene, or at least assess for a mental health problem. See Chapter 8 for more details regarding mental health.

Head injury

CASE STUDY 10.5 MADDIE

Maddie is a 14-year-old girl who sustained serious injuries after a fall on her farm. She was standing on the roof of a small shed when the roof gave way; she fell approximately 2 metres, landing on the ground. She sustained a closed head injury with a witnessed loss of consciousness for three minutes, fracture of the left femur, chest bruising, cuts and grazes. Maddie was initially assessed in a local hospital. On arrival, she was tachycardic with a heart rate of 120, and her blood pressure (BP) and respiratory rate were within limits for her age. Maddie's initial Glasgow Coma Scale (GCS) was 12 (eyes 3, verbal response 4 and motor response 5). The severity of her injuries indicated that she may require a computerised tomography (CT) scan of her brain (NICE, 2014; New South Wales Health, 2011). CT scanning was not available at Maddie's local hospital, so a decision was made to contact the relevant retrieval service. She was transferred to the high-dependency unit of a tertiary referral centre. On arrival in the unit, Maddie had a GCS of 14, vital signs within limits for age and was complaining of a persistent headache.

Most head injuries that occur to children and young people are minor, and most will not have significant intracranial pathology (Davis & Ings, 2015). However, any head injury can result in significant harm. It is therefore important to monitor and assess the child or young person closely after the event. The extent or degree of severity of head injury should determine the initial response. Head injuries traditionally are classified by severity into mild, moderate and severe (New South Wales Health, 2011). Maddie's injuries are consistent with a moderate head injury, as she had a GCS of 12 at the local hospital (New South Wales Health, 2011).

Head injuries can be categorised as internal (involving the skull or the brain) or external (involving the scalp). In Case study 10.5, Maddie's injury involved trauma to the brain; she did not suffer any injuries to her scalp. The likely severity of a head injury can be estimated according to risk factors (see Table 10.3) that would categorise the injury as high, intermediate or low risk. In Maddie's case, her injuries are consistent with an intermediate risk: the injury occurred as a result of a fall of 2 metres, there was a loss of consciousness of three minutes, she did not vomit and her behaviour is normal. She does have a persistent headache and a score on the Glasgow Coma Scale (GCS) of 14, however, and thus requires close observation and ongoing neurological assessment (Dunning, 2021; New South Wales Health, 2011).

Table 10.3 Risk groups in head injury

Signs and symptoms	Low risk (all features)	Intermediate risk (any feature/ not low or high risk)	High risk (chalice criteria) (any feature)
History			
Witnessed loss of consciousness	Nil	<5 minutes	>5 minutes
Anterograde or retrograde amnesia	Nil	Possible	>5 minutes
Behaviour	Normal	Mild agitation or altered behaviour	Abnormal drowsiness
Episodes of vomiting without other cause	Nil or 1	2 or persistent nausea	3 or more
Seizure in non-epileptic patient	Nil	Impact only	Yes
Non accidental injury (NAI) suspected	No	No	Yes
Headache	Nil	Persistent	Persistent
Comorbidities	Nil	Present	Present
Age	>1 year	<1 year	Any
Mechanism			
Motor vehicle accident (MVA) (pedestrian, cyclist or occupant)	Low speed	<60 km/h	>60 km/h
Fall	<1 m	1–3 m	>3 m
Force from a projectile or object	Low impact	Moderate impact or unclear mechanism	High-speed projectile or object
Examination			
Glasgow Coma Scale (GCS)	15	Fluctuating 14–15	<14 (or <15 if under 1 year of age)
Focal neurological abnormality (motor, sensory, coordination or reflex abnormality)	Nil	Nil	Present
Injury			High-risk features – for example, scalp haematoma in <1 year of age (see below)
Placement			
Observation area	Anywhere in ED	Acute area in ED	Acute or resuscitation bay
Observations			
• Respiratory rate, oxygen saturations • Pulse, blood pressure • Temperature	Hourly observations until discharge	Half-hourly observations for four to six hours until GCS 15 sustained for two hours, then hourly observations until discharge	Continuous cardio-respiratory and oxygen saturation monitoring BP and GCS every 15 to 30 minutes

Table 10.3 (*cont.*)

Signs and symptoms	Low risk (all features)	Intermediate risk (any feature/ not low or high risk)	High risk (chalice criteria) (any feature)
• GCS, pupillary response and size, limb strength • Pain assessment • Sedation score as necessary		Revert to half-hourly observations/continuous monitoring if signs of deterioration occur	

Notes: High-risk injury: a) penetrating injury, or suspected depressed skull fracture or base of skull fracture (e.g. blood or CSF leakage from ear or nose, panda eyes, Battle's sign, haemotympanum (blood in the middle ear), facial crepitus (cracking or popping sound under skin upon palpation) or severe facial injury); b) scalp bruise, swelling or laceration >5 cm, or tense fontanelle in infants <1 year of age.
Source: Adapted from New South Wales Health (2011, p. 8).

Assessment and management

Assessment – both at the time of the injury and over time – is a critical element in the nursing management of people who have sustained a head injury. A rapid neurological assessment of level of consciousness can be undertaken using AVPU: is the patient alert, verbal, responding to pain or unconscious? In addition to the rapid initial assessment of consciousness, a more in-depth assessment should be performed over time using the GCS. While a modified GCS is appropriate in children, in young people the standard GCS should be used. In addition to these assessment tools, clinicians should also consider the opinion of parents in neurological assessment. Parents know their children well, and are often the first to notice that all is not well. If a parent is concerned about a change in the behaviour of their child, then we should also be concerned. In addition to changes in behaviour, clinicians should also be alert to any signs of generalised or local seizure activity – clear signs the injury is severe or worsening. For more details on neurological assessment, including the AVPU and modified GCS, refer to Chapter 11 on recognising the signs of a deteriorating child.

Frequency of neurological assessment and the timeframe for close observation will be determined by the estimated severity of the head injury. Initially, at least hourly neurological and vital observations are required, though these should be more frequent if a higher severity of head injury is suspected. If the head injury is assessed as mild and observations are normal, most patients are discharged after approximately four hours. If there is concern that the injury is of moderate severity, a longer period of observations and a CT scan may be required. Children and young people may need to be kept nil by mouth initially, pending decisions about further investigations or surgery that may require administration of an anaesthetic.

Not surprisingly, head injuries can be painful; however, clinicians can be concerned about the use of analgesia in patients with head injury – especially analgesics with a known sedative effect. When considering what analgesia to give a patient with head injury, consideration should be given to factors such as the patient's clinical signs, the need for analgesia and the patient's pain score (Trauma Victoria, 2016). For mild pain, an oral analgesic (for example, paracetamol) that does not cause sedation may be appropriate. For more severe pain, consideration may be given to using opioids, but these should be administered with care. The sedative effects of opioids may mask deterioration in level of consciousness due to the head injury. The New South Wales

Clinical Practice Guidelines on management of patients with head injury (New South Wales Health, 2011) recommend that a sedation assessment be performed in addition to neurological assessments such as GCS to monitor the sedative effect of opioids administered in people with head injury.

Another very important aspect of assessment of head injury is the history of the injury. It is important that clinicians give consideration to whether the severity and location of the head injury accord with the history of the injury that is provided. Sadly, we have to consider that a head injury in a child or young person may be non-accidental. Clinicians need to maintain an open mind to this possibility during assessment. For further details on non-accidental injury, and child abuse and neglect, see Chapter 2.

For young people like Maddie, serious injuries incurred in a rural area usually result in retrieval to a city or regional hospital, distant from their home, as specialist neurological services are centrally located in cities. This can mean additional concerns for young people and their families, who are already frightened or anxious about the extent of the injury sustained. In addition, families in this situation incur additional costs associated with living away from home while they care for their child in a city hospital. In some instances, one parent may need to stay with the rest of the family at home while the other parent travels with their injured child. Nurses need to ensure that they support families in this situation. The importance of caring, flexible and understanding health professionals, facilities and resources to enable families to stay with their injured child, or the means for them to stay in contact from a distance, is vital. Preparing young people and parents for discharge after head injury is also important. Make sure that parents and young people are clear regarding signs that would require them to return for further assessment.

Musculoskeletal injuries

Musculoskeletal injuries are a frequent reason for children and young people to require hospital care. Musculoskeletal injuries that may occur include strains, sprains, joint dislocations and fractures. For young children, these injuries commonly arise from play equipment (Mulligan, Adams & Brown, 2016; Pointer 2014). It is interesting to note that with the introduction of trampoline parks, hospitals are seeing an increase in injuries sustained on trampolines (Kasmire, Rogers & Sturm, 2016; Mulligan, Adams & Brown, 2016). In older children and young people, the injury may arise from sport and recreational activities or from motor vehicle accidents (Pointer, 2014). In both children and young people, attention should be paid to correlation between the injury and the history of how the injury occurred. As mentioned previously, clinicians should always be mindful that an injury may be the result of physical abuse of the child or young person (Emalee et al., 2014). For further information about child abuse, see Chapter 2.

A fracture of the bone will occur when the force exerted on a bone is greater than the strength of the bone is able to resist. In younger children, bone formation is still immature. The bones are more porous and the periosteum is thicker, so the bone is compliant and thus less likely to completely break in response to a greater force. For these reasons, younger children and infants will be more likely to have an incomplete fracture, such as a greenstick injury. By early adolescence, the bone is much more dense and complete fractures are more likely (Curtis & Ramsden, 2016) (see Figure 10.1).

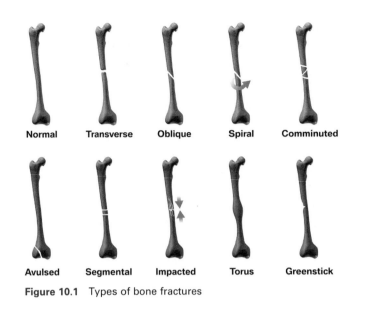

Normal   Transverse   Oblique   Spiral   Comminuted

Avulsed   Segmental   Impacted   Torus   Greenstick

Figure 10.1   Types of bone fractures

Assessment and management

When caring for children or young people with musculoskeletal injuries, it is import-ant to consider interventions such as splinting or elevating the limb to help reduce their pain. Applying splints, such as a backslab, to the injured limb reduces pain and prevents further damage to bone and soft tissues around the fracture (Curtis & Ramsden, 2016). Analgesia should be administered based on the severity of pain; this should be assessed using an appropriate age-based pain scale such as the Faces Pain Scale or a linear scale (New South Wales Health, 2016).

Infection control is an important consideration for management of children with an open fracture. The general principles of caring for a child with an open fracture include covering the wound with an appropriate dressing and the administration of a broad-spectrum antibiotic and tetanus prophylaxis. It is important that the wound site is thoroughly cleaned to prevent bacteria invading the fracture site; this is usually done under a general anaesthetic (Schaller & Calhoun, 2016). Depending on the nature of the fracture, open or closed reduction of the fracture and application of traction or plaster cast under anaesthetic may also be required, and therefore pre-operative and post-operative care should be considered.

Frequent and accurate neurovascular observations are an essential component of nursing assessment in the care of people with a fracture. These assessments are somewhat easier in young people than younger children, as young people are more likely to understand the questions put to them as part of the assessment. The main components of neurovascular assessment include the five Ps: pain, paralysis, paresthesia, pulses and pallor (Curtis & Ramsden, 2016; Shields & Clarke, 2011).

Regular pain assessment should be undertaken, as increasing pain can indicate neurovascular impairment. Increasing analgesic requirements can be one of the signs of compartment syndrome in children; this needs to be considered particularly in children who are not able to verbalise their pain accurately (Hosseinzadeh & Talwalkar, 2016). We also need to consider whether the pain is from the original injury and the need for appropriate analgesia to be administered as required. The child or young person should be asked to move their limb distal to the injury. Be aware that pain may inhibit movement, so it is important to ensure that adequate analgesia is administered. Sensation, pulses and colour should be assessed in the affected limb and compared with those in the unaffected limb. The limb pulses should be palpated for rate and quality at a site that is distal to the injury, traction or cast. If pulses are absent or unable to be assessed due to a plaster cast, then perform capillary refill assessment. Capillary refill time should be less than two seconds. The colour and swelling of the limb are also important indicators of vascular impairment – a swollen cool, pale or mottled limb is a concerning sign (Curtis & Ramsden, 2016; Shields & Clarke, 2011). The limb should be elevated and medical review should be requested.

Prior to discharge, young people and their parents should be given information about the signs of neurovascular impairment. In addition, if a plaster cast is applied, cast care instructions should be discussed, including protection from water, physical damage and the risk of the insertion of foreign objects into the cast.

Alcohol intoxication

CASE STUDY 10.6 RYAN

Ryan is a 14-year-old boy who has been at a party with a large group of friends. During the evening, Ryan smoked cannabis and consumed a large quantity of alcohol. Over time, he became disoriented, vomited and eventually passed out. His friends were unable to rouse him. One of his friends called an ambulance, and Ryan was assessed and transferred to the emergency department of the local hospital. On arrival at hospital, Ryan is lethargic, confused and difficult to rouse, responding only to painful stimuli, with a GCS of 11 (eyes 2, verbal response 4, motor response 5). His pupils are equal and reacting briskly to light. His vital observations include heart rate 115 per minute, respiratory rate 18 per minute, BP 90/50 mmHg and S_aO_2 96 per cent in room air. He smells strongly of vomit and alcohol. Bloods are taken, and the results reveal a blood alcohol level of 55 mmol/L.

According to the National Drug Strategy Household Survey of 2019, the most commonly used drugs in young people aged 12–17 years are cannabis, alcohol and tobacco (AIHW, 2020). This is similar to the data from New Zealand, where cannabis the most commonly used drug in youth aged up to 16 years (Ministry of Health, 2010). The age at which young people first use illicit drugs is increasing, with the current age for first time illicit drug use now on average 19.9 years, which is the oldest this age for initiation has been in nearly two decades (AIHW, 2020). Recent 2019 figures estimate that approximately 11.6 per cent of young people aged 14 years had used cannabis in the previous year (AIHW, 2020). This puts Ryan in Case study 10.7 in a younger age group than the average Australian. When it comes to alcohol, approximately three of every four Australian secondary students aged 12–17 years will have tried alcohol, and the rate of alcohol consumption increases with age. By the age of 16 years, approximately 13 per cent of young people report having experienced an episode of binge drinking in the past seven days, consuming more than four standard drinks on one day

(White & Bariola, 2012). In New Zealand, almost 90 per cent of children will have consumed alcohol by 14 years of age and one-third of secondary school students binge drink up to five drinks once a month (Ministry of Health, 2010). Consequently, some young people may consume harmful amounts of alcohol, resulting in alcohol intoxication and poisoning, and requiring acute care in a hospital setting. Additionally, they also present to emergency departments with injuries sustained while intoxicated or severe injuries as a result from violence with others.

During adolescence, the brain is still developing and young people can put themselves at risk of long-term deficits if they drink alcohol regularly. The ingestion of alcohol in this age group has been shown to lead to a decline in cognitive abilities such as memory loss and visuo-spatial abnormalities (Hanson et al., 2011; Risher et al., 2015). Alcohol can also lead to neurological deficits when it is ingested initially, as it causes central nervous system (CNS) depression. The sedative effects of alcohol, in addition to the risk of vomiting when intoxicated, mean that there is a significant risk of respiratory arrest.

Assessment and management

Immediate care of the young person with alcohol poisoning begins by maintaining a clear airway. In Case study 10.7, Ryan is at risk of aspirating vomit, and therefore should be positioned on his side in the recovery position. The next important priority is to monitor level of consciousness. We would expect this to improve over time, as Ryan has stopped ingesting alcohol and any residual alcohol in his blood will be metabolised. Administration of intravenous fluids may be required to maintain hydration and replace fluids lost from vomiting.

REFLECTION POINTS 10.5

People from different ethnic and cultural backgrounds often have different perspectives on adolescence, particularly in relation to social and emotional development. In countries such as Australia and New Zealand, with diverse multicultural populations, there can be a range of views on what might be appropriate behaviour, rules and expectations regarding adolescents. Take a few minutes to think about the following points:

- What is your ethnic and cultural background?
- In your family, would Ryan's drinking be accepted or tolerated, or neither?
- How might your background impact on your perception of Ryan's behaviour?
- If you found Ryan's behaviour confronting, what could you do to ensure that your personal judgement of this behaviour did not impede the care you provided to Ryan?

Once the initial acute phase has resolved, consideration needs to be given to psychosocial issues. Psychosocial screening can be undertaken, using a recognised framework such as the HEADSSS, which assesses home circumstances, engagement in education/employment, activities with peers, use of drugs, sexuality and mental health (suicide risk, self-harm and depression). The HEADSSS psychosocial screening tool is a useful framework in the assessment of adolescent risk and sources of support. The

Royal Children's Hospital in Melbourne provides a useful clinical guideline for engaging with adolescents, using the HEADSSS tool (RCHM, 2020).

Abuse of alcohol and illicit drugs can be an indicator of psychosocial or mental health problems in the young person. Some young people may use substances such as alcohol to deal with feelings of sadness, anxiety or despair. It is important that the young person's mental health and wellbeing are assessed prior to discharge. An admission related to alcohol abuse should be seen as an opportunity to provide education and support for a young person to deal with alcohol abuse and any related psychosocial issues and refer them to appropriate community-based services.

Paediatric perioperative care

Pre-operative care

Adequate preparation for operations is an essential and important role for nurses in the care of children and young people. For children and young people who require elective procedures, there is often sufficient time to support parents to be the main 'preparers' for the child or young person, or at least for parents to provide the initial explanation to their child about what will happen. Emergency procedures such as that required by Bo (see Case study 10.4) are often a shock to the parent, and they may be unable to take in, process and use the information we provide to explain to their child what is about to occur to an adequate level. In either event, the onus is on medical and nursing staff to ensure that everyone – the parents and the young person – is clear about what is required and what is likely to occur. Older children and adolescents may have a more sophisticated understanding of the workings of their insides than younger children; however, it is important to remember that the level of understanding can vary considerably between individuals when providing explanations about pre-operative procedures and post-operative care (Panella, 2016).

Apart from psychological preparation, physical preparation is also required. This may include nil by mouth for a period of time, showering prior to the procedure and dressing in a theatre gown. These procedures are very familiar to nurses used to caring for adults, but it is important to remember that, for most young people like Bo, this would be their first experience of surgery. Seemingly strange practices such as the requirement that patients do not wear any underwear to theatre can be unsettling for a young person who is modest and conscious of their body. A young person such as Bo may become quite anxious once the decision is made to operate, and therefore consideration may also be given to some form of pre-operative sedation. Obtaining informed consent for procedures is an important part of preparation. Details of the legal and ethical issues that arise in obtaining consent are dealt with in Chapter 2.

Parental presence during induction of anaesthesia

One key difference in perioperative care for children is parental presence during induction of general anaesthesia. For many parents, being able to support their child during induction is desirable and results in reduced parental anxiety and increased satisfaction (Yousef et al., 2018). This is a well-accepted practice in paediatric hospitals; however, its effectiveness depends on good preparation of the parent and support for the parent during and after the induction. This preparation is important to ensure safety, so parents are calm and know what to do to support and reassure their child (Luehmann, 2019).

Post-operative care

Emergence delirium (ED) – A dissociated state of consciousness where children, upon awakening from general anaesthesia, may be inconsolable, irritable, crying, incoherent and exhibit thrashing movements. They may be at risk of injury from dislodging intravenous lines, drains or dressings or from falling. Parental presence is thought to assist with ED.

Patient-controlled analgesia (PCA) – A form of analgesia where administration is controlled by the patient. In acute care settings such as paediatrics, it is usually intravenous analgesia administered via a special intravenous pump designed to administer medications by the patient, such as opioids, by bolus injection. This form of analgesia is well suited to patients older than 6 years, who have appropriate cognition regarding their pain and the use of the device.

The principles of post-operative care are similar for children, young people and adults. The priority of nursing care in the immediate post-operative period is to monitor for any adverse effects of the surgical intervention and/or anaesthesia, including airway obstruction and haemorrhage. Initially, continuous cardio-respiratory monitoring is indicated until the young person rouses. Once they are awake, frequent assessment of respiratory and cardiovascular status – including heart rate, respiratory rate, respiratory assessment, blood pressure and oxygen saturation – is required. The incision site should be observed for excess blood loss. As with parental presence during induction of anaesthesia, parents may often be invited in to the post anaesthesia care unit (PACU) to support their child following surgery. Their presence in the PACU can minimise anxiety relating to separation, and may even assist with the management of **emergence delirium** in paediatric patients (In et al., 2019). Pain management is an important component of post-operative care. By the time children reach early adolescence, they are able to describe and quantify pain with greater precision and detail. Pain-assessment tools, including the Faces Pain Scale or numerical rating scales, can be used with young people. Analgesics should be administered regularly to relieve pain and to facilitate early post-operative ambulation. **Patient-controlled analgesia (PCA)** is an excellent choice for young people and can help to give them a sense of control over their post-operative care. For further understanding on PCA for Pain Management Guidelines, refer to Forster and Kotzur (2018) in the Further reading section.

SUMMARY

- Acute viral infections are common in childhood. Although most cause only mild illness, some children will require nursing and medical care in a hospital setting.
- The approach to nursing assessment needs to take the developmental differences in infants and children into consideration.
- Fever, dehydration, hypoxia and pain are common reasons for children to require nursing care and intervention.
- Nursing care needs to consider the age and development of the infant, child and young person, as well as the needs of the family.
- Perioperative care of children differs from adult perioperative care, and paediatric nurses are well placed to support children and families both pre- and post-operatively.
- Adolescence is a time of transition for both the young person and their family.
- The healthcare needs of adolescents are different from those of young children and adults, and care should be tailored to their needs.
- Young people should be cared for in an environment that is best able to meet their special developmental needs.

- Injury is a common reason for hospitalisation of young people, and some will require admission to hospital for nursing care and medical treatment.
- Injuries may indicate underlying psychosocial or mental health issues in young people.

LEARNING ACTIVITIES

10.1 Clinical practice guidelines (CPG) or evidence-based practice guidelines (EBPG) are often used to guide practice in acute-care settings. These guidelines are developed by expert groups of clinicians and researchers, who have systematically reviewed and evaluated evidence for best practice. Following this, the expert groups have determined and then published the best recommendations, information and advice to assist health professionals to assess and intervene in the care and treatment of children with a range of conditions. In this chapter, you have read several case scenarios of children with different presenting symptoms. Undertake an internet and database search for local and international CPG and EBPG for the care of a child with one of these conditions.

- Read the guidelines. Are they similar or different?
- Do they address all aspects of the condition, including assessment, treatment, nursing care and after care?
- Which expert groups have contributed to their development?
- What level of evidence or literature review has been undertaken in the preparation of the guideline?

10.2 Read the case scenarios for the children in this chapter. For each child, consider your response to the following questions:

- What key assessments and observations would you perform?
- How often would you perform these assessments?
- What changes might indicate that the child's/young person's condition is deteriorating?
- What changes might indicate that the child's/young person's condition is improving?
- What interventions would you include to meet the child's/young person's emotional needs during hospitalisation?

FURTHER READING

Brown, N & Green, J 2018, Fluid balance and nutrition, in E Forster & JA Fraser (eds), *Paediatric nursing skills for Australian nurses*, Cambridge University Press, Melbourne, pp. 253–74.

Forster, E & Kotzur, C 2018, Pain assessment and management, in E Forster & JA Fraser (eds), *Paediatric nursing skills for Australian nurses*, Cambridge University Press, Melbourne, pp. 146–68

Forster, E, Maher, D & Patane, I 2018, Administration of medication in E Forster & JA Fraser (eds), *Paediatric nursing skills for Australian nurses*, Cambridge University Press, Melbourne, pp. 124–45.

Hutchinson, L & Fraser J 2018, Adolescent nursing skills, in E Forster & JA Fraser (eds), *Paediatric nursing skills for Australian nurses*, Cambridge University Press, Melbourne, pp. 81–100.

- The Centers for Disease Control and Prevention (CDC) is an internationally renowned, leading public health organisation in the United States, with responsibilities for the prevention of disease, injury and disability. The link below takes you to information about rashes and infectious diseases: https://search.cdc.gov/search/index.html?query=rashes%20and%20infectious%20diseases&dpage=1.
- Medicinenet is a reputable website based in the United States that provides detailed and relevant information about diseases, health and illness. The following link takes you to a slide show of images, including children with rashes: www.medicinenet.com/childrens_health_illnesses_pictures_slideshow/article.htm.
- Icon Pediatrics is a private paediatric practice based in the United States, with an excellent web page that contains resources about anaphylaxis and allergy: http://iconpediatrics.com/news-and-media/2015/09/severe-allergic-reactions-signs-symptoms-risks-treatment.
- The Ministry of Health in NSW provides a useful fact sheet on infectious diseases in childhood: www.health.nsw.gov.au/Infectious/factsheets/Factsheets/infectious_childhood.PDF.

REFERENCES

Agency for Healthcare Research and Quality (AHRQ) 2015, *Diagnosis of right lower quadrant pain and suspected acute appendicitis*, AHRQ, Sydney, viewed 30 August 2016, https://effectivehealthcare.ahrq.gov/ehc/products/528/2159/appendicitis-executive-151214.pdf

Ambuel, B, Hamlett, KW, Marx, CM & Blumer, JL 1992, Assessing distress in pediatric intensive care environments: The COMFORT scale, *Journal of Pediatric Psychology*, 17(1), pp. 95–109.

Ashkenazy, S & DeKeyser-Ganz, F 2011, Assessment of the reliability and validity of the Comfort Scale for adult intensive care patients, *Heart & Lung*, 40(3), pp. e44–e51.

Association of Paediatric Anaesthetists of Great Britain and Ireland (APAGBI) 2012, Good practice in postoperative and procedural pain management, *Pediatric Anesthesia*, 22(S1), pp. 1–79.

Australian Institute of Health and Welfare (AIHW) 2018, *Emergency department care 2017–2018 Australian hospital statistics*, cat. no. HSE 216, AIHW, Canberra.

—— 2020. *National Drug Strategy household survey 2019*, cat. no. PHE 270, AIHW, Canberra.

Australian Medicines Handbook 2017, viewed 20 February 2021, http://amhonline.amh.net.au

Bai, J, Hsu, L, Tang, Y & van Dijk, M 2012, Validation of the COMFORT Behavior scale and the FLACC scale for pain assessment in Chinese children after cardiac surgery, *Pain Management Nursing*, 13(1), pp. 18–26.

Balli, S & Sharan, S 2021, Physiology, fever, in *StatPearls*. Treasure Island, FL: StatPearls Publishing, viewed 30 August 2021, www.ncbi.nlm.nih.gov/books/NBK562334

Barson, WJ 2015, Pneumonia in children: Epidemiology, pathogenesis and etiology, *Up to Date,* viewed 21 March 2016, www.uptodate.com/contents/pneumonia-in-children-epidemiology-pathogenesis-and-etiology

Bearde, C & Greco, C 2011, Pain management in children, in GA Gregory & DB Andropoulous (eds), *Gregory's pediatric esthesia*, Wiley Blackwell, Hoboken, NJ, pp. 845–74.

Beltramini, A, Milojevic, K & Pateron, D 2017, Pain assessment in newborns, infants and children, *Paediatric Annals*, 46(10), pp. 387–95.

Bjornson, C et al. 2011, Nebulized epinephrine for croup in children, *Cochrane Database of Systematic Reviews*, 16(2), CD006619.

Bradbury, AW, Forsythe, JLR & Parkes, RW 2012, *Principles and practice of surgery*, Churchill Livingstone, London.

Brummelte, S, Oberlander, TF & Craig, KD 2014, Biomarkers of pain: Physiological indices of pain reactivity in infants and children, in PJ McGrath et al. (eds), *Oxford textbook of paediatric pain*, Oxford University Press, Oxford, pp. 391–400.

Butters, C, Curtis, N & Burgner, DP, 2020, Kawasaki disease fact check: Myths, misconceptions and mysteries, *Journal of Paediatrics and Child Health*, 56(9), 1343–5.

Children's Health Queensland Hospital and Health Service (CHQ) 2019, *Queensland Paediatric Emergency Guidelines*, viewed 8 July 2020, www.childrens.health.qld .gov.au/guideline-asthma-emergency-management-in-children

Crook, J 2010, Fever management: Evaluating the use of ibroprofens and paracetamol, *Paediatric Nursing*, 22(3), pp. 22–6.

Cullen, C. 2021, Febrile and first-time seizures, *Pediatric Emergency Medicine Reports*, 26(3), viewed 20 February 2021, http://search.proquest.com.libraryproxy.griffith .edu.au/trade-journals/febrile-first-time-seizures/docview/2493045452/se-2? accountid=14543

Curtis, K & Ramsden C 2016, *Emergency and trauma care for nurses and paramedics* (2nd ed.), Elsevier, Sydney.

Dalby-Payne, J & Elliott, E 2011, Gastroenteritis in children, *Clinical Evidence*, 7, p. 314.

Davis, T & Ings, A 2015, Head injury: Triage, assessment, investigation and early management of head injury in children, young people and adults (NICE guideline CG 176), *Archives of Disease in Childhood Education and Practice*, 100(2), pp. 97–100.

de Benedictis, FM, Kerem, E, Chang, AB, Colin, AA, Zar, HJ & Bush, A 2020, Complicated pneumonia in children, *The Lancet*, 396(10253), pp. 786–98.

Desai, DJ, Gilbert, B & McBride, CA 2016, Paediatric urinary tract infections: Diagnosis and treatment, *Australian Family Physician*, 45(8), pp. 558–63.

Doyle, L, Treacy, M & Sheridan, A 2015, Self-harm in young people: Prevalence, associated factors, and help-seeking in school-going adolescents, *International Journal of Mental Health Nursing*, 24, pp. 485–95.

Dunning, J. 2021 *CHALICE (Children's Head Injury Algorithm for the prediction of important clinical events) Rule*, viewed 20 February 2021, www.mdcalc.com/chalice-childrens-head-injury-algorithm-prediction-important-clinical-events-rule

El Hitti, DE 2020, Acute epiglottitis, *InnovAiT Education and Inspiration for General Practice*, 13(10), pp. 608–12.

Emalee, G, Flaherty, JM, Perez-Rossello, AL & William LH 2014, Evaluating children with fractures for child physical abuse, *Pediatrics*, 133(2), pp. e477–e89.

Fitzgerald, DA & Kilham, HA 2003, Croup: Assessment and evidence-based management, *Medical Journal of Australia*, 179(7), pp. 372–7.

Forbes, H 2013, Vital signs, in J Crisp, C Taylor, C Douglas & G Rebeiro (eds), *Potter and Perry's fundamentals of nursing*, 4th ed., Mosby Elsevier, Sydney, pp. 658–702.

Forster, E & Scaini-Clarke, L 2017, Respiratory nursing skills, in E Forster & JA Fraser (eds), *Paediatric nursing skills for Australian nurses*, Cambridge University Press, Melbourne, pp. 184–207.

Gates A, Gates M, Vandermeer B, Johnson C, Hartling L, Johnson DW & Klassen TP 2018, Glucocorticoids for croup in children. *Cochrane Database of Systematic Reviews*, 8, CD001955.

Griffin, E, Corcoran, P, Cassidy, L, O'Carroll, A, Perry, IJ & Bonner, B 2014, Characteristics of hospital-treated intentional drug overdose in Ireland and Northern Ireland, *BMJ Open*, viewed 28 December 2016, http://nsrf.ie/wp-content/uploads/journals/2014/Griffin%20et%20al%202014.pdf

Hanson, KL, Medina, KL, Padula, CB, Tapert, SF & Brown, SA 2011, Impact of adolescent alcohol and drug use on neuropsychological functioning in young adulthood: 10-year outcomes, *Journal of Childhood Adolescent Substance Abuse*, 20(2), pp. 135–54.

Haq, IJ, Battersby, AC, Eastham, K & McKean, M 2017, Community acquired pneumonia in children, *BMJ*, 356, p. j686.

Harrison, JE, Berry, JG & Jamieson, LM 2012, Head and traumatic brain injuries among Australian youth and young adults, July 2000–June 2006, *Brain Injury*, 26(7–8), pp. 996–1004.

Hobbs, M, Tomintz, M & Kingham, S 2019, *Investigating the rates and spatial distribution of childhood ambulatory sensitive hospitalisations in New Zealand*. University of Canterbury GeoHealth Laboratory, Christchurch, viewed 20 February 2021, https://ir.canterbury.ac.nz/handle/10092/16898

Hosseinzadeh, P & Talwalkar, VR 2016, Compartment syndrome in children: Diagnosis and management, *American Journal of Orthopedics*, 45(1), pp. 19–22.

Howell, JM et al. 2010, Clinical policy: Critical issues in the evaluation and management of emergency department patients with suspected appendicitis, *Annals of Emergency Medicine*, 55(1), pp. 71–116.

In, W et al. 2019, The effect of a parental visitation program on emergence delirium among postoperative children in the PACU, *Journal of PeriAnesthesia Nursing*, 34(1), pp. 108–16.

Kasmire, KE, Rogers, SC & Sturm, JJ 2016, Trampoline park and home trampoline injuries, *Pediatrics*, 138(3), pp. e2016–e36.

Kesson, AM, Benwell, N & Elliott, EJ 2010, Norovirus diarrhoeal disease in infants and children, *Medical Journal of Australia*, 192(2), pp. 108–9.

Klein, JO & Pelton, S 2015, Acute otitis media: Epidemiology, microbiology, clinical manifestations, and complications, *Up to Date*, viewed 10 March 2016, www.uptodate.com

Koller, D & Goldman, RD 2012, Distraction techniques for children undergoing procedures: A critical review of pediatric research, *Journal of Pediatric Nursing*, 27, pp. 652–81.

Luehmann, NC 2019, Benefits of a family-centred approach to pediatric induction of anesthesia, *Journal of Pediatric Surgery*, 54(1), 189–193.

Lux, AL 2010, Treatment of febrile seizures: Historical perspective, current opinions, and potential future directions, *Brain & Development*, 32(1), pp. 42–50.

Malviya, S, Voepel-Lewis, T, Burke, C, Merkel, S & Tait, AR 2006, The revised FLACC observational pain tool: Improved reliability and validity for pain assessment in children with cognitive impairment, *Paediatric Anaesthesia*, 16(3), pp. 258–65.

Manworren, RCB & Hynan, LS 2003, Clinical validation of FLACC: Preverbal patient pain scale, *Pediatric Nursing*, 29(2), pp. 140–6.

Mazza, D, Wilkinson, F, Turner, T, Harris, C & Health for Kids Guideline Development Group 2008, Evidence-based guideline for the management of croup, *Australian Family Physician*, 37(6), pp. 14–20.

Meremikwu, MM & Oyo-Ita, A 2009a, Paracetamol versus placebo or physical methods for treating fever in children, *Cochrane Database of Systematic Reviews*, 2, CD003676.

—— 2009b, Physical methods versus drug placebo or no treatment for managing fever in children, *Cochrane Database of Systematic Reviews*, 4, CD003676.

Merkel, SI, Voepel-Lewis, T, Shayevitz, JR & Malviya, S 1997, The FLACC: A behavioral scale for scoring postoperative pain in young children, *Pediatric Nursing*, 23(3), pp. 293–7.

Ministry of Health 2010, *Drug use in New Zealand: Key results of the 2007/08 New Zealand Alcohol and Drug Use Survey*, Ministry of Health, Wellington.

—— 2020, *Longer, healthier lives: New Zealand's Health 1990–2017*, Ministry of Health, Wellington.

Mitchell RJ, Curtis K & Foster K 2018, A 10-year review of child injury hospitalisations, health outcomes and treatment costs in Australia, *Injury Prevention* 24, pp. 344–50.

Monasta, L et al. 2012, Burden of disease caused by otitis media: Systematic review and global estimates, *PLoS ONE*, 7(4), p. e36226.

Mulligan, CS, Adams, S & Brown J 2016, Paediatric injury from indoor trampoline centres, *Injury Prevention*, 23(5), 352–4.

National Asthma Council Australia 2020, *Australian Asthma Handbook, Version 2.1*, National Asthma Council Australia, Melbourne.

National Health and Medical Research Council (NHMRC) 2010, *Australian guidelines for the prevention and control of infection in healthcare*, Commonwealth of Australia, Canberra, viewed 20 February 2014, www.nhmrc.gov.au/_files_nhmrc/publications/attachments/cd33_infection_control_healthcare.pdf

—— 2013, *The Australian immunisation handbook*, Commonwealth of Australia, Canberra.

National Institute of Clinical Studies 2011, *Emergency care acute pain management manual*, NHMRC, Canberra, viewed 1 September 2016, www.nhmrc.gov.au/_files_nhmrc/publications/attachments/cp135_emergency_acute_pain_management_manual.pdf

National Institute for Health and Care Excellence (NICE) 2009, *Diarrhoea and vomiting caused by gastroenteritis: Diagnosis, assessment and management in children younger than 5 years*, NICE, London, viewed 20 February 2014, www.nice.org.uk/nicemedia/live/11846/43817/43817.pdf

—— 2014, *Head injury: triage, assessment, investigation and early management of head injury in children, young people and adults. CG 176 Methods, evidence and recommendations*, viewed 17 August 2016, www.nice.org.uk/guidance/cg176/evidence/full-guideline-191719837

—— 2020, *Intravenous fluid therapy in children and young people in hospital (NG29)*, viewed 16 March 2021, www.nice.org.uk/guidance/ng29/resources/intravenous-fluid-therapy-in-children-and-young-people-in-hospital-pdf-1837340295109

New South Wales Health 2010, *Infants and children – Acute management of croup* (2nd ed.), NSW Health, Sydney, viewed 15 March 2016, www.health.nsw.gov.au/policies.

—— 2011, *Children and infants: Acute management of head injury*, NSW Health, Sydney, viewed 16 August 2016, www.health.nsw.gov.au/policies/pd/2011/pdf/PD2011_024.pdf

—— 2013, *Infants and children: Acute management of abdominal pain – clinical practice guideline* (2nd ed.), NSW Health, Sydney, viewed 2 September 2016, www .health .nsw.gov.au/policies/pd/2013/pdf/PD2013_053.pdf

—— 2015, *Standards for paediatric intravenous fluids: NSW Health,* NSW Health, Sydney, viewed 28 March 2016, www0.health.nsw.gov.au/policies/gl/2015/pdf/gl2015_008 .pdf

—— 2016, *Infants and children: Management of acute and procedural pain in the emergency department*, NSW Health, Sydney, viewed 19 August 2016, www 0.health.nsw.gov .au/policies/gl/2016/pdf/GL2016_009.pdf

Nilsson, S, Finnstrom, B & Kokinsky, E 2008, The FLACC behavioral scale for procedural pain assessment in children aged 5–16 years, *Paediatric Anaesthesia*, 18(8), pp. 767–74.

Ogoina, D 2011, Fever, fever patterns and diseases called 'fever': A review, *Journal of Infection and Public Health*, 4(3), pp. 108–24.

Paediatric Research in Emergency Departments International Collaborative (PREDIC) 2016, *Australasian bronchiolitis guideline*, viewed 20 February 2021, www.accypn.org.au/wp-content/uploads/PREDICT_Australasian_Bronchiolitis_Guideline_FINAL_7_Sept_2016.pdf

Panella, JJ 2016, Preoperative care of children: Strategies from a child life perspective, *AORN*, 104(1), pp. 12–19.

Penrose, S, Palozzi, L & Dowden, S 2013, *Managing acute pain in children*, in A Twycross, S Dowden & J Stinson (eds), *Managing pain in children: A clinical guide for nurses and healthcare professionals* (2nd ed.), John Wiley & Sons, Hoboken, NJ.

Piedra, PA & Stark, AR 2016, Bronchiolitis in infants and children: Treatment, outcome, and prevention, *Up to Date,* viewed 21 March 2016, www.uptodate.com

Pillai Riddell, RR et al. 2015, Non-pharmacological management of infant and young child procedural pain, *Cochrane Database of Systematic Reviews*, 12, CD006275.

Plotnick, L & Ducharme, F 2000, Combined inhaled anticholinergics and beta2-agonists for initial treatment of acute asthma in children, *Cochrane Database of Systematic Reviews,* 3, CD000060.

Pointer, S 2014, *Hospitalised injury in children and young people 2011–2012*, cat. no. INJCAT 167, AIHW, Canberra, viewed 10 August 2016, www.aihw.gov.au/WorkArea/DownloadAsset.aspx?id=60129549323

—— 2016, *Hospitalised injury in Aboriginal and Torres Strait Islander children and young people 2011–13*, cat. no. INJCAT 172, AIHW, Canberra.

Pringle, K et al. 2011, Comparing the accuracy of the three popular clinical dehydration scales in children with diarrhea, *International Journal of Emergency Medicine*, 4, p. 58.

Prisco A et al. 2020, How to interpret symptoms, signs and investigations of dehydration in children with gastroenteritis, *Archives of Disease in Childhood – Education and Practice*, 106(2), pp. 114–19.

Rang, HP, Dale, MM & Ritter, JM 2011, *Rang and Dale's pharmacology* (7th ed.), Churchill Livingstone, St Louis, MO.

Rathnayake, T 2012, Intravenous cannulation (paediatric): Clinician information, *[Joanna Briggs Institute] Evidence Summaries*, 1–4.

Risher, M, Sexton, HG, Risher, WC, Wilson, WA, Fleming, RL, Madison, RD, Moore, SD, Eroglu, C & Swartzwelder, HS 2015, Adolescent intermittent alcohol exposure: Dysregulation of thrombospondins and synapse formation are associated with decreased neuronal density in the adult hippocampus, *Alcoholism: Clinical and Experimental Research*, 39(12), pp. 2403–13.

Royal Children's Hospital Melbourne (RCHM) 2018, *Clinical practice guidelines: Asthma acute,* viewed 8 July 2020, www.rch.org.au/clinicalguide/guideline_index/Asthma_acute

—— 2019, *Clinical practice guidelines: Febrile child*, viewed 30 October 2019, www.rch.org.au/clinicalguide/guideline_index/Febrile_child

—— 2020, *Engaging with and assessing the adolescent patient*, viewed 13 October 2020, www.rch.org.au/clinicalguide/guideline_index/Engaging_with_and_assessing_the_adolescent_patient

Russell, K et al. 2011, Glucocorticoids for croup, *Cochrane Database of Systematic Reviews,* 1, CD001955.

Safekids Aotearoa 2015, *Child unintentional deaths and injuries in New Zealand, and prevention strategies*, Safekids Aotearoa, Auckland.

Santillanes, G, & Rose E 2018, Evaluation and management of dehydration in children, *Emergency Medicine Clinics of North America*, 36(2), 259–73.

Schaller, TM & Calhoun, JH 2016, Open fractures, *Medscape,* viewed 30 December 2016, http://emedicine.medscape.com/article/1269242-overview

Schomacker, H, Schaap-Nutt, A, Collins, PL & Schmidt, AC 2012, Pathogenesis of acute respiratory illness caused by human parainfluenza viruses, *Current Opinions on Virology*, 2, pp. 294–9.

Schreiber, S et al. 2013, Does EMLA cream application interfere with the success of venipuncture or venous cannulation? A prospective multicenter observational study, *European Journal of Pediatrics*, 172(2), pp. 265–8.

Shields, CJ & Clarke, S 2011, Neurovascular observation and documentation for children within accident and emergency: A critical review, *International Journal of Orthopaedic and Trauma Nursing*, 15(1), pp. 3–10.

Simpson J, Duncanson M, Oben G, Adams J, Wicken A, Pierson M, Lilley R & Gallagher S. 2017, *Te Ohonga Ake: The health of Māori children and young people in New Zealand*, New Zealand Child and Youth Epidemiology Service, University of Otago, Dunedin.

Srouji, R, Ratnaplan, S & Schneeweiss, S 2010, Pain in children: Assessment and management, *International Journal of Pediatrics,* article ID 474838.

Szajewska, H, Guarino, A, Hojsak, I, Indrio, F, Kolacek, S, Orel, R, Salvatore, S, Shamir, R, van Goudoever, JB, Vandenplas, Y, Weizman, Z & Zalewski, BM 2020, Use of probiotics for the management of acute gastroenteritis in children, *Journal of Pediatric Gastroenterology and Nutrition*, 71(2), 261–9.

Sydney Children's Hospital 2019, *Acute asthma – management: Practice guideline*, viewed 8 July 2020, www.schn.health.nsw.gov.au/_policies/pdf/2007-8358.pdf

Tibballs, J & Watson, T 2011, Symptoms and signs differentiating croup and epiglottitis, *Journal of Paediatrics & Child Health*, 47(3), pp. 77–82.

Trauma Victoria 2016, *Paediatric trauma,* viewed 28 December 2016, http://trauma.reach
.vic.gov.au/guidelines/paediatric-trauma/key-messages

van den Anker, JN 2013, Optimising the management of fever and pain in children,
International Journal of Clinical Practice, 67, pp. 26–32.

van Dijk, M et al. 2000, The reliability and validity of the COMFORT scale as a postoperative
pain instrument in 0- to 3-year-old infants, *Pain*, 84(2–3), pp. 367–77.

Venekamp, RP, Sanders, S, Glasziou, PP, Del Mar, CB & Rovers, MM 2015, Antibiotics for
acute otitis media in children, *Cochrane Database of Systematic Reviews*, 6,
CD000219.

Walsh, A, Edwards, H & Fraser, J 2008, Parents' childhood fever management:
Community survey and instrument development, *Journal of Advanced Nursing*,
63(4), pp. 376–88.

Watts, R & Robertson, J 2012, Non-pharmacological management of fever in otherwise
healthy children, *JBI Database of Systematic Reviews and Implementation
Reports*, 10(26), pp. 1634–87.

Wente, SJK 2012, Nonpharmacological pediatric pain management in emergency
departments: A systematic review of the literature, *Journal of Emergency Nursing*,
39(2), pp. 140–50.

White, V & Bariola, E 2012, *Australian secondary school students' use of tobacco, alcohol,
and over-the-counter and illicit substances in 2011,* Department of Health and
Ageing, Canberra, viewed 20 September 2016, www.nationaldrugstrategy.gov.au/
internet/drugstrategy/Publishing.nsf/content/BCBF6B2C638E1202CA257ACD00
20E35C/$File/National%20Report_FINAL_AS SAD_7.12.pdf

Willis, MHW, Merkel, SI, Voepel-Lewis, T & Malviya, S 2003, FLACC Behavioral Pain
Assessment Scale: A comparison with the child's self-report, *Pediatric Nursing*,
29(3), pp. 195–8.

Wood, JM & Vijayasekaran, S 2014, Acute otitis media in young children. Diagnosis and
management, *Medicine Today*, 15(7), pp. 12–22.

Woods, CR 2015, Croup: Clinical features, evaluation, and diagnosis, *Up to Date,* viewed
10 March 2016, www.uptodate.com

Woragidpoonpol, P, Yenbut, J, Picheansathian, W & Klunklin, P 2013, Effectiveness of non-
pharmacological interventions in relieving children's postoperative pain:
A systematic review, *JBI Database of Systematic Review & Implementation
Reports*, 11(10), pp. 117–56.

World Health Organization (WHO) & UNICEF 2013, *Ending preventable child deaths from
pneumonia and diarrhoea by 2025: The integrated Global Action Plan for Pneumonia
and Diarrhoea (GAPPD),* WHO, Geneva, viewed 20 April 2014, www.who.int/
maternal_child_adolescent/documents/global_action_plan_pneumonia_diarrhoea/en

Yousef, Y, Drudi, S, Sant'Anna, A & Sherif, E 2018, Parental presence at induction of
anesthesia: Perceptions of a pediatric surgical department before and after program
implementation, *Journal of Pediatric Surgery* 53(8), pp. 1606–10.

Zoorob, R, Sidani, M & Murray, J 2011, Croup: An overview, *American Family Physician*,
83(9), pp. 1067–73.

Recognising and responding to the sick child

Elizabeth Forster and Loretta Scaini-Clarke

LEARNING OBJECTIVES

In this chapter you will:

- Gain an understanding of normal assessment findings in the paediatric patient and those indicating deterioration
- Learn how to recognise a sick or deteriorating child using an appropriate framework
- Develop an understanding of how to respond to a sick or deteriorating child and provide appropriate respiratory and circulatory support
- Learn the elements of paediatric cardiopulmonary resuscitation
- Consider the importance of supporting families and parental presence during paediatric resuscitation

Introduction

As a nurse caring for paediatric patients, it is important for you to develop the ability to recognise and respond to a sick infant or child. The ability to do this is so important that a variety of projects have been undertaken, both internationally and throughout Australia and New Zealand, to ensure that nurses working with paediatric patients are able to recognise, respond promptly to and appropriately manage sick and deteriorating infants and children. Examples are the Between the Flags program or Standard Paediatric Observation Chart (SPOC) in New South Wales, the Victorian Children's Tool for Observation and Response (VICTOR), the Children's Early Warning Assessment Tool (CEWT) in Queensland and the Paediatric Early Warning Score (PEWS) in New Zealand. These programs aim to support the assessment skills of the clinician working with infants and children. **Paediatric early warning tools** help clinicians to recognise a deteriorating infant or child, and trigger an escalation in care to prevent further deterioration and achieve favourable outcomes. This chapter will provide you with a basic understanding and knowledge so that you will be able to recognise and respond to a sick and deteriorating child.

Paediatric early warning tools – Tools that assist nurses to recognise signs and symptoms indicating deterioration in paediatric patients; these include triggers and directions for escalations in management, including urgent medical review.

Clinical signs – a warning of deterioration – are often present in the paediatric patient as for as long as six to 12 hours before a catastrophic event. Failure to identify and treat these early warning signs can result in continued clinical deterioration until cardiopulmonary arrest. The poor outcomes associated with paediatric cardiopulmonary arrest emphasise the importance of being able to detect and respond to early signs of deterioration (McLellan & Connor, 2013).

The primary cause of paediatric cardiopulmonary arrest is respiratory in origin, and the second most common cause is circulatory failure (Jones, Wilmshurst & Graydon, 2017). In both situations, the child will display signs of respiratory or cardiovascular compromise prior to deteriorating into cardiac arrest. Timely intervention can treat or stabilise the child, preventing the progress of the condition. Sudden cardiac arrest is extremely rare in paediatrics, and is limited to a small number of uncommon conditions, such as hypertrophic cardiomyopathy, myocarditis, underlying congenital cardiac disease or arrhythmias such as long or short QT syndrome or drugs and/or stimulants (Scheller et al., 2016).

Paediatric characteristics that increase the risk of illness and deterioration

Understanding the causes of deterioration in the paediatric patient is important for enhancing early recognition of problems. Due to their stage of development, paediatric patients have anatomical, physiological and behavioural differences that underpin their predisposition to develop illness and their ability to respond to the stress of disease. Table 11.1 reviews some of the significant respiratory and cardiovascular differences.

Table 11.1   Respiratory and cardiovascular differences in paediatric patients

Paediatric respiratory characteristics that increase risk of respiratory compromise	
Characteristic	**Relationship to increased risk of compromise**
Infants are obligatory nose breathers	Respiratory difficulties if the nares become blocked with secretions.
Narrow airways	Even a small amount of swelling or secretion results in a large increase in airways resistance, impacting the work of breathing.
Soft, collapsible airways • Submucosal glands in airway larger than in adults • Lower pH of airway lining	In newborns, airway cartilage is not fully developed and it is thus more susceptible to collapse. Avoid over-extension of the head. Smaller diameter increases airflow resistance when narrowed. Possible hyperactivity of mucous production. May be linked to dysfunction of epithelial cells of respiratory tract, impaired mucocillary clearance and viscosity of secretions.
Large tongue and adenoids	Lead to an increased risk of airway obstruction. Adenoids are often problematic around 2 years of age.
Stiff, omega-shaped epiglottis	Difficult to view the glottic opening during intubation.
Cricoid cartilage is narrowest point of the airway (infants)	Increases the risk for trauma to the subglottic region during insertion of an endotracheal tube.
Horizontal, cartilaginous ribs due to lack of ossification of the ribs	The chest wall collapses inwards when the infant increases their work of breathing. This is seen as intercostal, sternal and subcostal recession, and often results in decreased air entry. The compliant and soft chest wall and likelihood of collapse during anaesthesia can increase risk for atelectasis and oxygen desaturation.
Immature intercostal and accessory muscles	Primarily use the diaphragm to breathe. The lack of type II muscle fibres results in early fatigue of the infant's respiratory muscles. Increased work of breathing results in head bob, seesaw movement between the chest and abdomen.
Less alveolar surface area available for gas exchange	By approximately 8–12 years of age, a child has nine times the alveoli that were present at birth.
Large head and an inability to reposition	Infants have a large occiput that can push the head forward and obstruct the airway. They lack the muscle strength or developmental ability to reposition themselves to aid breathing.
Higher metabolic rate	Greater need for oxygen to support metabolic processes, and consequently higher respiratory rates. Greater need for oxygen leads to rapid oxygen desaturation if apnoea occurs.
Developmental stage of placing objects into the mouth or nose	Upper airway obstruction due to foreign objects is common, and can be life-threatening in toddlers and young children.
Paediatric cardiovascular characteristics that increase risk of cardiovascular compromise	
Characteristic	**Relationship to increased risk for compromise**
Immature myocardium	Limited ability to increase contractility, making stroke volume relatively fixed. Cardiac output is increased by increasing the heart rate.
70–80 mL/kg blood volume	Low total blood volume – 240 mL for a newborn. Small losses can result in shock.

Table 11.1 *(cont.)*

Paediatric cardiovascular characteristics that increase risk of cardiovascular compromise	
Characteristic	**Relationship to increased risk for compromise**
Ability to maintain blood pressure	Compensatory increased heart rate and systemic vascular resistance mean that hypotension is a very late sign of cardiovascular compromise. Earlier signs of compromise are increased HR, capillary refill, decreased peripheral perfusion. Urine output must be observed, as it will decrease with a fall in renal perfusion.
Changes from foetal circulation may continue for several weeks	Undiagnosed congenital cardiac structural defects may present within the first weeks of life.
Increased risk for fluid depletion	Large surface area increases the risk of insensible losses. Reduced ability to concentrate urine during infancy. Larger percentage of total body fluids.
Limited metabolic and physiological reserve	If left unsupported, infants and children may become exhausted from their disease states. This may manifest as a reduction in respiratory rate or slowing of the heart rate. These are indicators that the child is rapidly approaching cardiorespiratory arrest.

Source: Adapted from Hsu & Fiadjoe (2020); Santillanes & Gausche-Hill (2008); Walsh, Hood & Merritt (2011).

Structured assessment of the paediatric patient

The use of a structured assessment framework can assist with your ability to perform a patient assessment (Munroe et al., 2013). Assessment frameworks can assist clinicians to prioritise assessment of critical body systems and ensure that these are methodically assessed. We will discuss two commonly used assessment approaches here: the **Paediatric Assessment Triangle** and the **Primary Assessment Framework**.

The Paediatric Assessment Triangle

Figure 11.1 represents the Paediatric Assessment Triangle (Dieckmann, Brownstein & Gausche-Hill, 2010), a rapid-assessment framework used to perform an initial assessment and to quickly identify a sick and deteriorating child.

The Paediatric Assessment Triangle works via rapid assessment of three components: the child's appearance, work of breathing and circulation to the skin (Dieckmann, Brownstein & Gausche-Hill, 2010).

The child's appearance relates to:

- *tone* – includes whether the child moves spontaneously, resists being examined, sits or stands (age appropriate)
- *interactiveness* – includes whether the child appears alert and engaged with clinicians/caregivers, interacts with people and environment, reaches for toys, objects
- *consolability* – includes whether the child stops crying with holding/comforting by caregiver or has differential response to caregiver versus examiner

Paediatric Assessment Triangle – A tool that can be used to complete a rapid 'hands-off' 30-second (approximately) assessment of the paediatric patient. The tool assesses the child's appearance, work of breathing and circulation to the skin.

Primary Assessment Framework – An assessment framework that provides a 'first look' at body systems – for example, respiratory, cardiovascular and neurological. If an abnormality is detected, it should be addressed immediately.

- *look/gaze* – includes whether child makes eye contact with clinician, tracks visually
- *speech/cry* – includes whether the child has a strong cry/uses age-appropriate speech.

The child's work of breathing relates to:

- abnormal airway sounds (including snoring, muffled or hoarse speech, stridor, grunting, wheezing)
- abnormal positioning (sniffing position, tripoding or preference for seated posture)
- retractions (supraclavicular, intercostal or substernal retractions, head bobbing in infants)
- flaring of the nares on inspiration
- respiratory rate (fast or slow respirations for age of child).

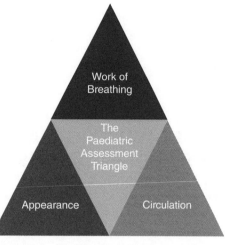

Figure 11.1 The Paediatric Assessment Triangle
Source: Adapted from Dieckmann, Brownstein & Gausche-Hill (2010).

The child's circulation relates to characteristic abnormal features such as:

- pallor (white or pale skin or mucous membranes)
- mottling (patchy skin discoloration due to varying degrees of vasoconstriction)
- cyanosis (bluish discoloration of skin and mucous membranes).

The Paediatric Assessment Triangle provides clinicians with a rapid 'hands-off' 30-second (approximately) assessment that can be completed prior to the hands-on primary survey. It means that life-saving treatments can be initiated immediately if necessary.

The Primary Assessment Framework

We will now discuss the ABCD, primary survey or Primary Assessment Framework for assessing the paediatric patient. The Primary Assessment Framework approach to assessment uses an ABCD assessment framework for paediatric patients. Many of the early warning tools use a variation of the primary survey in guiding the initial assessment of the paediatric patient.

The Primary Assessment Framework is designed to assist in assessing and managing clinical deterioration in order of priority. When completing a primary assessment, if life-threatening conditions are identified they must be managed prior to continuing with the assessment. The following is a brief description of the primary assessment framework:

A *Airway:*   assessed for patency and security
B *Breathing:*   work and rate of breathing and the effectiveness of breathing to achieve adequate oxygenation and air entry
C *Circulation:* heart rate, skin perfusion and evidence that the body is achieving sufficient adequate blood flow

D *Disability:*   mental status and level of consciousness. You will be able to use your beginning understanding of the primary assessment framework when you consider Case study 11.1, which concerns Maggie, an infant with respiratory distress.

CASE STUDY 11.1 MAGGIE: AN INFANT WITH RESPIRATORY DISTRESS

Maggie, a 6-month-old infant, has a three-day history of a respiratory tract infection. She has been admitted to the paediatric ward diagnosed with bronchiolitis (suspected to be Respiratory Syncitial Virus [RSV]). Upon assessment, Maggie is pale and lethargic. She has a moist cough and thick, creamy rhinorrhoea. Her respiratory rate is 55 breaths per minute and she has moderate intercostal and subcostal recession and tracheal tug. Bilateral wheeze can be heard upon auscultation. Her oxygen saturations (S_pO_2) in room air are 91 per cent. Her heart rate is 154 beats per minute and her temperature is 37.9°C.

Maggie's mother reports that she has been 'not feeding well' over the past few days. She last changed a wet nappy at 5.00 am (six hours ago).

Applying the Primary Assessment Framework

By utilising the Primary Assessment Framework when performing Maggie's assessment, as Maggie's nurse you are able to collect the data in systematic manner.

- Airway:
  - maintaining own airway; no upper airway noises
  - thick nasal secretions potential for obstructing nasal breathing.
- Breathing:
  - respirations are 55 breaths per minute
  - increased work of breathing evidenced by intercostal and subcostal recession
  - wheeze
  - reduced oxygen saturations in room air: 91 per cent (impaired gas exchange).
- Circulation:
  - heart rate of 154 beats per minute
  - pallor, peripheries cool
  - peripheral pulses present
  - blood pressure 100/52
  - reduced urine output
  - reduced oral intake.
- Disability:
  - lethargic
  - responses to voice on AVPU score
  - uninterested in feeding.

Recognition of clinical deterioration using a Primary Assessment Framework

You already have a beginning understanding of the elements of the Primary Assessment Framework, and you have applied this to collect assessment data about Maggie in Case study 11.1. In this section, we will utilise the Primary Assessment Framework to provide you with a systematic and detailed review of a paediatric assessment. In most instances, a rapid assessment should be undertaken to identify the need for emergency care prior to performing a more comprehensive assessment. If, however, immediately life-threatening conditions present during the primary assessment, then they must be managed immediately.

A – Airway

In the primary survey, A represents airway assessment. For the paediatric patient, you need to consider whether the patient can maintain their own airway. Is the airway clear or is it obstructed? An inability to maintain a patent airway is immediately life-threatening and needs to take priority in the management of the patient. The child's ability to vocalise or speak provides a rapid assessment of airway patency.

There are a number of anatomical and behavioural developmental factors that increase the paediatric patient's risk for compromised airway. Some of these factors include having a large tongue, a soft floor of the mouth that is easily compressible, a large head that tends to flex the neck when lying in a neutral or supine position and a small-sized mid-face (Hsu & Fiadjoe, 2020; Miller & Nagler, 2019; Cullen, 2012a). In a child with decreased or a loss of consciousness, the large tongue could easily obstruct the airway. When artificial support is given, care should be taken to hold any mask along the jawline so as not to compress the soft floor of a child's mouth, further contributing to airway compromise. The large head with a predominant occiput can result in the child's neck becoming flexed and obstructing the airway (Hsu & Fiadjoe, 2020; Miller & Nagler, 2019).

The child's upper airway is narrow and cone-shaped, with the cricoid cartilage being the narrowest point. This anatomy places the child at increased risk of upper airway obstruction due to swelling associated with infections such as 'croup' (laryngotracheobronchitis).

Another important cause of airway obstruction in young children is a foreign body. Inhalation of small objects, including toys, batteries or pieces of food, can partially or completely obstruct the upper airway.

Characteristics of partial upper airway obstruction may include:

- difficulty breathing with increased work of breathing
- upper respiratory tract noises such a stridor or snoring sounds
- drooling or inability to swallow secretions
- the child positioning their neck or head to open their airway
- a history of illness or choking on a foreign object
- decreased air entry and impaired oxygenation in severe cases.

Rapidly assessing the child for the cause and degree of respiratory compromise is essential to ensure appropriate management and referral. For example, a child with a partially obstructed airway following anaesthesia may require the application of a simple airway opening manoeuvre such as jaw thrust until they are more awake. However, a child with a severe episode of croup may require urgent medical attention.

Children with complete upper airway obstruction will quickly deteriorate into cardiac arrest and require an urgent emergency airway. The management of any child with acute upper airway obstruction is therefore critical. It is important that a doctor who is able to perform a difficult paediatric intubation is notified.

Children at risk of airway obstruction should be observed continuously and never left unattended.

It is important to remember that severe airway obstruction can occur without changes to oxygenation. Falling oxygen levels are a sign of decompensation and require immediate medical attention.

B – Breathing

In the primary survey, B represents breathing – that is, assessment of the adequacy of breathing, and therefore oxygenation. In the paediatric patient, this incorporates a variety of assessment parameters, including:

- respiratory rate, which will vary depending upon the age of the infant or child, and the presence of fever or coexisting health conditions (see Table 11.2 for usual paediatric respiratory rates)
- symmetry and excursion of chest wall movement
- work of breathing, including the presence of signs such as nasal flaring and head bobbing in infants, recession or retractions, and diaphragmatic movement in conjunction with chest wall movement.
- respiratory pattern, regular or irregular breathing, apneas, long expiratory phase
- central colour.

Chest recession or retractions

The assessment of chest recession or retractions is important, as normally there is minimal chest wall movement in the child because they rely upon diaphragmatic abdominal breathing. Any respiratory issue that causes increased airway resistance therefore results in the generation of increased negative intrathoracic pressure needed to produce inward airflow during inspiration causes recession (Agbim, Wang & Moon, 2018).

While the presence of increased labour of breathing is an important sign, consideration should be made for children unable to generate significant work of breathing. This includes children too fatigued to continue to generate increased respiratory effort, those with neuromuscular disorders such as muscular dystrophies and children with a reduced level of consciousness.

Breath sounds and air entry

Breath sounds and air entry, or the absence of breath sounds, can be an important element of breathing assessment in the paediatric patient. Breath sounds can alert the clinician to the nature of the respiratory issue – for example, wheezing indicates fluid or swelling in the lower airways, and stridor indicates narrowing, oedema or obstruction of the trachea and upper airway. Stridor and wheeze may be audible. Using a stethoscope to auscultate the chest can provide more detailed information about the quality and sounds of air entry. Air entry should be heard equally, bilaterally. The inability to hear breath sounds on auscultation is a life-threatening sign.

Grunting may be heard in infants with severe respiratory distress, and indicates an effort to increase end expiratory pressure during respiration to promote gas exchange (Agbim, Wang & Moon, 2018).

Children may also alter their position and assume the tripod position (sitting upright and learning forward slightly while supporting their upper body with arms on their thighs or on the bed) to try to optimise the use of their thoracic and abdominal muscles when in respiratory distress (Agbim, Wang & Moon, 2018).

Oxygen saturation

Oxygen saturations are a measure of the oxygen saturation of haemoglobin and provide valuable information about the child's oxygenation status. Pulse oximeters are commonly used to measure the oxygen saturation in peripheral blood (S_pO_2). Normal S_pO_2 should be greater than 97 per cent in room air (O'Meara & Watton, 2012).

A variety of factors impact the accuracy of readings in the paediatric patient, including movement, peripheral perfusion and skin pigmentation (Fouzas, Priftis & Anthracopoulos, 2011). This means it is important to look at oxygen saturation values in conjunction with the general clinical appearance of the child and other assessment data collected.

Table 11.2 shows the respiratory rate parameters for paediatric age groups and factors that may influence respiratory rate.

Central cyanosis is a clinical sign of low oxygen saturation requiring the administration of oxygen and/or respiratory support. Cyanosis can be seen as a bluish

Table 11.2 Respiratory rate parameters for paediatric age groups

Age	Respiratory rate breaths per minute	Consider factors that may affect respiratory rate
Term newborn (0–28 days)	25–60	Fever Comorbidities (e.g. congenital respiratory or heart disease) Seizure activity Neurological injury pH imbalances Fear, emotional upset, anxiety
Infant (3 months)	25–60	
Infant (6 months)	20–55	
Toddler (1–3 years)	20–45	
Child (4–6 years)	16–30	
Child (6 –12 years)	15–25	
Adolescent (13 years and over)	14–25	

Source: Adapted from RCHM (2020a).

colouration of the lips, mucus membranes and around the mouth as a result of increased deoxygenated (blue) haemoglobin. Cyanosis cannot be easily equated to a particular oxygen saturation; however its presence is associated with significantly reduced oxygen saturation (McMullen & Patrick, 2013). Children with low haemoglobin levels require lower oxygen saturations before they will display signs of cyanosis than children with normal haemoglobin. This may be an important consideration for post-operative or chronically unwell children.

It is important to remember that decreasing respiratory effort and respiratory rate are a sign of fatigue and decompensation. Without immediate support, the child can progress to respiratory arrest.

C – Circulation

In the primary survey, C represents your assessment of the adequacy of circulation in the paediatric patient, and involves assessing:

- heart rate and rhythm
- peripheral pulses and perfusion
- colour
- urine output
- blood pressure.

Assessing paediatric circulation requires an understanding of the way the sick infant or child responds to altered and inadequate circulatory or cardiovascular function. The sick infant or child with cardiovascular compromise will trigger compensatory mechanisms as the body attempts to maintain blood pressure and ensure that vital organs are perfused.

A reduced pressure within the circulatory system will trigger the release of catecholamines (adrenaline and noradrenaline) and hormones (angiotensin and anti-diuretic hormone) that result in an increased heart rate, vasoconstriction of peripheral blood vessels and retention of sodium and water by the kidneys. These responses enable the sick infant or child to maintain blood pressure and circulation to the heart, lungs and brain. However, if the circulatory compromise is not corrected, these compensatory mechanisms will no longer be able to sustain sufficient perfusion of the vital organs and blood pressure will no longer be able to be maintained. This pre-terminal stage will be evident in a drop in blood pressure and decreased level of consciousness.

Table 11.3 shows the heart rate parameters for paediatric age groups and the factors to consider that may influence heart rate and rhythm.

Heart rate and rhythm

During childhood, the heart rate is faster and the stroke volume continues to increase from birth until 5 years of age and then stabilises (Top, Tasker & Ince, 2011). Normal heart rates and blood pressure values are presented in Table 11.3 and are based between the 5th and 95th percentile values for each paediatric age group (RCHM, 2020a). During early childhood, cardiac muscle fibres are immature and lack the ability to increase the strength of myocardial contractility. Stroke volume – the volume of blood ejected with each ventricular contraction – is therefore relatively fixed.

Table 11.3 Heart rate and systolic blood pressure parameters for paediatric age groups

Age	Heart rate (beats per minute)	Systolic blood pressure (mmHg)	Consider factors that may affect heart rate/ rhythm
Newborn (0–28 days)	70–190	60–95	Hypoxia, fever
Infant (3 months)	115–180	60–105	Comorbidities (e.g. congenital respiratory or heart disease)
Infant (6 months)	110–180	75–105	
Toddler (1–3 years)	95–180	70–105	Dehydration Pain
Child (4–6 years)	75–150	75–115	Fear, emotional upset, anxiety
Child (6–12 years)	65–140	80–120	
Adolescent (13 years and over)	60–115	90–130	

Source: Adapted from RCHM (2020a).

In children – particularly infants – cardiac output is increased primarily by increasing the heart rate. The child's dependence on heart rate to manipulate cardiac output makes heart rate one of the most important observations in the paediatric cardiovascular assessment. Observation of trends in heart rate can provide signs of cardiovascular improvement or deterioration. However, while heart rate is a very sensitive sign of cardiovascular status, it is not a very specific sign. The child's heart rate may be increased due to other factors such as temperature, pain or anxiety. Therefore, it is essential to evaluate the heart rate in the context of other clinical observations.

Bradycardia is an important sign of cardiorespiratory decompensation. This may occur in children who have become physiologically exhausted from respiratory or cardiac illness.

For infants under 12 months of age, a heart rate of less than 60, accompanied by signs of impaired perfusion, will require cardiopulmonary resuscitation.

In the paediatric patient, stroke volume may be evaluated by assessing the volume and strength of pulses, and systemic vascular resistance may be evaluated via assessment of the child's peripheral skin perfusion.

Blood pressure

Normal blood pressure is not a reliable sign of a child's cardiovascular status. Severe cardiovascular compromise and inadequate tissue perfusion can be present despite normal blood pressure. However, performing a paediatric blood pressure assessment is important because hypotension is poorly tolerated and needs to be addressed urgently.

The paediatric patient's compensatory mechanisms in the event of hypovolaemia work towards the maintenance of blood flow to the vital organs despite falling cardiac output due to decreased stroke volume (Hobson & Chima, 2013; Mendelson, 2018). The paediatric patient's blood pressure is maintained by increasing heart rate and systemic vascular resistance through peripheral vasoconstriction until shock is severe.

Tachycardia, delayed capillary refill time and diminished peripheral pulses are indicative of these compensatory mechanisms, and when these mechanisms fail hypotension occurs and thus a drop in blood pressure is considered a late and pre-terminal sign (Hobson & Chima, 2013; Mendelson, 2018). It is therefore important that early signs of circulatory compromise are detected. Clinicians must assess and interpret heart rate, colour, perfusion, skin temperature, capillary refill times and level of consciousness to ensure that early intervention and circulatory support are initiated. In sick infants, assessing the blood pressure in the upper and lower limbs can provide information about undiagnosed congenital cardiac conditions such as coarctation of the aorta.

Note: The size of the blood pressure cuff is important to ensure accuracy of the measurement (see Figure 11.2). The cuff bladder should encircle 80–100 per cent of the mid-upper arm circumference (Ostchega et al., 2014). Table 11.4 provides a guide for appropriate blood pressure cuff sizes and Figure 11.3 indicates the correct BP cuff size on the infant's left arm (white-coloured BP cuff) and the incorrect cuff size and application on the infant's right arm (navy-coloured BP cuff).

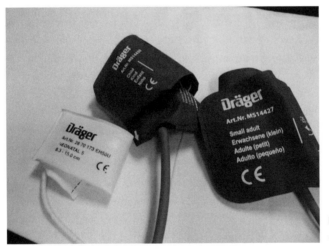

Figure 11.2 Blood pressure cuffs

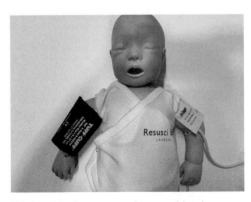

Figure 11.3 Incorrect and correct blood pressure cuff

Peripheral pulses and perfusion

Pulses should be checked both centrally and peripherally, and evaluated for differences. Marked variation in intensity of pulses may be indicative of blood being directed towards central organs and away from the peripheries. This is a compensatory mechanism that can occur in conditions such hypovolaemia.

Table 11.4 Blood pressure cuff sizes

Patient	Cuff width	Cuff length	Maximum arm circumference
Infant	6 cm	12 cm	15 cm
Child	9 cm	18 cm	22 cm
Adolescent	10 cm	24 cm	26 cm

Source: Adapted from the National High Blood Pressure Education Program Working
Group on High Blood Pressure in Children and Adolescents (2004); Ostchega et al. (2014).

The strength and volume of the pulse provide information about stroke volume. A weak or thready pulse – especially if found centrally – is a worrying sign of poor cardiac output. This may be present in a child with severe vasoconstriction and/or impaired cardiac function.

The carotid pulse can be used to assess a central pulse in children. Because infants often have short, chubby necks, the most reliable locations to palpate central pulses in infants are the brachial and femoral arteries. Absent or weak femoral pulses may be indicative of undiagnosed congenital cardiac conditions where upper limb pulses are adequate.

The colour and temperature of skin can reflect the adequacy of peripheral perfusion and provide information about systemic vascular resistance. Skin mottling has been demonstrated to be a reliable measure of skin hypoperfusion and is responsive to changes in peripheral vasoconstriction (Ait-Oufella et al., 2013).

Peripheral vasoconstriction is part of the compensatory response designed to maintain blood pressure during cardiovascular compromise, and is therefore an indirect measure of cardiovascular function. Severe alterations in peripheral perfusion, such as mottling, pale, cold skin and decreased peripheral pulses, are indicative of serious cardiovascular dysfunction.

When assessing skin temperature and perfusion, it is valuable to identify the level of skin involvement so that reassessment for change is possible. For example, the skin may be cool and mottled to the level of the child's knee. Factors such as low environmental temperatures and fever can also cause peripheral vasoconstriction, resulting in pale or cool skin. Therefore, it is important to apply your assessment finding to the clinical context.

Capillary refill

Capillary refill is often used to assess skin perfusion in the paediatric patient. It refers to the amount of time for the capillary bed to return its colour after pressure has been applied to cause the area to blanch (Pickard, Karlen & Ansermino, 2011). A variety of factors may affect capillary refill time, including:

- *age* (with neonates having an upper limit of three seconds and children having an upper limit of two seconds)
- *environmental, skin and core temperature* – capillary refill time tends to increase with cooler ambient temperature and decrease with warmer environments, such as when

radiant heaters are used; skin temperature also affects capillary refill time, and reductions in skin temperature tend to be reflected in an increased capillary refill time; core temperature also influences capillary refill time with each $1°C$ rise in core temperature, resulting in a shorter capillary refill time (Pickard, Karlen & Ansermino, 2011)

- *duration* of application and *location of pressure* applied.

There is no consensus about the correct duration of pressure application prior to measuring capillary refill time, and the variables range from three to seven seconds – or sufficient time to cause blanching. Recent paediatric studies recommend using your index finger to apply enough pressure to cause the skin to turn pale and applying pressure for five seconds and timing how long it takes for the original colour to return, which has improved reliability of this measure (Crook & Taylor, 2013; Fleming et al., 2016).

A variety of sites have been used for testing capillary refill, including the forehead, sternum, nail bed of fingers or toes, or pulp or pads of fingertips and heels. The location used may affect the capillary refill time – for example, the capillary refill time at the heel may show a longer time than at the finger, and fingertip capillary refill time is faster than the sternum capillary refill time (Crook & Taylor, 2013). Therefore, when testing capillary refill in practice, it is important to use a consistent site for measurement, to time the duration of refill time with a watch for accuracy and reliability, and to interpret your findings in conjunction with your overall assessment of the paediatric patient. Paediatric advance life-support groups recommend performing capillary refill centrally, on the sternum, to assist with consistency and reliability of this assessment in the unwell child (Samuels & Wiesteska, 2016).

Urine output

A normal urine output for a child is approximately $1\,mL/kg/hour$. The normal urine output for an infant is $>2\,mL/kg/hour$, which equates to approximately six to eight wet nappies per day. An infant with no wet nappy for more than four to six hours may have a decreased urine output. Weighed nappies (see Figure 11.4) can be used to calculate urine output more accurately. If infants have diarrhoea and evidence of dehydration, an indwelling catheter may be needed to accurately assess urine output.

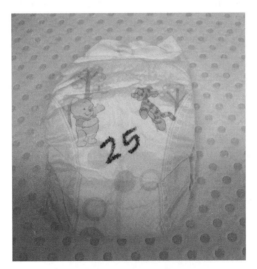

Figure 11.4 Weighed disposable nappy

The colour and concentration of the urine also provide information about the child's hydration status. A reduction in urine output with concentrated urine is often associated with hypovolaemia. As part of the compensatory mechanism, increased concentrations of antidiuretic hormone, angiotensin and aldosterone act on the kidneys to promote reabsorption of water and sodium into the body and reduce the volume of urine produced. Renal blood flow may also be decreased, resulting in further decreases in urine output.

It is important to remember that some paediatric conditions that may cause hypovolaemia may have increased urine output – for example, diabetic ketoacidosis, diabetes insipidus and adrenal insufficiency (Hobson & Chima, 2013). In these conditions, urine output may continue to be high despite the child's depleted intravascular volume. Performing a urinalysis and specific gravity can provide more information. During the neonatal period, infants have a reduced capacity to concentrate urine, and may be at greater risk of dehydration.

It is important to remember that hypotension in children is a late sign of cardiovascular decompensation and requires immediate management.

CASE STUDY 11.2 ROBERT: A CHILD WITH CIRCULATORY COMPROMISE

Robert is a 7-year-old boy who fell from his bicycle yesterday. He sustained a contusion and laceration to his liver. Robert was admitted to the paediatric ward for observation. When you assess Robert, you notice that he looks pale, his heart rate has increased to 140 beats per minute and his peripheral pulse is difficult to feel and thready. You assess his peripheries to be cool up to his elbows. His central capillary refill time is three seconds and his respiratory rate is 22 breaths per minute. When you take his blood pressure, it has fallen minimally from 105/55 to 100/54 mmHg.

Robert is displaying clinical signs of circulatory compromise due to blood loss from his liver injury. His tachycardia and vasoconstriction demonstrate physiological attempts to compensate for the blood loss; however, if Robert does not receive urgent medical treatment he will quickly decompensate into cardiovascular collapse.

D – Disability

The assessment of disability relates to the assessment of the patient's neurological status. It requires a focus on the general appearance, consciousness level and responsiveness of the child. Alteration in neurological status may be in response to a primary neurological condition or as a secondary response to other disease processes.

A sick or deteriorating child will often be listless or uninterested in their surroundings, have inappropriate responses to the parents or caregivers, or have a decreased level of consciousness. Reduced level of consciousness in children with respiratory or cardiovascular compromise is a marker of poor cerebral perfusion and signals the need for urgent cardiorespiratory support.

Muscle and limb tone may provide information about the child's neurological status. Hypotonia may be present in the exhausted or seriously ill child. Abnormal posturing, such as decorticate (upper limb flexion, lower limb extension) or decerbrate (upper and lower limb extension posturing), is indicative of raised intracranial pressure and serious brain dysfunction (O'Meara & Watton, 2012). Hypertonia or tonic-clonic movements are associated with seizures in children after infancy. Infant seizures are often subtle and easily missed, possibly presenting as apnoeas or subtle movements such as tongue thrusting, lip smacking or bicycling leg movements (Kim, Brousseau & Konduri, 2009).

During illness, increased metabolism and disruption to feeding can often cause hypoglycaemia, which can result in alterations in neurological status, including jitteriness, hypotonia, lethargy and seizures (DePuy et al., 2009; Hoops et al., 2010). It is important that a blood glucose level is included in the assessment of sick infants and young children (O'Meara & Watton, 2012).

Up to 12 months of age, an infant will have an open anterior fontanel. A tense or bulging fontanel is indicative of raised intracranial pressure: a normal fontanel should be rounded, soft and pulsatile. Performing a paediatric neurological assessment is challenging because of the different cognitive abilities at each developmental stage. In addition, there can be significant variations in ability within each developmental stage, making it difficult for clinicians to determine what the child's normal behaviour would be. Psychological factors such as fear of strangers and anxiety often alter a child's behaviour, adding a further challenge to the neurological assessment.

Parents and caregivers are often able to provide valuable information regarding alterations from their child's usual behaviour. When they present with their sick child, caregivers will often report that the child is not their usual self or has been behaving abnormally. Engaging the child's caregivers to assist in neurological assessment is especially important to assist with achieving an accurate assessment.

Changes in pupil size and reactivity can provide important information about the neurological status. In an unconscious child, large and non-reactive pupils are an important sign of life-threatening intracranial hypertension. Pinpoint pupils may indicate ingestion or use of narcotic medications (O'Meara & Watton, 2012).

Paediatric neurological assessment tools

Two commonly used paediatric neurological assessment tools, the AVPU and Paediatric Glasgow Coma Scale (GCS), will be discussed in this section to help you gain an understanding of this important aspect of assessing the paediatric patient.

A quick tool that may be used to assess the paediatric patient's level of consciousness is the AVPU (Cullen, 2012a):

A   Alert
V   responds to **V**oice
P   responds to **P**ain
U   **U**nresponsive

This tool is very useful, as it enables the clinician to quickly assess whether the neurological status is normal, slightly abnormal or seriously abnormal. If a child is only responding to painful stimuli, this indicates that the neurological status is seriously abnormal and that the child may no longer be able to protect their own airway.

Medical staff able to intubate the child should be involved in assessing and managing the child. Any child with an altered level of consciousness or mental status needs close and regular monitoring because they are at risk of further deterioration.

The GCS (see Table 11.5) is also used for the assessment of neurological status. It provides a more comprehensive assessment than the AVPU. The GCS has been modified for infants and children to accommodate for the developmental differences. A GCS of 8 is a seriously low score and is associated with the need for clinical interventions to provide airway protection. A GCS of 8 is approximately equivalent to a 'P' on the AVPU scale.

Table 11.5 Glasgow Coma Scale

Response	Paediatric GCS	Infant <1 year	Child 1–5 years
Eye opening	4	Spontaneous	Spontaneous
	3	To verbal stimuli	To verbal stimuli
	2	To pain	To pain
	1	No response to pain	No response to pain
Best motor response	6	Spontaneous movements	Follows/obeys commands
	5	Withdraws to touch	Localises pain
	4	Withdraws from pain	Withdraws from pain
	3	Abnormal flexion to pain (decorticate)	Abnormal flexion to pain (decorticate)
	2	Abnormal extension to pain (decerebrate)	Abnormal extension to pain (decerebrate)
	1	No response to pain	No response to pain
Best verbal response	5	Alert, babbles, coos, smiles	Oriented, converses with appropriate words, phrases
	4	Cries and inconsolable	Inappropriate words
	3	Persistent inappropriate crying or screaming	Persistent crying or screaming
	2	Grunts, agitated or restless	Grunts or groans
	1	No response to pain	No response to pain

Source: Adapted from Teasdale et al. (2014).

It is important to remember that neurological changes are sensitive indicators of deterioration in children and should *never* be ignored.

REFLECTION POINTS 11.1

- Early warning tools have been developed to assist clinicians to recognise signs of deterioration in a paediatric patient and trigger an escalation in care, such as an urgent medical review. Consider your clinical experiences in the acute paediatric setting and the early warning tools you have seen or used. What did you find most

(cont.)

helpful in relation to the tools? What further learning did they stimulate for you in relation to the care of acutely ill children?

- We have now reviewed two structured paediatric assessment tools: the Paediatric Assessment Triangle and the Primary Assessment Framework for the paediatric patient. What are some of the differences between these approaches – for example, does one approach precede the other?

- The Primary Assessment Framework assesses airway, breathing, circulation and disability. Airway assessment includes history and ability to maintain a clear airway – considering anatomical, physiological and developmental characteristics that increase the paediatric patient's risk for airway compromise, as well as signs of airway compromise, such as inability to speak, manage oral secretions, work of breathing, abnormal breath sounds, posturing in an attempt to open airway and decreased air entry upon auscultation and impaired oxygenation. Why is urgent management of a compromised airway critical in the paediatric patient?

- Breathing assessment incorporates respiratory rate, symmetry of chest wall movement, colour, air entry and breath sounds, and signs that indicate increased work of breathing, including recession or nasal flaring, or head bobbing and marked diaphragmatic movement in the infant. Oxygen-saturation measurements will also complement this data. Why should paediatric nurses look at oxygen-saturation readings in conjunction with their complete respiratory assessment?

- The assessment of circulation involves evaluating heart rate and rhythm, peripheral pulses and perfusion, colour and urine output. It is essential to understand the child's normal response and compensatory mechanisms that operate in response to compromised circulatory or cardiovascular function. How might these mechanisms affect heart rate and blood pressure? Why is it important to assess peripheral pulses, perfusion, capillary refill and urine output?

- Disability assessment equates to neurological assessment, and we have reviewed two tools that can assist in this assessment the AVPU and the paediatric GCS. If you detected a deterioration in a child's conscious level or responsiveness, what immediate actions would you take?

CASE STUDY 11.3 ANGELA: AN ADOLESCENT WITH NEUROLOGICAL COMPROMISE

Angela is a 14-year-old girl who presents to the emergency department accompanied by her mother. She had been generally unwell for the previous day and her parents had taken her to the family general practitioner, who had prescribed amoxicillin. Yesterday evening, Angela complained of severe headache and when Angela's parents turned her light on in her room this morning, Angela screamed at them to turn it off. Her mother reports she was 'really aggressive and confused as to where she was and not her usual self'.

Angela is brought into the emergency room to be assessed. Responding to the AVPU method, Angela intermittently opens her eyes when you call her name, consistently withdraws from painful stimuli and continually moans, 'My head is killing me!', appears agitated and moves about the bed continuously. She does not want to cooperate with your examination and her mother states, 'This is not like her at all.' She starts vomiting as you take her vital signs. Her heart rate is 105, respiratory rate 22, temperature 39.5°C and blood pressure 90/51 mmHg. Angela has no visible rash; however, her capillary refill time is slowed. Her mother reports that she hasn't passed urine this morning.

Angela displays serious signs of neurological compromise. She needs to be closely monitored, should receive urgent fluid resuscitation and must be assessed further to ensure that she is able to adequately protect her airway. Angela is stabilised and transferred to the paediatric intensive care unit. She is diagnosed with bacterial meningitis and sepsis.

Responding to the sick child

A timely response to the sick child generally requires a team approach. The severity of illness generally will indicate the urgency of treatment. Early warning tools incorporate the activation of timely responses to clinical assessment findings. This supports the clinician's decision-making and reinforces the need to activate prompt clinical reviews.

Similar to assessment, a structured framework can be used to guide the management of the seriously sick child. Following an A, B, C, D approach, any serious or life-threatening problems must be addressed before continuing with the assessment. For example, if breathing is found to be inadequate, action must be taken to support the breathing before continuing on to assess the circulation.

There has been a significant amount of research into systems that improve the coordination and delivery of emergency care. Often, poor communication or inadequate communication systems have been found to create barriers to the effective delivery of timely care. Nurses need to understand the communication processes for individual clinical settings and how to effectively activate a timely clinical review or call for help in an emergency – for example, when and how to initiate a Medical Emergency Team (MET) response.

Paediatric emergency equipment should be available in all clinical areas where children are cared for. As a nurse caring for children, it is important that you are familiar with this equipment and know how to select the appropriate size. There are many resources and algorithms available to assist with paediatric emergency procedures. One example is the Australian and New Zealand Committee on Resuscitation (ANZCOR) approved guidelines, which are available at http://resus.org.au.

Respiratory support
Airway and breathing

Respiratory support comprises both airway and breathing support. Some children may require assistance in one of these areas, while others will require it in both.

Secretions can block the child's airway. Infants primarily breathe through their noses, so suctioning nares that are blocked with secretions can quickly relieve airway obstruction. Oropharyngeal suction can be useful if children are unable to remove oral secretions that pool at the back of the oropharynx. It is advisable to perform oral suction under direct vision to avoid pushing a foreign body back into the airway and causing further obstruction. Appropriate personal protective equipment (PPE) should be utilised when performing this procedure, and would include gloves, mask and goggles.

The COVID-19 pandemic has highlighted the importance of PPE considerations, especially during performance of oxygenation and cardiopulmonary resuscitation. Although children are more likely to arrest from causes other than COVID-19 and seem to be less likely to transmit the virus, first responders should wear, masks, gloves and eye protection to initiate CPR until a clinician with airborne precaution PPE can take over (Advanced Paediatric Life Support, 2020). Airborne precautions include a N95 mask, gown, gloves and eye protection, and when intubation is to occur a face shield should be added. Airborne precautions are needed as a variety of procedures involved in resuscitation may increase aerosolising the virus, including bag valve mask ventilation, suctioning, intubation including laryngeal mask airway insertion and performance of cardiac compressions (Advanced Paediatric Life Support, 2020; RCHM, 2020b). In addition to donning airborne precaution PPE, these procedures should be performed in the highest level of isolation environment available. These levels of isolation may move from the lowest level – that is, a curtained cubicle with curtains closed – through to single rooms with curtains closed, single rooms with doors closed or the highest level of isolation, which is a negative pressure room (RCHM, 2020b).

Supporting a child's airway can be achieved by effective positioning of the head. For infants, the neutral position optimally opens the airway, while a slightly extended position described as 'sniffing' is used for children over 1 year of age. It is important to avoid neck extension (which would be used in an adult) because this collapses the soft airways, resulting in airway obstruction. Young babies do not have the muscle strength to reposition their heads. Care should be taken when positioning an infant to ensure that the head is supported to avoid airway obstruction. Using a small towel or roll under the shoulders can effectively align the infant in the neutral position aiding airway management.

Children at risk of airway obstruction should be observed continuously and never left unattended. In cases where a child has a partially obstructed airway due to swelling or a foreign body, it is prudent to avoid upsetting the child to prevent exacerbating respiratory distress (Fitzgerald & Kilham, 2003). Strategies include leaving a toddler sitting on the parent/caregiver's lap and avoiding unnecessary invasive procedures if at all possible until someone is present who can confidently manage the airway. Continuous observation and preparation of emergency airway equipment are required because the airway may deteriorate suddenly.

Adrenaline nebulisers may be prescribed and used to relieve the symptoms of upper airway swelling. The administration of adrenaline causes vasoconstriction to reduce airway swelling, which improves airflow and therefore provides temporarily relief. It is important to monitor these children closely, as the airway obstruction may return as the adrenaline effect wears off, usually within a two-hour period (Elder & Rao, 2019). If required, adrenaline nebulisers can be repeated. The use of adrenaline can be very effective in providing time for suitably skilled staff to attend the child. The recommended dose of nebulised adrenaline is 0.5 mL/kg of the 1:1000 solution, up to maximum of 5 mL (Fitzgerald & Kilham, 2003; Shann, 2014). Given the approximate two-hour duration of clinical effect, it is important to continually assess the child to see whether an additional dose/s of adrenaline is necessary (Elder & Rao, 2019).

A lowered level of consciousness can result in airway obstruction due to the child's tongue falling back into the oropharynx. Performing a 'chin lift' or 'jaw thrust' manoeuvre lifts the tongue from the posterior oropharynx to open the airway. Nasopharyngeal or oropharyngeal airways can be used to assist in maintaining an open airway. An oropharyngeal airway is only suitable in an unconscious patient because the device could stimulate a gag reflex in a conscious or semi-conscious person.

Oropharyngeal airways (Figure 11.5) must be sized (angle of the mandible to the middle of the lips/incisors) and inserted into the oropharynx with the concave side against the tongue. Incorrect sizing and insertion can cause trauma and/or further obstruct the airway. Sizing for a nasopharyngeal airway is from the nare to the tragus of the ear, then gently inserted into the nare.

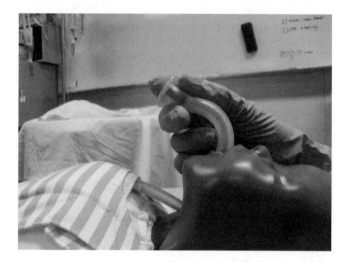

Figure 11.5 Insertion of oropharyngeal airway

A small number of children may present to hospital with a tracheostomy tube in situ. Paediatric tracheostomy tubes have a very small diameter and therefore can block easily. Ensuring patency of the tracheostomy tube is an essential element in the airway management of these children. Passing a suction catheter to suction into the tracheostomy tube can both remove secretions and assess the patency of the tube. If the tracheostomy is blocked, a tube change is required. Children presenting to hospital with a tracheostomy tube in situ should have their own supply of appropriately sized tracheotomy tubes with them. Their caregivers will have experience in changing the tracheotomy tube. Consider utilising these resources if required.

Oxygenation

Oxygen should be an early intervention for any sick or deteriorating paediatric patient. For patients with decreased oxygen saturations in room air, oxygen therapy can be applied using a paediatric Hudson mask with a minimum flow rate of 4 L/min. If required, higher percentages of oxygen can be delivered using a paediatric non-rebreathing mask with a reservoir bag. Using an appropriately sized mask and flow rate is important to prevent the retention and rebreathing of carbon dioxide. Nasal prongs can also be used to deliver lower flows of oxygen (see Figure 11.6). High flow nasal cannula oxgyenation is often used clinically to provide respiratory support to paediatric patients in respiratory distress/at risk of acute respiratory failure. You can read more about high-flow cannula oxygenation in the Learning activity. Generally, in paediatric patients, the prongs are taped in place using a protective hydrocolloid dressing under the tape to protect the skin.

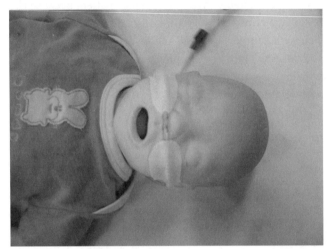

Figure 11.6   Nasal prongs

Inadequacy of breathing needs to be supported with bag and mask ventilation. If the child has an inadequate respiratory rate or effort, without support they will progress to cardiorespiratory arrest. Correct bag and mask sizing and attaching high flow oxygen achieves best results for bag mask ventilation.

If the child is still taking some spontaneous breaths, bag and mask ventilation should be administered carefully. This includes squeezing the bag in time with the child's own respirations to enable airflow to the child. Due to the resistance in a self-inflating bag-valve mask, children will be unable to breathe if the self-inflating bag and mask is just held over the face without providing breaths. If the child is breathing adequately, an oxygen mask is preferable to a bag-value mask for oxygen delivery.

Circulatory support

Vascular access is important for paediatric patients, and will often be obtained via the insertion of a peripheral cannula upon admission and before problems occur, as the peripheral vasoconstriction that occurs in response to hypovolaemia, for example, can make the already small peripheral veins of an infant or child even more difficult to cannulate. In infants and children, vascular access may be obtained via peripheral veins, including the dorsum of the hand, wrist, forearm and the antecubital fossa, as well as the foot and ankle where the long saphenous vein may be accessed (ANZCOR, 2016c). In infants, a scalp vein is also sometimes used.

If a child is seriously ill and deteriorating, intravenous access should be attempted for no more than 60 seconds (ANZCOR, 2016a). Failure to obtain access in this period requires alternative access to be attempted. If a suitably skilled person is available to insert a central venous line, this may be used. Alternatively, the intraosseous route may be used to gain emergency vascular access.

Intraosseous needles are usually used in infants and children up to approximately 6 years of age, as changes to the vascularity of the bone marrow and thickening of the bone after this age make it harder to obtain access. However, if an intraosseous drill is available, the intraosseous route may be used for older children and adults (Cullen, 2012b). The location for insertion of an intraosseous needle in infants and young children is the anterior and medial surface of the tibia, approximately 1–2 cm below the tibial tuberosity (see Figure 11.7) (Cullen, 2012b). The intraosseous route can be used for medications and fluids. Fluids cannot run via gravity but must be injected or administered via an infusion pump.

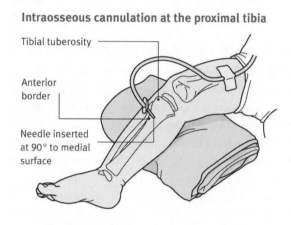

Intraosseous cannulation at the proximal tibia

Tibial tuberosity

Anterior border

Needle inserted at 90° to medial surface

The site of needle insertion is 1–3 cm (children) or 0.5–1 cm (babies) below and just medial to the tibial tuberosity on the flat, medial aspect of the tibia where the bone lies subcutaneously. Support the leg on a firm surface, grasping the thigh and knee above and lateral to the site of insertion. Insert the needle at right angles to the coronal plane, directing the needle tip slightly caudally and away from the tibial growth plate. To prevent dislodgement, carefully immobilize the cannula and splint the limb

Figure 11.7 Intraosseous cannulation site in children
Source: Reproduced from Cullen (2012b).

Once vascular access has been obtained, fluid resuscitation and/or medications may be administered. If hypovolaemia is suspected as a cause of circulatory compromise, then the administration of an initial 20 mL/kg bolus of a crystalloid solution such as 0.9 per cent sodium chloride is recommended and the child's response to this initial bolus is then assessed (ANZCOR, 2016b). Further boluses of crystalloid solutions or colloids such as 4 per cent albumin may then be ordered by the physician. If bleeding is the cause of hypovoleamia then prompt administration of blood should be the priority. Most health services have a protocol for accessing blood for this purpose and protocols for massive haemorrhage management.

Collection of relevant blood samples should be considered at the time of obtaining vascular access. These could include venous blood gas, glucose level, electrolytes, full blood count, cross match, blood cultures and coagulation profile depending on the patient's presentation or diagnosis.

A practical method for quickly and accurately administering fluid resuscitation in children is to use 50 mL syringes to draw up and inject the fluid bolus.

After administration of a fluid bolus, it is important to reassess the child's circulation observations to determine the effect of the fluid in improving the cardiovascular state. Providing adequate fluid resuscitation is critical; equally, though, excessive fluid resuscitation can be harmful, so it is imperative to continue to monitor the child's response to fluid resuscitation (Myburgh & Finfer, 2013).

Paediatric sepsis

Sepsis – A serious condition where the body's response to infection results in organ dysfunction. Sepsis can rapidly progress to shock. In septic shock, cardiovascular dysfunction results in hypotension and hypoperfusion and can lead to organ failure and death (Australian Sepsis Network, 2021).

Globally, **sepsis** remains the leading cause of paediatric mortality and morbidity, often as a result of diarrhoeal or respiratory infections (Rudd et al., 2020). Children under 5 years of age account for 40 per cent of sepsis cases internationally, and Aboriginal, Torres Strait Islander, Pacific Islander and Māori children are at greater risk (Australian Sepsis Network, 2021).

Early recognition and management of sepsis is essential and can be lifesaving. Early recognition by parents and emergency personnel in the community is important for prompt intervention (Harley et al., 2021). Parents' concerns should be taken seriously by clinicians to avoid delays in diagnosis and treatment. Paediatric nurses also need to recognise signs of sepsis to ensure prompt review and intervention.

According to Weiss and Pomerantz (2020) there are a number of red flags that may alert clinicians to paediatric sepsis. These include:

- fever > 38.3°C in paediatric patients older than 3 months or >38°C in infants younger than 3 months
- hypothermia (core temperature < 36°C)
- tachycardia
- tachypnoea
- abnormal (diminished, weak or bounding) pulse
- abnormal capillary refill (>3 seconds or flash refill <1 second)
- hypotensive (note however that this is a late and pre-terminal sign)
- abnormal mental status (irritability, inappropriate crying, drowsiness, or interaction with caregiver, difficult to rouse (lethargic or obtunded) confused or disorientated
- purpura anywhere or petechiae below the nipple line
- signs of infection – for example, toxic or ill appearance, dehydration, rigors, low tone in infants, abnormal or decreased breaths sounds as in pneumonia, distended or tender abdomen, warmth, swelling, and/or erythema of an extremity or joint suggestive of osteomyelitis and/or septic arthritis
- macular erythema with mucosal changes (e.g. strawberry tongue and conjunctival infection).

Additional factors increase the risk of sepsis, including neutropenia or altered immune status, indwelling lines, catheters or devices, recent injury, trauma, surgery or disruption to skin integrity. For a more detailed table of red flags, please visit the companion website.

Sepsis flow charts or screening tools for identifying and treating sepsis are linked to improved outcomes when incorporated into sepsis management (Nutbeam & Daniels, 2021; Weiss et al., 2020). Because sepsis can be a rapidly progressing condition, management is time-critical. Priorities and timelines for management differ between sepsis and septic shock. However, in both cases treatment should not be delayed.

Priorities for treatment include:

- airway: maintain a secure airway
- breathing: provide oxygen and breathing support if required
- circulation: obtain vascular access and bloods
- administer broad spectrum antimicrobials within one hour in septic shock and within three hours in sepsis associated organ dysfunction without shock
- fluid resuscitation (10–20 mL/kg isotonic crystalloid boluses over first hour to maximum of 60 mL/kg in PICU or maximum 40 mL/kg in non PICU settings) (NSW Government, 2021; Nutbeam & Daniels, 2021; Weiss et al., 2020).

Careful and continuous monitoring of cardiac output and response to fluid resuscitation needs to occur (heart rate, blood pressure, capillary refill, level of consciousness and urine output) to ensure fluid resuscitation is sufficient to correct deficits and maintain cardiac output without causing overload.

Paediatric basic and advanced life support

So far, we have discussed strategies to provide respiratory and circulatory support to the deteriorating child. We will now provide an overview of paediatric cardiopulmonary resuscitation, which may be required if the initial measures of respiratory and circulatory support are not successful in averting further deterioration. It is important to distinguish between **basic life support** and **advanced life support**. Basic life support refers to efforts made to restore or maintain airway, breathing and circulation that do not require adjunct equipment such as airways and masks. Advanced life support involves basic life support with the addition of more invasive measures such as advanced airway management, intubation, intravenous access and defibrillation.

We have already discussed some basic airway support manoeuvres and establishing intravenous access. We will now provide an overview of cardiopulmonary resuscitation and some more invasive respiratory support measures. Table 11.6 provides a summary of the latest guidelines for paediatric cardiopulmonary resuscitation and cardiac compression delivery site and depth, and ratio of cardiac compression to ventilation.

In situations where the infant or child has stopped breathing or respiration is insufficient, the child should be supported by providing bag and mask ventilation. In most cases, this should be provided by using a paediatric self-inflating bag **attached to oxygen** and with an appropriately sized face mask. A correctly sized mask covers the mouth and nose, and achieves a seal when held gently on the child's face. To effectively hold the mask, the thumb and index finger form a 'C' around the mask, while the other

Basic life support – Efforts made to restore or maintain airway, breathing and circulation or masks. An example of resuscitation in a public area that does not require adjunct equipment such as airways would be a first responder performing cardiopulmonary resuscitation.

Advanced life support – Incorporates basic life support as well as more invasive measures such as advanced airway management, intubation, intravenous access and defibrillation.

Table 11.6   Paediatric cardiopulmonary resuscitation

Child age	Infant <1 year	Child 1–8 years	Older child >8 years or adult
Pulse check	Australian resuscitation guidelines now recommend check for no pulse or 'signs of life'/response for all age groups		
Head tilt position	Neutral position	Slightly extended sniffing position from 1 year For older child, semi- to full-extension head tilt with chin lift	Semi- to full-extension head tilt with chin lift
Compression site	Centrally on the lower half of the sternum	Centrally on lower half of sternum	Centrally on lower half of sternum
Compression delivery method	Pressure with two thumbs or two fingers In the two-thumb technique, hands encircle chest and thumbs compress the sternum	Pressure with heel of one hand	Pressure with heel of one hand with other hand superimposed
Compression depth	4 cm or approximately one-third depth of anterior posterior dimension of the chest	4–5 cm or approximately one-third depth of anterior-posterior dimension of the chest	5 cm or approximately one-third depth of anterior-posterior dimension of the chest
Basic life support rescue by one or two rescuers Compression: Ventilation ratio ECC rate/minute Time for one cycle	15:2 Compression rate irrespective of age or ratio is approximately 100–120 compressions per minute One compression every 0.6 seconds or almost two per second five cycles in two minutes		
Advanced life support rescue by two healthcare rescuers Compression: Ventilation ratio ECC rate/minute Time for one cycle	15:2 Compression rate irrespective of age or ratio is approximately 100–120 compressions per minute Five cycles per minute		

Source: Adapted from ANZCOR (2016a).

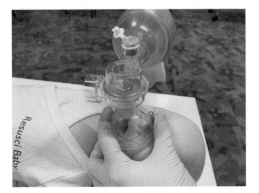

Figure 11.8 Correct-size mask and seal and correct C shape of finger placement

fingers are placed along the jawline (see Figure 11.8). For newborns and small neonates, there is a 250 mL self-inflating bag, for infants greater than 1 month of age normally a 500 mL self-inflating bag is used and for older infants and children a 1500 mL size is available.

When providing bag and mask ventilation, you should observe the rise and fall of the chest. Excessive pressure will result in air being forced into the stomach, which in turn can splint the diaphragm, inhibiting effective air entry. The insertion of a nasogastric tube can be useful to decompress the stomach.

While not discussed here, post-resuscitation care is important following cardiopulmonary resuscitation, and continuous respiratory and haemodynamic monitoring will normally be undertaken in the PICU.

It is worthwhile obtaining paediatric mannequins to be able to practise basic life support with a peer or colleague. Your university clinical laboratory on campus or the clinical educator in the paediatric setting will be able to assist you to engage in this important preparation for paediatric cardiopulmonary resuscitation.

Parental presence during resuscitation

COVID-19 restrictions limited the number of personnel and family present during resuscitation procedures due to the aerosol-generating nature of many procedures during resuscitation, and it is unclear when these restrictions will be relaxed. The pandemic required health professionals to traverse a fine line between limiting exposure to the virus and supporting the needs of family members (Frampton, Agrawal & Guastello, 2020). In the United States, guidelines have been developed for preserving family presence during challenging times, and these considerations include determining the need for restrictions based on available evidence, communicating proactively with families regarding restrictions and whether there is any compassionate exceptions to restrictions available (Frampton, Agrawal & Guastello, 2020).

Historically, it has been recognised that parents may wish to be present during resuscitation of their child and the COVID-19 pandemic limited family presence during resuscitation with flow-on effects on communication with parents and emotional support (Hiu Yan Law et al., 2020). In the event of paediatric resuscitation, whether family members are directly present or nearby, it is very important to have an experienced staff member available to support the family. Some nurses may worry that witnessing resuscitation could be distressing for parents; however, a pivotal Australian study of families whose child required resuscitation in the paediatric intensive care unit found that parents who did not witness their child's resuscitation experienced greater distress than the parents who stayed (Maxton, 2008). Since this study, it is now accepted that parents may wish to be present during resuscitation, and a recent integrative review found that the published literature supports parental preference to be present during their child's resuscitation (Mark, 2020).

Family members such as siblings will also need to be supported at an appropriate location and, depending on the circumstances, may be cared for by another family member in the patient lounge or ward play area. In some settings, such as paediatric intensive care units, a nurse or other member of the multidisciplinary team not directly involved in the resuscitation may be available to talk with older siblings who, although not present for the resuscitation, may want to discuss their concerns.

As a nurse caring for paediatric patients, your ability to provide safe care is paramount. Recognising the sick infant or child and responding promptly can prevent deterioration and life-threatening respiratory and circulatory collapse. From your reading and reflection on the case studies in this chapter, you should now be well equipped with the ability to assess an infant or child using appropriate assessment frameworks and tools, to be able to detect signs of deterioration and to be able to respond quickly and effectively to escalate the need for an urgent medical review of the patient, and provide respiratory and circulatory support if needed to prevent further deterioration.

REFLECTION POINTS 11.2

- We have now reviewed responding to the sick child with respiratory and circulatory support. What are two ways in which you can support the airway and circulation for a paediatric patient?
- Paediatric basic life support has differences between infants (up to 1 year), children (1–8 years) and older children (over 8 years) in terms of head tilt, compression site, delivery and depth. Summarise these differences and consider what the best site would be to perform the pulse check for these age groups.
- Parental presence during paediatric resuscitation is considered to be an important part of caring for the deteriorating paediatric patient and their family members. Having an experienced health professional who can explain things and provide support to parents is essential. Have you ever participated in or witnessed a resuscitation in the acute setting? Can you recall how the health professional supported family members? What elements of their support would you like to incorporate into your own practice?

SUMMARY

- Paediatric patients have distinct developmental, anatomical and physiological characteristics that increase their susceptibility to respiratory and circulatory compromise. Respiratory and heart rates vary according to age, and the assessment of airway, breathing, circulation and disability involves obtaining and evaluating key assessment data within each element of the primary survey in order to detect abnormalities and signs of deterioration that necessitate an escalation in care and medical review.
- Early-warning tools such as the Paediatric Early Warning Score (PEWS), the Cardiac Children's Hospital Early Warning Score (CCHEWS) or Between the Flags may be used in paediatric nursing practice to assist nurses to identify a child who is deteriorating and who warrants an urgent and appropriate response.
- A deteriorating child may require airway and breathing and/or circulatory support, so it is essential that paediatric nurses know how to support the child's airway and to provide appropriate oxygenation using suitable devices (high-flow nasal prong oxygen, masks, or bag and mask ventilation). Circulatory support requires vascular access, either through intravenous or intraosseous routes. If intravenous access is not obtained and there is an urgent need for fluid resuscitation and medications, the intraosseous route is used. Initial fluid resuscitation for hypovolaemia is generally a 20 mL/kg bolus of 0.9 per cent normal saline.
- If initial measures to support respiration and circulation are unsuccessful, then cardiopulmonary resuscitation may be required. The correct head tilt position, appropriate mask, compression site, depth and ratio of compression to ventilation will depend on

whether the patient is an infant, child or adolescent, and the number of rescuers. Paediatric nurses need to practise resuscitation skills regularly to ensure their competence in this area.

- Support for the family is integral to effective care for the sick and deteriorating child, and family members should have a designated support person during resuscitation to answer questions and provide information and emotional support. Parental presence during paediatric resuscitation can be achieved provided there is adequate support available but will also be an individual family's choice.

LEARNING ACTIVITY

Case study 11.1 introduced you to Maggie, a 6-month-old infant with suspected RSV bronchiolitis. This learning activity encourages you to explore the nursing assessment and management of Maggie. Read the information below, then answer the questions that follow.

Nasopharyngeal suctioning and bronchiolitis

Routine nasopharyngeal (NP) suctioning is no longer recommended for managing infants with bronchiolitis, although superficial nasal suction may be helpful in infants such as Maggie to assist with feeding (O'Brien, 2019). Deep nasal suctioning is not recommended (O'Brien, 2019).

High-flow nasal cannulae therapy and bronchiolitis

High-flow nasal cannulae oxygen in bronchiolitis can be administered to hospitalised infants with bronchiolitis who have hypoxia (oxygen saturations less than 92 per cent) (O'Brien et al., 2019). High-flow nasal cannulae (HFNC) therapy provides respiratory support for infants and children by delivery of warmed and humidified air/oxygen blend at high flow rates. HFNC therapy can be effective in decreasing work of breathing. When it has been used for paediatric patients with bronchiolitis, the need for invasive respiratory support such as intubation and mechanical ventilation has been avoided. Research is continuing to emerge regarding HFNC (Moreel & Proesmans, 2020), and a large multi-centre paediatric study is currently underway in Australia and New Zealand to determine the efficacy of HFNC compared with standard oxygen in the treatment of bronchiolitis (Franklin et al., 2015). Early research indicates that paediatric patients generally respond to HFNC within one to two hours of initiation, demonstrating a reduction in heart rate and respiratory rate towards a normal range, and those infants who did not respond could be escalated to alternative respiratory support (Mayfield et al., 2014).

Our understanding of the mechanism of respiratory support in HFNC is growing, and it is thought that the high flow provides some continuous positive airway pressure (CPAP), which facilities an opening of the airways to promote gas exchange (Beggs et al., 2012; Schibler et al., 2011). This is achieved during expiration, when patients expire 'against' the high flow oxygen, which creates a resistance and therefore positive end expiratory pressure (Pham et al., 2015; Schibler & Franklin, 2016). The heat and humidification of HFNC enhance conductance and pulmonary compliance, and reduce rebreathing of carbon dioxide by washing out of nasopharyngeal anatomical dead space during expiration (Schibler &

Franklin, 2016). Furthermore, HFNC has been shown to reduce the work of breathing in infants, as indicated by a reduction in workload of the diaphragm (Pham et al., 2015). When expiration occurs against resistance provided by the high flow, this splints the airways, keeping them open; therefore, respiratory muscles such as the diaphragm do not need to work so hard, and fatigue of respiratory muscles is reduced (Morley, 2016).

11.1 Based on your reading in this chapter, what assessment data in the case study indicate that Maggie is experiencing respiratory distress?

11.2 Considering that infants are obligatory nose breathers, and that bronchiolitis results in copious nasal secretions that increase airway resistance and respiratory distress, what nursing interventions could you implement to address this issue for Maggie and promote feeding?

11.3 What is HFNC therapy, and why is it used in infants with bronchiolitis?

11.4 What additional concerns (other than respiratory distress) are significant for Maggie?

FURTHER READING

Akre, M et al. 2010, Sensitivity of the Pediatric Early Warning Score to identify patient deterioration, *Pediatrics*, 125, pp. e763–e770. This article provides an overview of the PEWS and includes an image of the tool.

Bressan, S et al. 2013, High-flow nasal cannula oxygen for bronchiolitis in a paediatric ward: A pilot study, *European Journal of Pediatrics*, 1–8, pp. 1649–56. This article can be accessed to enhance your understanding of high-flow nasal cannulae oxygen therapy for infants with bronchiolitis.

Paul, SP 2013, Managing children with raised intracranial pressure: Part one (introduction and meningitis), *Nursing Children and Young People*, 25(10), pp. 31–6. This article provides an overview of brain anatomy, intracranial pressure, and meningitis assessment and management in paediatric patients.

Schibler, A, Pham, TM, Dunster, KR, Foster, K, Barlow, A, Gibbons, K & Hough, JL 2011, Reduced intubation rates for infants after introduction of high flow nasal prong oxygen delivery, *Intensive Care Medicine*, 37(5), pp. 847–52.This article can be accessed to enhance your understanding of high-flow nasal cannulae oxygen therapy for infants with bronchiolitis.

REFERENCES

Advanced Paediatric Life Support 2020, *Paediatric advanced life support (with COVID-19 considerations),* viewed 20 March 2021, www.apls.org.au/algorithm-paediatric-advanced-life-support-covid-considerations

Agbim, CA, Wang, N & Moon, L 2018, Respiratory distress in pediatric patients, *Pediatric Emergency Medicine Reports*, 23(4), viewed 20 March 2021, http://search.proquest.com.libraryproxy.griffith.edu.au/trade-journals/respiratory-distress-pediatric-patients/docview/2017930473/se-2?accountid=14543

Ait-Oufella, H et al. 2013, Alteration of skin perfusion in mottling area during septic shock, *Annals of Intensive Care*, 31(3), viewed 20 March 2014, www.annalsofntensivecare.com/content/3/1/31.

Australian and New Zealand Committee on Resuscitation (ANZCOR) 2016a, *ANZCOR guideline 12.2 – advanced life support for infants and children: Diagnosis and management,* ARC, Canberra, viewed 4 October 2020, www.resus.org.au

—— 2016b, *ANZCOR guideline 12.4 – medications and fluids in paediatric advanced life support,* ARC, Canberra, viewed 4 October 2020, www.resus.org.au

—— 2016c, *ANZCOR guideline 12.6 – Introduction to paediatric advanced life support techniques in paediatric advanced life support*, ARC, Canberra, viewed 4 October 2020, www.resus.org.au

Australian Sepsis Network 2021, *Paediatric sepsis*, ARC, Canberra, viewed 20 March 2021, www.australiansepsisnetwork.net.au

Beggs, S, Wong, ZH, Kaul, S, Ogden, KJ & Walters, JAE 2012, High-flow nasal cannula therapy for infants with bronchiolitis (protocol), *Cochrane Database of Systematic Reviews*, 2, CD009609.

Crook, J & Taylor, RM 2013, The agreement of fingertip and sternum capillary refill time in children, *Archives of Disease in Childhood*, 98, pp. 265–8.

Cullen, PM 2012a, Paediatric trauma: Continuing education in anaesthesia, *Critical Care and Pain*, 12(3), pp. 157–61.

—— 2012b, Intraosseous cannulation in children, *Anaesthesia & Intensive Care Medicine*, 13(1), pp. 28–30.

Dieckmann, RA, Brownstein, D & Gausche-Hill, M 2010, The Pediatric Assessment Triangle: A novel approach for the rapid evaluation of children, *Pediatric Emergency Care*, 26(4), pp. 312–15.

DePuy, A, Coassolo, K, Som, D & Smulian, J 2009, Neonatal hypoglycemia in term, nondiabetic pregnancies, *American Journal of Obstetrics and Gynecology*, 200(5), pp. e45–e51.

Elder, AE & Rao, A 2019, Management and outcomes of patients presenting to the emergency department with croup: Can we identify which patients can safely be discharged from the emergency department? *Journal of Paediatrics & Child Health*, 55(11), 1323–8.

Fitzgerald, D & Kilham, H 2003, Croup: Assessment and evidence-based management, *Medical Journal of Australia*, 179, pp. 372–7.

Fleming, S, Gill, PJ, Van den Bruel, A & Thompson, M 2016, Capillary refill time in sick children: A clinical guide for general practice, *British Journal of General Practice*, 66(652), 587–8.

Fouzas, S, Priftis, KN & Anthracopoulos, MB 2011, Pulse oximetry in pediatric practice, *Pediatrics*, 128, pp. 740–52.

Frampton, S, Agrawal, S & Guastello, S, 2020, Guidelines for family presence policies during the COVID-19 pandemic, *JAMA Health Forum*, doi:10.1001/jamahealthforum.2020.0807

Franklin, D et al. 2015, Early high flow nasal cannula therapy in bronchiolitis: A prospective randomized control trial (protocol): A Paediatric Acute Respiratory Intervention Study (PARIS), *BMC Pediatrics*, 15, pp. 183–91.

Harley, A, Schlapbach, LJ, Johnston, ANB & Massey, D 2021, Challenges in the recognition and management of paediatric sepsis – the journey, *Australasian Emergency Care*, doi:10.1016/j.auec.2021.03.006

Hiu Yan Law, B, Cheung, P, Aziz, K & Schmolzer, GM, 2020, Effect of COVID-19 precautions on neonatal resuscitation practice: A balance between healthcare provider safety, infection control, and effective neonatal care, *Frontiers in Pediatrics*, 18(8), p. 478.

Hobson, MJ & Chima, RS 2013, Pediatric hypovolemic shock, *The Open Pediatric Medicine Journal*, 7(Supp. 1), pp. 10–15.

Hoops, D et al. 2010, Should routine peripheral blood glucose testing be done for all newborns at birth?, *American Journal of Maternal Child Nursing*, 35(5), pp. 264–70.

Hsu, G & Fiadjoe, JE 2020, The pediatric difficult airway, *Anesthesiology Clinics*, 38(3), 459–75.

Jones, H, Wilmshurst, SL & Graydon, C 2017, Aetiology and outcome of paediatric cardiopulmonary arrest, *Anaesthesia and Intensive Care Medicine*, 18(11), 537–40.

Kim, U, Brousseau, D & Konduri, G 2008, Evaluation and management of the critically ill neonate in the emergency department, *Clinical Pediatric Emergency Medicine*, 9, pp. 140–8.

Mark, K 2020, Family presence during paediatric resuscitation and invasive procedures: The parental experience: An integrative review, *Scandinavian Journal of Caring Sciences*, 35, pp. 20–36.

Maxton, FJ 2008, Parental presence during resuscitation in the PICU: The parents' experience. Sharing and surviving the resuscitation: A phenomenological study, *Journal of Clinical Nursing*, 17(23), pp. 3168–76.

Mayfield, S, Jauncey-Cooke, J, Hough, J, Schibler, A, Gibbons, K & Bogossian, FE 2014, High-flow nasal cannula therapy for respiratory support in children, *Cochrane Database of Systematic Reviews*, 3, CD009850.

Mendelson, J 2018, Emergency department management of pediatric shock, *Emergency Medicine Clinics of North America*, 36(2), pp. 427–40.

McLellan, MC & Connor, JA 2013, The Cardiac Children's Hospital Early Warning Score (CCHEWS), *Journal of Pediatric Nursing*, 28, pp. 171–8.

McMullen, S & Patrick W, 2013, Cyanosis, *The American Journal of Medicine*, 126(3), 210–12.

Miller, KA & Nagler, J 2019, Advances in emergent airway management in pediatrics, *Emergency Medicine Clinics of North America*, 37(3), 473–91.

Moreel, L & Proesmans, M 2020, High flow nasal cannula as respiratory support in treating infant bronchiolitis: A systematic review, *European Journal of Pediatrics*, 179(5), pp. 711–18.

Morley, SL 2016, Non-invasive ventilation in paediatric critical care, *Paediatric Respiratory Reviews*, 20, pp. 24–31.

Munroe, B, Curtis, K, Considine, J & Buckley, T 2013, The impact structured patient assessment frameworks have on patient care: An integrative review, *Journal of Clinical Nursing*, 22, pp. 2991–3005.

Myburgh, J & Finfer, S 2013, Causes of death after fluid bolus resuscitation: New insights from FEAST, *BMC Medicine*, 11, pp. 67–70.

National High Blood Pressure Education Program Working Group on High Blood Pressure in Children and Adolescents 2004, The fourth report on the diagnosis, evaluation, and treatment of high blood pressure in children and adolescents, *Pediatrics*, 114(Suppl. 2), pp. 555–76.

NSW Government, Clinical Excellence Commission 2021, *Paediatric sepsis pathway,* viewed 22 April 2021, www.cec.health.nsw.gov.au/__data/assets/pdf_file/0008/343475/NH700131-Paediatric-Sepsis-Pathway.pdf

Nutbeam, T & Daniels, R on behalf of the UK Sepsis Trust 2021, *UK Sepsis Trust Screening and Action Tools,* viewed 22 April 2021, https://sepsistrust.org/professional-resources/clinical-tools

O'Brien, S 2019, Australasian bronchiolitis guideline, *Journal of Paediatrics & Child Health*, 55(1), pp. 42–53.

O'Meara, M & Watton, DJ (eds) 2012, *Advanced paediatric life support: The practical approach* (5th ed.), Blackwell, London.

Ostchega, M et al. 2014, Mid-arm circumference and recommended blood pressure cuffs for children and adolescents aged between 3 and 19 years: Data from the National Health and Nutrition Examination Survey, 1999–2010, *Blood Pressure Monitoring*, 19(1), pp. 26–31.

Pham, TMT, O'Malley, L, Mayfield, S, Martin, S & Schibler, A 2015, The effect of high flow nasal cannula therapy on the work of breathing in infants with bronchiolitis, *Pediatric Pulmonology*, 50, pp. 713–20.

Pickard, A, Karlen, W & Ansermino, JM 2011, Capillary refill time: Is it still a useful clinical sign?', *Anesthesia and Analgesia*, 113(1), pp. 120–3.

Royal Children's Hospital Melbourne (RCHM) 2020a, Acceptable ranges for physiological variables, viewed 22 April 2021, www.rch.org.au/clinicalguide/guideline_index/ Normal_Ranges_for_Physiological_Variables

—— 2020b, Resuscitation: Hospital management of cardiopulmonary arrest COVID-19, viewed 22 April 2021, www.rch.org.au/clinicalguide/guideline_index/Resuscitation_ COVID-19

Rudd, K et al. 2020, Global, regional, and national sepsis incidence and mortality, 1990–2017: Analysis for the Global Burden of Disease Study, *The Lancet*, 395(10219), pp. 200–11.

Samuels, M & Wieteska, S 2016 *Advanced paediatric life support: A practical approach to emergencies* (6th ed.). John Wiley & Sons, Chichester.

Santillanes, G & Gausche-Hill, M 2008, Pediatric airway management, *Emergency Clinics of North America*, 26, pp. 961–75.

Scheller, RL, Johnson, L, Lorts, A & Ryan, TD 2016, Sudden cardiac arrest in pediatrics, *Pediatric Emergency Care*, 32(9), pp. 630–6.

Schibler, A & Franklin, D 2016, Respiratory support for children in the emergency department, *Journal of Paediatrics and Child Health*, 52, pp. 192–6.

Schibler, A, Pham, TM, Dunster, KR, Foster, K, Barlow, A, Gibbons, K & Hough, JL 2011, Reduced intubation rates for infants after introduction of high flow nasal prong oxygen delivery, *Intensive Care Medicine*, 37(5), pp. 847–52.

Shann, F 2014, *Drug doses RCH intensive care unit* (16th ed.), Royal Children's Hospital, Melbourne.

Teasdale, G, Maas, A, Lecky, F, Manley, G, Stocchetti, N & Murray, G 2014, The Glasgow Coma Scale at 40 years: Standing the test of time, *Lancet Neurology*, 13(8), pp. 844–54.

Top, APC, Tasker, RC & Ince, C 2011, The microcirculation of the critically ill paediatric patient, *Critical Care*, 15, pp. 213–19.

Walsh, BK, Hood, K & Merritt, G 2011, Pediatric airway maintenance and clearance in the acute care setting: How to stay out of trouble, *Respiratory Care*, 56(9), pp. 1424–44.

Weiss, SL & Pomerantz, WJ 2020, Septic shock in children: Rapid recognition and initial resuscitation (first hour), *UpToDate,* viewed 22 April 2021, www.uptodate.com/ contents/septic-shock-in-children-rapid-recognition-and-initial-resuscitation-first-hour

Weiss, SL et al. 2020, Executive summary: Surviving Sepsis campaign international guidelines for the management of septic shock and sepsis-associated organ dysfunction in children, *Pediatric Critical Care Medicine*, 21(2), pp. 186–95.

12

Evidence-based care of children with complex medical needs

Nicola Brown

With acknowledgement to Donna Waters and Helen Stasa for the second edition

LEARNING OBJECTIVES

In this chapter you will:

- Explore common chronic health conditions and their origins in children and young people with complex medical needs
- Consider current evidence regarding the critical role of families in supporting the care and development of children with complex medical needs
- Develop an understanding of nursing assessments and interventions used in the care of children and young people with complex medical needs
- Explore the challenges facing children and young people with complex conditions and their families, as they transition from paediatric to adult healthcare services

Introduction

As a nurse caring for children and young people, you will encounter children with chronic health conditions that require complex daily management and intervention. Your initial contact with the child and their family may be at the time of the diagnosis of the condition or during the course of the child's illness. You may be part of a team that intervenes to manage the acute exacerbation of the child's longer-term medical condition – such as a child with cerebral palsy, who is experiencing respiratory distress due to infection.

While most of the time children with chronic conditions with complex needs are cared for at home by their parents, with support from ambulatory services, the child may require frequent admission to hospital, frequent medical follow-up, and nursing or allied healthcare in the community to maintain health and continue in the activities of daily life, such as school. As such, children with complex medical needs and their families are important and frequent consumers of healthcare services.

Children and young people who are dependent on medical technology have a higher risk of severe acute illness and are more likely to require admission to an intensive-care unit. Furthermore, some illnesses may be life-limiting, resulting in premature death in childhood, adolescence or early adulthood. Some children, young people and their families may require palliative care services towards the end of their illness.

It can be difficult to determine when a child can be defined as having **complex medical needs** (Cohen et al., 2011). What one family finds complex, another family may adapt to more easily. One child with a particular condition may have less severity and more function than another child with the same or a similar condition. Furthermore, the discussion around the care of children with complex medical needs has often used different terms for similar things – care that is 'medically complex', or children who are 'technology dependent' or 'medically frail'.

In this chapter, we will explore some of the causes of complex medical needs in children and young people, and discuss related nursing care and interventions. The important and central role of parents, caregivers and families in the care of children with complex needs will also be considered.

> **Complex medical needs** – Refers to infants and children with complex and chronic conditions, functional limitations, high health and family needs, and high levels of health service use (Cohen et al., 2011).

Chronic health conditions associated with complex medical needs

Diseases that might result in a child having complex medical needs are generally rare; however, the range of diseases defined as 'rare' is vast. There are approximately 8000 rare diseases that affect 6–10 per cent of the population (Elliott & Zurynski, 2015), and these rare disorders may be evident at birth or may emerge during childhood. Children with such diseases may have mild to profound disability, and may have complex medical needs. It is beyond the scope of this chapter to explore all conditions that might require a child and family to receive complex medical care. Instead, some examples are provided to highlight the more 'common' of the 'rare' conditions.

Congenital anomalies (also known as birth defects) – Health problems or physical anomalies that are present at birth and may result in long-term disability, morbidity or death.

Congenital anomalies are a major cause of hospitalisation during infancy and childhood in Australia; however, the collation and reporting of data specific to the experience of children and young people with these conditions is not routine. There is also limited reporting of the major personal, social, community and economic consequences of caring for children and young people with congenital conditions. The Australian Congenital Anomalies Monitoring System (ACAMS) is supported by the Australian Institute of Health and Welfare (AIHW) as a register of congenital anomalies or birth defects across all Australian states and territories, with the exception of the Northern Territory. The last report (Abeywardana & Sullivan, 2008) collated data from 2002–03, and noted that hypospadias – a condition characterised by the opening of the urethra on the ventral side of the male penis – is the most commonly reported congenital condition in Australia (Abeywardana & Sullivan, 2008). According to this report, the overall rate of hypospadias, regardless of the severity of the condition, is approximately 23.8 per 10 000 births, or 46.4 per 10 000 male births.

Neural tube defects occur in approximately 4.2 per 10 000 live births, but it is estimated that up to 76 per cent of affected pregnancies may be terminated or die in utero (Abeywardana & Sullivan, 2008). Other congenital anomalies associated with chronic conditions of children and young people include spina bifida, cleft lip or palate, intestinal and cardiac anomalies, and limb-reduction deficits.

Chromosomal birth defect – A birth defect caused by an alteration in the number or structure of chromosomes (extra copies or missing copies of specific chromosomes), or having chromosomes with missing or extra pieces. Chromosomes are the genetic structure of a cell that carries DNA.

Children with **chromosomal birth defects** or abnormalities are born with either an irregular number of chromosomes or with one or more chromosomes that have an irregular structure, such as a duplication or deletion. Trisomy 21, or Down syndrome, is characterised by minor or major congenital malformations associated with excess chromosomal material (all or part of a third copy) or translocations of chromosome 21. Down syndrome is the second most commonly reported congenital condition in Australian children, occurring more commonly with advancing maternal age and at a rate of 11.1 per 10 000 live births. It is estimated that approximately 64 per cent of foetuses affected by this chromosomal abnormality are either managed by termination or die in utero, making the actual rate for trisomy 21 closer to 26.3 per 10 000 pregnancies (Abeywardana & Sullivan, 2008: 140). Other common chromosomal conditions in Australia are Klinefelter syndrome (which affects boys), Turner syndrome (which affects girls), and Prader-Willi and Angelman syndromes.

Gene defects – Mutations or alterations to chromosomes (the genetic structure of a cell that carries DNA), causing abnormalities in the genome. These defects cause genetic disorders that are present from birth (congenital).

Single **gene defects** describe conditions for which defects in a certain (single) gene have been identified as the cause of a disorder. Single gene defects have predictable inheritance patterns and can be classified as recessive, dominant or X-linked. Neurofibromatosis is caused by an autosomal dominant gene defect (only one copy of the changed gene is required to be affected by the disease), with the mild form occurring in one per 2500 to 4000 live births in Australia. Recessive disorders can only occur when both parents are carriers of the recessive gene and the child inherits two copies of the mutated gene. Cystic fibrosis is one of the more common (autosomal recessive) single gene defects, and because symptoms affect a range of body systems, paediatric nurses are very likely to encounter children and young people affected by this condition. Other single gene defects cause Huntington disease, phenylketonuria (PKU), sickle cell disease, Tay-Sachs disease, thalassaemia and Duchenne muscular dystrophy (an X-linked condition affecting boys).

CASE STUDY 12.1 MAX AND AHMED

Max and Ahmed are new friends – 6-year-old boys who have recently started school. Each boy has complex medical needs. Max and Ahmed attend a school for children with high-support needs, with teachers who specialise in the education of children with special needs and additional support staff to assist with the care needs of the children.

Max has a rare protein metabolism condition and requires feeding with a specialised formula via a gastrostomy button. In early infancy, Max began to have seizures, and in later infancy his parents noticed that he was not developing as quickly as his older siblings had done. He was slower to sit, crawl and walk. At 6 years of age, Max has difficulty standing and walking, and has begun to use a walker to assist with mobility. Jo, Max's mother, is his full-time carer, and has been a single mother since Theo, Max's dad, left. Theo has had little subsequent contact with the family.

Ahmed has cerebral palsy. Ahmed was born prematurely at 32 weeks and required admission to a special care nursery. One of the earliest indicators that Ahmed may have had a physical disability was identified by the child and family health nurse when Ahmed still had problems with head control at 4 months. Now Ahmed uses a wheelchair for mobility, as he has a significant motor impairment due to bilateral spastic quadriplegia. The level of motor impairment means that Ahmed needs considerable physical care, including urinary catheterisation, gastrostomy feeding, transferring and hygiene care. Ahmed has difficulties communicating, and is using a picture board to assist with this. Ahmed lives at home with his parents, Rameen and Aamil, grandparents and two older siblings. His mother and grandmother are his main carers.

Both boys have required admissions to hospital for acute illness in the past. Most recently, Max suffered a fall during a seizure, and sustained a mild concussion when his head hit the kerb. Ahmed has had admissions to hospital for management of respiratory distress due to pneumonia after upper respiratory tract infections.

Cerebral palsy (CP) is an umbrella term for non-progressive but often changing motor impairment that occurs before or soon after birth (Eunson, 2012) and is the most common physical disability in childhood. In recent years, the prevalence of children with CP has declined from 2.1 to 1.4 children with CP per 1000 live births, potentially due to improvements in the care of women during pregnancy and infants requiring neonatal intensive care (Australian Cerebral Palsy Register Group, 2018). However, there are proportionately more Aboriginal and Torres Strait Islander children with CP, including with more severe motor and other disabilities (Australian Cerebral Palsy Register Group, 2018).

For the majority of children, the brain injury associated with CP is most likely to have occurred during pre-natal and perinatal development (Australian Cerebral Palsy Register Group, 2018; Eunson, 2012). No two children or young people with CP are the same. CP can impact an individual's physical or intellectual function, activities of daily living and participation in community life (Novak et al., 2013).

Cerebral palsy (CP) – A non-progressive motor impairment that occurs before or soon after birth.

As the standard of antenatal and perinatal care has improved significantly over recent decades, it was anticipated that the prevalence of cerebral palsy might decline. However, as prevalence has declined, the survival rates of children with more severe types of CP have improved as medical interventions for children born prematurely or disabled have also improved (Eunson, 2012). Current risk factors associated with CP include prematurity, low weight for gestational age, multiple pregnancy and maternal genitourinary infections (Australian Cerebral Palsy Register Group, 2018; Eunson, 2012). The majority of children with CP (including Ahmed) have spasticity (86.6 per cent) and may have other impairments in addition to motor impairment, including epilepsy or intellectual, speech, visual or hearing problems (Australian Cerebral Palsy Register Group, 2018).

CASE STUDY 12.2 CALEB

Caleb is a 10-year-old boy who attends a mainstream public primary school with support from a teacher's aide.

Caleb was diagnosed with Duchenne muscular dystrophy at 4 years of age. Caleb's parents had noticed that he took longer to start walking than other children, and at 4 years of age, Caleb could not run well, jump or ride a tricycle. As his dystrophy progressed, Caleb needed to start wearing orthotic braces and began using a motor scooter at school and home. At age 10, Caleb uses a wheelchair to mobilise, but can still stand and bear weight for short periods, transferring himself with support from chair to bed. He is able to feed himself and can write and communicate independently. Caleb lives with his parents in a regional town, and the family often has to travel to the city for outpatient treatment at a tertiary-level referral paediatric hospital. The paediatric hospital employs a clinical nurse consultant (CNC) who specialises in children with degenerative conditions. The CNC is an important healthcare professional who works in collaboration with the specialist medical team, and the local general practitioner, physiotherapist, occupational therapist and community nursing services in Caleb's town, and often helps these local healthcare professionals to support the family while at home.

Caleb's parents have decided not to have any more children. They do not wish to risk having another child with muscular dystrophy and want to devote their efforts to caring for Caleb.

Muscular dystrophies – A group of neuromuscular genetic disorders that result in the progressive deterioration of muscle strength and function.

Muscular dystrophies are a group of neuromuscular genetic disorders that result in the progressive deterioration of muscle strength and function – another significant cause of physical disability in children and young people. The most serious impacts of this deterioration include diminished respiratory function and immobility (Mercuri & Muntoni, 2013). Most forms are diagnosed in children, although some children are not diagnosed until later in life.

Detection and diagnosis of muscular dystrophy can take some time. Usually, parents detect some delay in motor milestones and seek advice during the toddler and preschool years. Various clinical signs such as motor delay, serum creatinine kinase, muscle biopsy and genetic screening are used to determine the presence and type of dystrophy (Mercuri & Muntoni, 2013).

The most common form of muscular dystrophy in children is Duchenne muscular dystrophy, an X-linked recessive gene affecting male children such as Caleb. Duchenne dystrophy is a life-limiting condition; however, survival into early adulthood has improved with increasing access to mechanical ventilation and the use of antibiotics to treat respiratory infections (Yiu & Kornberg, 2015). As a result, the number of adolescents with Duchenne dystrophy who require support during transition from paediatric to adult services has increased. Longer survival time is associated with increased likelihood of cardiac muscle involvement. Severe ventricular arrhythmia may eventuate and sudden death may be the first indication of this (Mercuri & Muntoni, 2013).

There are many different types of metabolic conditions, some of which result in developmental disability and may also require specialist care and alternative nutrition. Many of these conditions are detected soon after birth through the newborn screening program (Wilcken & Wiley, 2015). All infants born in Australia have newborn screening: a heel-prick blood sample taken and tested for the presence of a number of metabolic and genetic conditions, including inborn errors of metabolism such as **phenylketonuria (PKU)**, hypothyroidism and cystic fibrosis (Royal Australasian College of Physicians, 2015). For some children, such as Max, the metabolic condition may not be detected until after birth. Metabolic and genetic conditions may be detected by parents and healthcare professionals when there are concerns about delays in development or regressed development, or idiopathic seizures.

Some children may have complex, chronic respiratory conditions, often associated with **premature birth** or respiratory complications in the neonatal period. Examples include chronic neonatal lung disease or subglottic stenosis. The impact of these respiratory conditions may lessen as the child develops and the respiratory tract becomes larger. Depending on the nature of the condition, these children may require an artificial airway (usually a tracheostomy) and/or oxygen therapy in the early years of life.

Phenylketonuria (PKU) –
A genetic condition resulting in a failure to metabolise phenylalanine, an amino acid found in proteins and some artificial sweeteners. If not detected and treated, this can lead to intellectual disability and seizures.

Premature birth – The live birth of an infant before 37 weeks' gestation (WHO, 2015).

CASE STUDY 12.3 TOBIAS

Tobias is a 4-month-old boy born to Karen and Zane. Tobias is their first child, and was born with Down syndrome and an atrioventricular septial defect. Karen and Zane knew before Tobias was born that he had Down syndrome and a heart problem, as these had been detected as part of prenatal screening.

Tobias was born by caesarean section at 39 weeks and needed admission to the intensive care unit with initial breathing difficulties. Once these settled, Tobias was transferred to the special care nursery. Tobias had difficulty feeding as he easily became tired and did not have a strong suck, and therefore needed nasogastric feeding. Prior to discharge, Karen and Zane learned how to prepare and administer nasogastric feeds, and prepare and administer Tobias's cardiac medications; they also practised inserting a nasogastric tube under the supervision of the nurses. Karen and Zane will need to bring Tobias to the outpatient department regularly to see the cardiac specialists, and plan for Tobias's heart surgery to correct his heart defect.

Down syndrome

Down syndrome, a disorder of chromosome 21, is one of the more common chromosomal disorders, and can be detected through maternal screening prior to birth. Usually we are born with two copies of chromosome 21, but most children with Down syndrome have three copies (standard trisomy 21). There are two other less common forms of Down syndrome: mosaicism, where some cells have trisomy 21 but others do not; and translocation, where part of chromosome 21 has attached to another chromosome. Children with mosaicism exhibit some but not all of the characteristics of trisomy 21. Children with trisomy 21 or translocation will present with all the characteristics of Down syndrome. Approximately one in 1100 births, or approximately 290 babies each year, are born with Down syndrome in Australia each year (Down Syndrome Australia, 2020).

It is not fully understood why the different errors of chromosome 21 might occur. Historically, Down syndrome was more likely to be associated with older maternal age; however, due to increased screening of older mothers, the prevalence is currently higher in infants born to younger women (Diamandopoulos & Green, 2018).

All women are offered initial screening in the first trimester, and may elect to terminate the pregnancy if the risk of the syndrome is high. Some women and their families decide to continue and give birth to a child with Down syndrome. Prenatal screening in the first trimester consists of serum human chorionic gonadatrophin and pregnancy associated plasma protein (9–12 weeks) and a **nuchal translucency scan** by ultrasound (12 weeks) (Diamandopoulos & Green, 2018). If these preliminary screening tests indicate a higher risk of Down syndrome, the woman will be offered further investigations for prenatal diagnosis, including **chorionic villi sampling** or **amniocentesis**.

Nuchal translucency scan – An ultrasound of the nuchal fold, performed around 12 weeks of pregnancy. The width of the nuchal fold at the back of the foetal neck is measured to estimate fluid build-up that may be indicative of a higher risk of Down syndrome.

Chorionic villi sampling – The sampling of chorionic cells from the developing placenta for diagnosis of chromosomal abnormalities in the foetus. Usually performed during the first trimester, at around 8–10 weeks.

Amniocentesis – the sampling of amniotic fluid via the abdominal wall for the purpose of detecting and diagnosing chromosomal disorders in the foetus. Usually performed during the second trimester, at around 12–14 weeks.

Characteristics of Down syndrome

Babies and children with Down syndrome have a distinct physical appearance due to specific physical characteristics of the disorder. Physical characteristics include:

- hypotonia (floppy, relaxed muscle tone)
- laxity of the joints, simian line (single deep crease across the palm of the hand)
- epicanthal folds (extra skin fold on the inner corner of the eyes)
- protruding tongue
- smaller, abnormally shaped ears
- a flat, broad nose and face
- wider spacing between the first and second toes and fingers
- a smaller head (Down Syndrome Australia, 2016).

Children will have some degree of intellectual disability with considerable individual variation, ranging from mild to profound intellectual disability. Children with Down syndrome also have a significantly higher likelihood of other complex illnesses and problems, including congenital heart defects, leukaemia, atlantoaxial instability, growth delay, thyroid dysfunction, ophthalmic and ear, nose and throat conditions. However, not all children will have all or any of these conditions (Diamandopoulos & Green, 2018).

Like Tobias, infants born with Down syndrome often have difficulty feeding. This is due to the hypotonia associated with Down syndrome, which means the infant is less able to latch to a teat or nipple, and may lack a strong suck. When the infant has a cardiac condition as well, they tire more easily during feeding. For these reasons, Tobias was unable to consume the amount of infant formula he needed, so the decision was made to use enteral feeding via a nasogastric tube. Once Tobias has his heart problem corrected, he may tolerate oral feeding better.

Families and children with complex medical needs

In most situations, children with complex medical needs are ultimately cared for by parents and family members at home. However, in many cases infants and children are cared for a prolonged period of time in hospital prior to discharge into the care of their family (Elias, Murphy & Council on Children with Disabilities, 2012; Noyes et al., 2014). Prior to discharge, parents and caregivers often need to learn new skills and gain new knowledge in order to care for their child at home and integrate the care into the day-to-day life of the family.

Children are now frequently sent home for care, with an ongoing need for interventions such as oxygen, tracheostomies, ventilation, enteral feeding, care of intravenous devices and complex medication regimes (to name just a few) (ten Haken et al., 2018). It is important to remember that not every child who requires complex medical care will end up at home with their family. Different families have different levels of health literacy, resources and capacity to support a child with complex medical needs. Some children may eventually live in out-of-home care, either in a foster family or in a long-term care unit.

Models of care are changing for families of children with complex healthcare needs. An evidence-based practice approach to the development of models of care is increasingly used to inform new service delivery and integrated care models as these demonstrate improved quality of life and cost savings for services (Wolfe et al., 2020). As parent access to technology improves, there is great potential to provide better support via video over the internet, especially to families living in rural and regional areas. One example is the Chronic Pain Team at Sydney Children's Hospital Network, which provides support to families of children with chronic pain.

When children with complex needs become acutely unwell and need admission to hospital, it is critical to remember that the parents or the child's primary caregiver(s) are often the experts in the care of their child. They know their child best, and often detect subtle changes in the child's behaviour or response before expert clinicians would. Parents may have had many years of experience in continuously caring for a child with a particular condition. If their child is dependent on technology, they often have a very good understanding of that technology and have developed practical 'know-how' about the finer nuances of their child's equipment. In these situations, healthcare professionals can be somewhat intimidated by parents' expertise! The best thing we can do is acknowledge and draw on that expertise to provide the best possible care for the child in partnership with the parents or caregiver(s).

Caring for a child with complex medical needs increases the burden of care for parents and family members. There is a lack of research to inform the best way in which to support parents as they learn to manage the equipment and exercise clinical judgement in relation to the care of their child at home (ten Haken et al., 2018). A systematic review published in 2015 provides some evidence of the value of an individualised approach to planning parent education that takes into account parent learning preferences (Nightingale, Friedl & Swallow, 2015).

It can be difficult to assess the extent of the burden of care for a family. Each family has different capacity for function, and each child has different characteristics as an individual that can make caring for that child at home easier or more difficult (Pangilinan & Hornyak, 2013). Depending on the nature of the child's needs, there may be considerable time requirements for care and the need to learn a range of new skills and master new areas of knowledge (ten Haken et al., 2018). To some extent, it is likely to be easier for families to adapt to managing a child's illness at home when there are less demanding levels of care, skill or technology required, or the condition is non-life-threatening. When planning care, the cultural and social practices of the family should be considered, as these may impact on parents' beliefs and values about the management of their child's health.

Depending on the level of care required, parents may need to reconsider their commitments outside the home, which can result in increased social isolation, a potential decrease in income and increased costs for the care of their child (Cockett, 2012). Mothers are often the primary caregivers of children with complex needs, so may be at a higher risk of depression due to the burden of care (Toly, Musil & Carl, 2012).The nature of the child's condition may also mean that the child requires frequent hospitalisation, outpatient appointments and/or invasive procedures that may be intrusive on family life, cause pain and suffering for the child and increase the stress on parents and families. Wherever possible, it is best to provide services to support children to remain at home with their families and within their communities, to enhance their opportunity to participate in normal, day-to-day life – for example, school, leisure activities and family life (WHO, 2012). However, while it may be ideal to discharge a child with complex needs to their own home as soon as possible, social, financial and environmental issues can delay discharge and prolong hospitalisation. For families such as Caleb's, which live in rural or regional areas, access to specialist paediatric services can be a challenge. Outreach nursing services such as the CNC working with Caleb's family act as an important link in the collaboration between specialist and local healthcare services for Caleb's care.

Respite care – Temporary care provided to children with complex needs by another, to provide parent(s) or primary caregiver(s) with the opportunity for a break from the demands of care.

Caring for a child with complex needs can be demanding for parents, and some families may choose to take a break from the demands of caring for a child with complex needs. **Respite care** may be provided for brief periods of time at home or overnight – either within the home or in another venue – by extended family, trained carers in the home or specific respite care organisations. Some parents may view an admission to hospital as a form of respite. Parents of children with complex needs can find it difficult to access community-based respite care that meets the needs and expectations of the child and the family (Teo, Kennedy-Behr & Lowe, 2018).

Many children with complex health needs will have life-limiting conditions. For example, children like Caleb, with Duchenne's muscular dystrophy, may die in adolescence or early adulthood. Families such as Caleb's will know this soon after a diagnosis is made and will experience feelings of sadness and grief before Caleb passes away. **Anticipatory grief** can help parents, siblings and other loved family and friends to prepare and adjust for the time when their child is gone. For further discussion about palliative care, end-of-life care and grieving, see Chapter 13.

Anticipatory grief – The experience of the grief response when the child or person is expected to die at some point in the future as a result of illness or disability.

REFLECTION POINTS 12.1

The proportion of children who survive childhood and adolescence with complex healthcare problems is increasing due to advances in medical treatments and technologies. What are the implications of this trend for:

- families
- paediatric healthcare professionals
- community healthcare services for children
- school and education services?

Nursing assessment and interventions

A broad scope of conditions is associated with complex medical needs, and therefore the discussion of the range of likely nursing interventions is considerable and beyond the scope of this chapter. Instead, the more common nursing assessment and care issues are discussed, including respiration, mobility, nutrition and communication.

Respiration

Children with chronic and complex conditions may have impaired respiration and oxygenation related to features of their medical condition, such as respiratory function, central nervous system, neuromuscular factors and/or abnormalities of the anatomy of their respiratory system (Chiang & Amin, 2017). Some children will require respiratory support as part of their condition, or as their condition progresses. This can take several forms, depending on the nature of the respiratory impairment, including the need for a tracheostomy, ventilation, suction and/or oxygen therapy.

Children with chronic lung disease are at higher risk of respiratory infections and are more likely to require hospitalisation when unwell. They may not be able to cough effectively or may have an impaired capacity to swallow their own saliva, increasing the risk of **aspiration**. Acute episodes of aspiration can result in pneumonia and airway obstruction, while frequent, chronic aspiration can lead to chronic damage to the lung

Aspiration – Inhalation of fluid, food or saliva below the subglottis and into the airways.

(Chiang & Amin, 2017). Symptoms of aspiration can include coughing, wheezing, choking and moist/wet inspiratory sounds.

Some of these difficulties with swallowing of fluids, food and saliva can benefit from speech therapy. The speech therapist can use a range of evidence-based techniques to improve oral motor skills such as mouth closure and swallowing coordination and efficacy (Chiang & Amin, 2017). An essential aspect of care is to ensure that parents can help encourage their child to practise speech therapy exercises and to recognise the signs and symptoms of aspiration, requiring medical assessment.

Oxygen therapy

Children with hypoxia requiring long-term oxygen therapy may have conditions associated with lung disease as a result of premature birth, interstitial lung disease or congenital cardiac disease. The decision to prescribe oxygen therapy for long-term use at home, in the community, is generally made on assessment of oxygenation and respiratory effort over time, during a range of daily activities, including sleep, feeding and exercise. Depending on the level of need for supplementary oxygen, it is most likely to be administered through nasal prongs or a cannula. The oxygen may be supplied in smaller portable oxygen cylinders or an oxygen concentrator system may be provided.

Parents and caregivers need to be provided with education and training in the safe use of oxygen. This will include providing instruction on how to set up the oxygen cylinder, use and regulate oxygen flow via a flow meter.

Depending on the nature of their condition, some children may eventually 'outgrow' their need for oxygen. This can include those children who were born prematurely, or children who have their underlying cardiac condition treated or repaired surgically. For children who have been receiving oxygen in the long term, weaning from oxygen may need to occur in hospital under supervision.

Tracheostomy and ventilation

Some children who are unable to maintain a patent airway may require the creation of a tracheostomy and insertion of a tracheostomy tube. Indications for a tracheostomy may include airway obstruction, difficulty maintaining a patent airway or the need for long-term ventilation (Chiang & Amin, 2017). The creation of a tracheostomy requires the creation of a stoma in the neck and trachea, which is then kept patent with a tube.

One issue with the creation of a tracheostomy is that the insertion of an airway into the trachea bypasses the upper airway. In normal respiration, the upper airway humidifies and filtrates the air before it reaches the lower airway, reducing the risk of infection. As a result, children with a tracheostomy tube would usually have a 'Swedish nose', or heat moisture exchanger, in place to help humidify and filter air.

Caleb will eventually require ventilation support as his respiratory muscles weaken. Initially, Caleb may only require non-invasive ventilation such as continuous positive airway pressure (CPAP) at night, to reduce the likelihood of nocturnal hypoventilation (Chiang & Amin, 2017). As his condition deteriorates, he may require insertion of a tracheostomy tube and continuous long-term ventilation. An increasing number of children requiring long-term ventilation are cared for in the community.

Preparing families to care for their child requiring long-term ventilation at home is a considerable undertaking for the family and supporting healthcare services. Current practice guidelines (Sterni et al., 2016) recommend that a comprehensive plan is developed in consultation with the family, and acute and community-based healthcare services, which addresses critical elements, including:

- assessment of preparedness for care in the home and provision of appropriate equipment including a work, health and safety plan, provision of all equipment for ventilation, suctioning, oxygenation, management of the tracheostomy and tube, and a maintenance plan for all equipment
- a comprehensive training program for family members and community-based carers, that includes an ongoing education plan to reinforce and support skills and knowledge of respiratory assessment, care of the tracheostomy tube, management of ventilation and maintenance of airway patency. It is essential that parents and healthcare professionals know the child's baseline parameters when they are well, are attuned to the signs of increasing respiratory effort and infection, and are trained in cardiopulmonary resuscitation. Additionally, parents and families need a clear plan for managing illness at home, and should know when and where to seek help from acute healthcare services, including the ambulance service.

Mobility

Children who have motor impairment may have difficulty with mobility. It is important to bear in mind that the extent of motor impairment associated with different conditions can vary. For example, although Ahmed requires a wheelchair, not all children with CP will need one. On the other hand, motor impairment will get worse over time in some children with progressive conditions, as it has done for Caleb with muscular dystrophy. Regardless of the condition or prognosis, the main aim for children with motor impairment is to maintain function, and independence where possible, for as long as possible.

The care required by a child with motor impairment includes several priorities and a range of nursing interventions. One of the most important priorities is the prevention or delay of contractures and maintaining posture, as these factors are key to maintaining current level of motor function (Eddy, 2013). Physical therapy is an important intervention in terms of maintaining function, and requires a multidisciplinary approach from a range of healthcare practitioners, including physiotherapists, occupational therapists and orthopaedic specialists. Nurses and parents may be required to assist children in passive range of motion exercises, the application of splints, positioning to promote best posture, and prevention or delay of scoliosis, which can result in difficulties with respiration as well as problems with mobility. Depending on the extent of the impairment, children may require assistance with transferring or use of walkers, wheelchairs or standing boards. Any child with impaired mobility is at risk of skin breakdown and has a higher risk of falls. Nursing staff need to assess the level of risk for both skin breakdown and falls, and institute appropriate nursing interventions (Crisp et al., 2016).

Children with impaired mobility may require nursing assistance or have specialist intervention to meet their hygiene and elimination needs. Some children may not have bladder or bowel control, and may use nappies or incontinence pads, or need assistance to use a toilet or commode. Others may require intermittent urinary catheterisation or have an indwelling urinary or suprapubic catheter.

Whether it is nurses, other healthcare professionals or parents who are assisting children with mobility problems, it is important to adhere to the principles of manual handling. Carers can often become fatigued by the physical demands of lifting and transferring children, and time should be made for rest.

Nutrition and hydration

Ideally, it is better for children to maintain hydration and nutrition by feeding orally. Eating is a pleasurable experience and contributes to language development. The sharing of meals is an important part of our social and family lives. Many children with chronic and complex needs will require some assistance to meet their nutritional and hydration needs (Burdall et al., 2017). These children may have difficulty with oral feeding due to neurological impairments, and may not be able to chew and swallow easily or safely. Some children may be able to take oral food and fluids, but may require assistance with drinking and feeding. Other children may have difficulty with swallowing, and may require pureed or mashed foods. In each of these instances, children should be supervised during meals to monitor for any signs of choking or aspiration. For other children, enteral feeding via a nasogastric or nasojejunal tube, or gastrostomy, may be required.

When children are dependent on others for their nutrition, it is essential that their level of nutrition and hydration is monitored – both by regular measurements of height and weight to monitor growth, and by observing for signs of inadequate nutrition and hydration such as constipation and decreased urine output.

Enteral feeding

Nasogastric tubes are usually used as a short-term form of enteral feeding, as may be the case with Tobias, the baby boy with Down syndrome in Case study 12.3. Children who require long-term or permanent enteral feeding are more likely to have a gastrostomy created and a gastrostomy tube or button inserted.

A gastrostomy is created via a surgical procedure under general anaesthetic (ACI & GENCA, 2015). A puncture site (stoma) is inserted through the abdomen and into the stomach. Either a tube or button device is inserted into the stoma and may be secured with a suture. The tube or button device maintains patency of the stoma and acts as a conduit for fluid and formula. Similar to a nasogastric tube, the position of the tube or device is confirmed by aspirating gastric fluid and testing with litmus paper.

Depending on the reason for enteral feeding, children may require bolus feeding during the day and continuous overnight feeds. In order to meet their metabolic needs for growth, children may have high-calorie feeds. Some children may require different types of formula, depending on their conditions.

Even though feeding via gastrostomy may be required long term to avoid risks of aspiration and maintain nutrition and hydration needs in children with complex needs, there are still risks associated with these methods. These can range from relatively minor complications such as infection, granulation of tissue and leakage at the site, to internal injury, bowel obstruction or fistula between the colon, stomach and insertion site. The tube can migrate through the stomach and into the bowel, causing obstruction. Gastric secretions can ooze around the site, causing skin irritation (Burdall et al., 2017).

Parents and carers will require support, education and training in the use and care of gastrostomy. In addition to the safe preparation, storage and administration of enteral feeding solutions, parents will need to learn how to recognise problems with the tube, and how best to trouble shoot, including blockage and accidental removal of the tube (Burdall et al., 2017).

Some children with complex medical conditions of the gastrointestinal tract may not be able to digest or absorb food and fluids. For these children, nutrition may need to be provided intravenously (parenteral nutrition), usually via a central venous access device (CVAD). Their need for parenteral nutrition may be temporary or permanent.

Communication

Some children with complex medical needs may have problems with speech, language or intellectual capacity. Any of these problems can reduce or interfere with their communication and understanding. Children with impairment in speech may use a variety of devices in order to communicate with others, from simple pictures to sophisticated computer-assisted devices.

Developing skills in communication with children who are well and developing normally can be challenging for healthcare professionals, and it can be more complex when the child has difficulty communicating. The principles of interpersonal communication are equally important for children with communication difficulties. Our body language, the way we position ourselves to communicate, the tone of voice we use, the simplicity of the language we use – all of these are valuable ways to enhance communication with children.

REFLECTION POINTS 12.2

Families vary in their cultural and social beliefs and values. For some families, their beliefs about people with complex medical needs will be influenced by their cultural background. Part of preparing to care for children with complex needs and disability means examining our own cultural beliefs, values and attitudes about children with disability, and being open and flexible towards people from different cultural backgrounds and their views.

- Do you have specific beliefs about the care of children or adults with complex medical needs?
- How might these beliefs influence the care you provide to a child with complex needs and their family?

Again, parents are often a very good source of advice, as they understand the particular ways in which their individual child communicates their needs to the world. This can be particularly important when caring for children with communication impairment when they are unwell. Parents are often able to interpret their child's unique ways of communicating pain, fear or distress (Burkitt, Breau & Zabalia, 2011;

Solodiuk et al., 2010). In addition to parent reporting, there are some specific pain-assessment tools that can be used when caring for children with severe disability, including the Non-Communicating Children's Pain Checklist, the FLAAC tool and the Paediatric Pain Profile (McKay & Clarke, 2012).

Transition to adult care

Many complex conditions will persist from childhood through adolescence and into adulthood. Individuals who experience these conditions and who survive to reach adulthood will face the important developmental task of transitioning to adult care. The process of transition has been identified for some time as the 'purposeful planned movement of adolescents and young adults with chronic physical and medical conditions from a child-centred to adult orientated healthcare system' (Bloom et al., 2012, p. 213).

Transitioning from paediatric to adult care is a complex process that often takes several years. There is no 'right' time for transition, but setting a target transfer age may potentially help the young person and their family, and the multidisciplinary healthcare team, to plan and prepare for the future. Transition will usually commence in adolescence, between the ages of 16 and 18 years (Fegran et al., 2014), or when a young person leaves secondary school, but this will depend upon the service organisations, the availability of their resources, the maturity and knowledge of the individual with the chronic condition, the level of family support they have, the nature and severity of their condition, the country in which care is being delivered and their personal preferences (Wisk et al., 2015).

The successful transition of young adults to adult services also requires attention to their physical, emotional and psychosocial needs. In order to be successful, it also requires engagement with their parents, who have an important role in helping to scaffold and facilitate increasing independence of the young person (Heath, Farre & Shaw, 2017). A transition process that focuses solely on the illness and its treatment is unlikely to meet the needs of the young person (ACI, 2014). It is essential that the individual developmental needs of the young person are taken into account.

Important considerations during transition

Let's consider Case study 12.4. Ellen had graduated from the children's hospital 'transitional care program', but naturally held some reservations about moving to the adult hospital.

The move from paediatric to adult healthcare services is characterised by a number of assumptions that are often not made explicit. Of particular importance is the assumption that the client will take a greater level of individual responsibility for managing their care in an adult service (Fegran et al., 2014; White & Cooley, 2018). Parents or caregivers who may previously have played a significant role in decision-making are designated to a more peripheral role (White & Cooley, 2018), their deep contextual and historical knowledge lost. Some young people find this new responsibility for decision-making intimidating or overwhelming – especially if they have not been prepared adequately. Some parents also find it difficult to disengage from a role they may have held for a long time (Heath, Farre & Shaw., 2017). Other assumptions include the giving of support, orientation and advice to help the young person 'way-find' in their new environment, to use different technologies for appointment and results notifications, and to manage personal electronic health records (Begley, 2013).

CASE STUDY 12.4 ELLEN

Ellen is a 16-year-old young woman with CF. She has now transitioned to the adult CF clinic. Ellen was late for her first appointment because her mum couldn't work out where to park and Ellen had to walk a long way to the clinic, arriving hot, tired, breathless and coughing. Ellen did not recognise any of the other patients in the waiting room, and some of them looked really sick. There was not a single staff member she knew. She went to the coffee shop, but she missed seeing her friend Sharon behind the service counter. By the time her mother arrived, Ellen had been taken in to see the registrar, who was in the process of asking her to recite her entire medical and surgical history from when she was a baby. Ellen said, 'Don't you have my notes from the other hospital? Can't you just read them?' The registrar then asked Ellen's mum to leave the room while she undertook a clinical examination. Ellen decided that she did not want to share any of her previous history with this person – if this new doctor didn't care enough to read her notes and the referral letter from her pediatrician, why should she waste her time?

The movement from paediatric to adult services also requires getting used to a new healthcare team and negotiating new relationships. The young person moves from specialist paediatric service providers (for instance, a paediatric endocrinologist, paediatric nurses, educators and dietitians) to adult service providers who may be used to delivering services to much older patients and who are practising within a different organisational context, and possibly in a different location. The young person (either in consultation with their paediatric team or independently) will need to find a suitable adult healthcare provider, and work towards establishing rapport and understanding with a new healthcare team that will rarely have the same extensive understanding of their previous history and may include new members such as genetic counsellors, surgeons or obstetricians (McInally, 2013; Oswald et al., 2013).

Young people with conditions that impact on their cognitive function will have special needs as part of the transition to adult services. Diminished cognitive function mean that their capacity to fully participate in decision-making will be affected (White & Cooley, 2018). The parents of these young people will have special concerns about their care. In such situations, consideration may need to be given to longer term guardianship of the young person to assist and support their autonomy in healthcare decisions.

Successful transition

A successful transition is promoted by healthcare providers who listen to, and who are sensitive and supportive of, the needs of the transitioning clients (Okumura et al., 2014). In their study of young people with type 1 diabetes, Ritholz et al. (2014) found that the transition process often raises a variety of emotions, including sadness and reluctance to separate from providers who have often been a part of the young person's life for a significant period of time. Consequently, it is important for adult providers to be aware of and sensitive to these emotions.

It is also recognised that health education, policy and research have failed to keep pace with rapid growth in the numbers of young people with often complex chronic conditions moving to adult care (White & Cooley, 2018). Adult healthcare providers are often unaware that young people who are moving from a paediatric to an adult service will have insights into their own condition and needs that are different from those of adult clients who have not previously been involved with healthcare systems. Contrast the experience of Ellen (Case study 12.4) with that of a young adult presenting to an adult respiratory clinic for the first time. Throughout the transition process, young people may experience feelings of not belonging and of being redundant (Fegran et al., 2014). Adult healthcare professionals need to understand, respect and actively acknowledge the years of personal insight and comprehensive knowledge that chronically ill young people have developed about their own bodies and their own disease.

Good preparation is another important factor in ensuring a successful transition to adult care (Jermyn, 2013). Talking about transition should ideally commence early in the teenage years (around 14 years of age), progressing over the next few years with a view to moving care completely to adult providers by 18 years of age (Fegran et al., 2014). Throughout, there must be active consultation between the young person, their family and both the paediatric and adult care facilities. Many healthcare facilities have introduced formal transition programs to aid movement from paediatric to adult care, although there is a wide discrepancy in their availability and success across different health conditions, and across states and countries (Fegran et al., 2014; Okumura et al., 2014). There is evidence that the inclusion of a dedicated local transition facilitator, with responsibility for the coordination of the transition and the people involved, has a positive impact (ACI, 2014). Advance planning and encouraging young people to gradually take on more of the responsibility for their healthcare decision-making can also make the transition process smoother (White & Cooley, 2018).

Factors known to contribute to the successful transition of young people with chronic conditions to adult care, and therefore useful to include in transition programs, are:

- clear communication between paediatric and adult healthcare providers at the transitioning institutions
- early planning of the transition process over a period of time (years rather than months)
- involving all stakeholders including the current main carer, GP and/or family in the process
- gradually encouraging more involvement of young person in healthcare decision-making

- a local transition case manager or facilitator for each individual
- transition clinics (hybridisation of paediatric and adult service) and introduction to peers who have successfully made the transition
- access to practical and online resources (checklists, maps, parking, names, contact details, who does what, social media, apps, chat rooms and blogs)
- flexibility and consideration of timing of other life events (such as final year at school)
- maintaining contact after the transition (ACI, 2014; White & Cooley, 2018).

Despite best intentions, the planning process for transitioning young people with a chronic condition to adult care is still often neglected (Fegran et al., 2014). Service gaps of six months or more are commonly reported between young people leaving the paediatric provider and establishing consistent relationships with adult care providers (Garvey et al., 2012), especially when young people and their families are left to locate the adult service themselves (Fegran et al., 2014). Ineffective transition and loss of young people to follow-up can be responsible for unnecessary morbidity, excess mortality, preventable emergency room attendances and expensive investigations. The flow-on effects for the young person are a potential loss of earnings, reduction in reproductive potential and negative impact on relationships. In one study of young people with type 1 diabetes, fewer than half of the respondents reported receiving a recommendation for an adult provider, and fewer than 15 per cent reported having a transition preparation visit or receiving written transition materials (Garvey et al., 2012).

The scarcity of healthcare professionals in the adult care sector with specific experience in childhood chronic conditions, and problems finding an adult specialist, are on their own sufficiently understandable reasons for young people's dissatisfaction with transitioning to adult care (Hilliard et al., 2014; Oswald et al., 2013; White & Cooley, 2018). Anticipated future needs include the establishment of specialist facilities and resources for appropriate transitioning, education and training for healthcare professionals in the prevention and treatment of acquired complications associated with improved survival in previously life-limiting paediatric conditions, and developing appropriate models of care for young adults seeking lifelong physical and emotional support from healthcare teams.

REFLECTION POINTS 12.3

- In your work as a paediatric nurse, how have you contributed to preparing young people with chronic conditions for their transition to adult healthcare?
- Do you know whether a transition to an adult healthcare program is part of the service offered by the organisation for which you work? If so, what defining features of the program make it a success? How is success of the program measured?
- Parents and carers play a vital role in planning for transition. What three things can you suggest to parents or carers to prepare their young person with a chronic condition for this process? (*Hint:* encourage the young person to keep a journal and write down questions.)

SUMMARY

- Children with complex healthcare needs are frequent consumers of acute and outpatient paediatric healthcare services.
- Although the different types of conditions that result in complex medical needs are 'rare', they are 'common' in the children who require paediatric healthcare services.
- The impact of complex medical needs on the day-to-day life of children and families is individual and complex.
- Parents and primary caregivers of children with complex healthcare needs have special expertise regarding their child, and often have specialist knowledge of the condition as it relates to their child.
- There is considerable variation between children with special healthcare need and their individual nursing needs; however, commonly nursing interventions for issues associated with impairment of respiration, mobility, nutrition and communication may be required.
- Children with complex healthcare conditions who are expected to survive until early adulthood or older will need to make the transition to adult healthcare services at some point during their adolescence or early adulthood. This transition requires a coordinated, person-centred approach from both paediatric and adult health services.

LEARNING ACTIVITY

It is useful for paediatric nurses and other healthcare professionals to have an understanding of the availability of resources for families of children with complex needs and to know where to locate this information.

In this activity, use the internet to undertake a search of resources in your area for children with a specific complex medical need and their family. Use Table 12.1 as a template to help you get started, but you may have additional information that you want to add to your search. An example (based on the Carer Allowance) is provided.

Table 12.1   Resources for children with complex medical needs

Resource		Funding source	Details	Source/link
Financial support	Carer Allowance	Commonwealth Government	Criteria: The carer must be caring for one or more children under 16 years with a recognised disability/medical condition lasting 12 months or longer and receiving care in home or hospital. A $250 000 annual family income test threshold applies.	www.dss.gov .au/disability-and-carers/ benefits-payments/ carer-allowance

Table 12.1   *(cont.)*

Resource	Funding source	Details	Source/link
Medications			
Equipment			
Disease/ condition support network			
Other			

FURTHER READING

- Rare diseases in Australia – the Steve Waugh Foundation. Approximately 8000 different or 'rare' conditions affect up to 300 000 children in Australia. Access to support from parents and clinicians normally available through disease/disorder specific support groups is more difficult when the condition is rare. Former Australian cricket captain Steve Waugh has established a charitable foundation to assist families of children with rare conditions: see www.stevewaughfoundation.com.au/about/rare-diseases

- The NSW Agency for Clinical Innovation (ACI) Transition Care Network is one example of a state-based organisation aiming to improve the continuity of care for young people with chronic and complex health conditions as they transition from paediatric to adult health services: see www.aci.health.nsw.gov.au/networks/transition-care/about/transition-care-service#:~:text=The%20NSW%20Agency%20for%20Clinical%20Innovation%20(ACI)%20Transition%20Care%20Service,services%20to%20adult%20health%20services.

- Having a child with complex medical needs is a challenge in many different ways. In the following recent study, parents recounted their experiences over the course of the first 12 months of their child having a tracheostomy. Their stories provide some insights into the perspectives of these parents and how they learned to manage and adapt. See:
  Flynn, A, Whittaker, K, Donne, AJ, Bray, L & Carter, B 2020, Holding their own and being resilient: Narratives of parents over the first 12 months of their child having a tracheostomy, *Comprehensive Child and Adolescent Nursing*, doi:10.1080/24694193.2020.1785046

REFERENCES

Abeywardana, S & Sullivan, EA 2008, *Congenital anomalies in Australia*, AIHW National Perinatal Statistics Unit, Sydney.

Agency for Clinical Innovation (ACI) 2014, *Key principles for transition of young people from paediatric to adult health care*, ACI, Sydney, viewed 5 July 2020, www.trapeze.org.au/sites/default/files/Transitional_Principles_Document.pdf

Agency for Clinical Innovation & Gastroenterological Nurses College of Australia (ACI & GENCA) 2015, *A clinician's guide: Caring for people with gastrostomy tubes and devices – from pre-insertion to ongoing care and removal*, ACI, Sydney, viewed 19 June 2020, www.aci.health.nsw.gov.au/__data/assets/pdf_file/0017/251063/gastrostomy_guide-web.pdf

Australian Cerebral Palsy Register Group 2018, *Australian Cerebral Palsy Register: Report 2018*, viewed 17 June 2020, www.cpregister.com/wp-content/uploads/2019/02/Report-of-the-Australian-Cerebral-Palsy-Register-Birth-Years-1995-2012.pdf

Begley, T 2013, Transition to adult care for young people with long-term conditions, *British Journal of Nursing*, 22(9), pp. 506–11.

Burdall, OC, Howarth, LJ, Sharrard A & Lee ACH 2017, Paediatric enteral tube feeding, *Paediatrics and Child Health,* 27(8), pp. 371–7.

Bloom, SR, Kuhlthau, K, Van Cleave, J, Knapp, A, Newacheck, P & Perrin, J. 2012, Health care transition for youth with special health care needs, *Journal of Adolescent Health*, 51(3), pp. 213–19.

Burkitt, CC, Breau, LM & Zabalia, M 2011, Parental assessment of pain coping in individuals with intellectual and developmental disabilities, *Research in Developmental Disabilities*, 32(5), pp. 1564–71.

Chiang, J & Amin, R, 2017, Respiratory care considerations for children with medical complexity, *Children*, 4, p. 41.

Cockett, A 2012, Technology dependence and children: A review of the evidence, *Nursing Children and Young People*, 24(1), pp. 32–5.

Cohen, E et al. 2011, Children with medical complexity: An emerging population for clinical and research initiatives, *Pediatrics*, 127(3), pp. 529–38.

Crisp, J, Taylor, C, Douglas, C & Rebeiro, G (eds) 2016, *Potter & Perry's fundamentals of nursing (5th ed.)*, Elsevier, Sydney.

Diamandopoulos, K & Green, J, 2018, Down syndrome: An integrative review, *Journal of Neonatal Nursing,* 24(5), pp. 235–41.

Down Syndrome Australia 2016, Down Syndrome in detail, viewed 9 September 2016, www.downsyndrome.org.au/down_syndrome.html

—— 2020, Down syndrome – statistics, viewed 17 June 2020, www.downsyndrome.org.au/about-down-syndrome/statistics

Eddy, LL (ed.) 2013, *Caring for children with special health-care needs and their families: A handbook for healthcare professionals*, Wiley-Blackwell, Malden, MA.

Elias, ER, Murphy, NA & Council on Children with Disabilities 2012, Home care of children and youth with complex health care needs and technology dependencies, *Pediatrics*, 129(5), pp. 996–1005.

Elliott, EJ & Zurynski, YA 2015, Rare diseases are a 'common problem' for clinicians, *Australian Family Physician*, 44(9), pp. 630–3.

Eunson, P 2012, Aetiology and epidemiology of cerebral palsy, *Paediatrics and Child Health*, 22(9), pp. 361–6.

Fegran L, Hall, EOC, Uhrenfeldt L, Aagaard H. & Ludvigsen MS 2014, Adolescents' and young adults' transition experiences when transferring from paediatric to adult care: A qualitative metasynthesis. *International Journal of Nursing Studies*, 51(1), pp. 123–35.

Garvey, KC, Wolpert, H, Rhodes, E, Laffel, L, Kleinman, K, Beste, M, Wolfsworth, J & Finkelstein, J 2012, Health care transition in patients with type 1 diabetes: Young adult experiences and relationship to glycemic control, *Diabetes Care*, 35(8), pp. 1716–22.

Heath, G, Farre, A & Shaw, K 2017, Parenting a child with chronic illness as they transition into adulthood: A systematic review and thematic synthesis of parents' experiences, *Patient Education and Counseling*, 100(1), pp. 76–92.

Hilliard, ME et al. 2014, Perspectives from before and after the pediatric to adult care transition: A mixed-methods study in type 1 diabetes, *Diabetes Care*, 37(2), pp. 346–54.

Jermyn, V 2013, 'You can't stay here!' Transition from paediatric to adult health care management for liver transplant recipients, *Transplant Journal of Australasia*, 22(3), pp. 15–18.

McInally, W 2013, Lost in transition: Child to adult cancer services for young people, *British Journal of Nursing*, 22(22), pp. 1314–18.

McKay, M & Clarke, S 2012, Pain assessment tolls for the child with severe learning disability, *Nursing Children and Young People*, 24(2), pp. 14–19.

Mercuri, E & Muntoni, F 2013, Muscular dystrophies, *The Lancet*, 381(9869), pp. 845–60.

Nightingale, R, Friedl S & Swallow, V 2015. Parents' learning needs and preferences when sharing management of their child's long-term/chronic condition: A systematic review, *Patient Education and Counseling*, 98(11), pp. 1329–38.

Novak, I et al. 2013, A systematic review of interventions for children with cerebral palsy: State of the evidence, *Developmental Medicine & Child Neurology*, 55(10), pp. 885–910.

Noyes, J, Brenner, M, Fox, P & Guerin, A 2014, Reconceptualizing children's complex discharge with health systems theory: Novel integrative review with embedded expert consultation and theory development, *Journal of Advanced Nursing*, 70(5), pp. 975–96.

Okumura MJ et al. 2014, Improving transition from paediatric to adult cystic fibrosis care: programme implementation and evaluation, *BMJ Quality and Safety*, 23(Suppl. 1), pp. i64–i72.

Oswald, DP, Gilles, D, Cannady, MS, Wenzel, DB, Willis, JH & Bodurtha, JN 2013, Youth with special health care needs: Transition to adult health care services, *Maternal and Child Health Journal*, 17(10), pp. 1744–52.

Pangilinan, PH & Hornyak, JE 2013, Rehabilitation of the muscular dystrophies, *Handbook of Clinical Neurology*, 110, pp. 471–81.

Ritholz, MD et al. 2014, Patient–provider relationships across the transition from pediatric to adult diabetes care: A qualitative study, *Diabetes Educator*, 40(1), pp. 40–7.

Royal Australasian College of Physicians 2015, *Newborn screening in Australia. Position statement May 2015*, viewed 5 July 2020, www.racp.edu.au/docs/default-source/advocacy-library/newbornscreeninginaustraliapositionstatement.pdf

Solodiuk, JC et al. 2010, Validation of the Individualized Numeric Rating Scale (INRS): A pain assessment tool for nonverbal children with intellectual disability, *Pain*, 150(2), pp. 231–6.

Sterni, LM et al. 2016, Official American Thoracic Society Clinical Practice Guideline: Pediatric Chronic Home Invasive Ventilation. *American Journal of Respiratory and Critical Care Medicine*, 193(8), pp. e16–e35.

ten Haken, I Ben Allouch, S & van Harten, WH 2018, The use of advanced medical technologies at home: A systematic review of the literature, *BMC Public Health*, 18, p. 284.

Teo, C, Kennedy-Behr, A & Lowe J 2018, Contrasting perspectives of parents and services providers on respite care in Queensland, Australia, *Disability & Society,* 33(9), pp. 1503–27.

Toly, VB, Musil, CM & Carl, JC 2012, A longitudinal study of families with technology dependent children, *Research in Nursing & Health,* 35(1), pp. 40–54.

White, PH and Cooley, WC 2018, Supporting the health care transition from adolescence to adulthood in the medical home, *Pediatrics,* 142(5), p. e20182587.

Wilcken, B & Wiley, V 2015, Fifty years of newborn screening, *Journal of Paediatrics and Child Health,* 51, pp. 103–7.

Wisk, LE et al. 2015, Predictors of timing of transfer from a pediatric to adult-focused primary care, *JAMA Pediatrics,* 169(6), pp. e150951–e150951.

Wolfe, I et al. 2020, Integrated care models and child health: A meta-analysis, *Pediatrics,* 145(1), p. e20183747.

World Health Organization (WHO) 2012, *Early childhood development and disability: A discussion paper,* viewed 11 September 2016, http://apps.who.int/iris/bitstream/10665/75355/1/9789241504065_eng.pdf

—— 2015, *Preterm birth,* World Health Organization fact sheet, viewed 10 September 2016, www.who.int/mediacentre/factsheets/fs363/en

Yiu, E & Kornberg, A 2015, Duchenne muscular dystrophy, *Journal of Paediatrics and Child Health,* 51(8), 759–64.

End-of-life and palliative care in paediatric care settings

Elizabeth Forster

13

LEARNING OBJECTIVES

In this chapter you will:

- Develop an understanding of the physical and psychological problems experienced by children in end-of-life care
- Develop an understanding of some of the strategies used to address or manage these problems in paediatric end-of-life care
- Consider the importance of communication with the child/young person, parents, siblings and grandparents in paediatric end-of-life care
- Explore ways to support parents, siblings and grandparents in paediatric end-of-life care
- Consider self-care and personal and professional boundaries in paediatric end-of-life care

Introduction

Although most children in Australia and New Zealand enjoy a long life expectancy and high level of wellbeing, paediatric death remains a sad reality for some families, and end-of-life care for children presents an important and challenging area of paediatric nursing practice.

The rate of child mortality in Australia more than halved from 20 to 10 deaths per 100 000 between 1998 and 2017, and the mortality rate has stabilised since 2011 to 10–12 deaths per 100 100 (AIHW, 2020). Among children aged 1–14 years between 2015 and 2017, the leading causes of death included injury (33 per cent), cancer (19 per cent) and nervous system diseases (10 per cent) (AIHW, 2020). In New Zealand, medical conditions are the leading cause of death among children and young people, followed by unintentional injury (usually transport related) and lastly intentional injury from suicide or assault (CYMC, 2019). It is also important to note that there is a disparity in child mortality between Indigenous and non-Indigenous children in both Australia and New Zealand, with Aboriginal and Torres Strait Islander children and Māori and Pacific Islander children having higher mortality rates than their non-Indigenous counterparts (AIHW, 2020; CYMC, 2019; QFCC, 2019).

As a beginning paediatric nurse, it is important that you understand that the terms **paediatric palliative care** and **paediatric end-of-life care** are conceptualised differently, despite some overlap. Paediatric palliative care begins when a disease is first diagnosed and continues throughout the illness trajectory. It therefore includes, but is not limited to, end-of-life care (Crozier & Hancock, 2012). The majority of paediatric palliative care is delivered by hospital-based or community teams in the last six months of a child's life (Crozier & Hancock, 2012). Paediatric end-of-life care is provided to the child and family towards the end of a child's life and includes care of the child's body and support for the family following the child's death. Although there are distinctions between the two terms, in this chapter they will be used interchangeably.

The World Health Organization (WHO, 1998) definition of palliative care for children was developed in recognition that paediatric palliative care, although related to adult palliative care, is a distinct and specialised area. The WHO (1998) definition includes the following principles:

- Palliative care for children is the active total care of the child's body, mind and spirit, and also involves giving support to the family.
- It begins when illness is diagnosed, and continues regardless of whether or not a child receives treatment directed at the disease.
- Health providers must evaluate and alleviate a child's physical, psychological and social distress.
- Effective palliative care requires a broad multidisciplinary approach that includes the family and makes use of available community resources; it can be implemented successfully even if resources are limited.
- It can be provided in tertiary care facilities, in community health centres and even in children's homes.

Central to paediatric end-of-life care are the frequent and comprehensive assessment and management of physical and psychological symptoms, facilitating effective and

Paediatric palliative care – The multidisciplinary care of the child's physical, psychosocial and spiritual needs, which encompasses the illness trajectory from diagnosis until death and includes end-of-life care. This care and support extends to the child's family.

Paediatric end-of-life care – The multidisciplinary care of the child's physical, psychosocial and spiritual needs, and the care and support of the child's family at end of life and beyond.

developmentally appropriate communication with the child and family, individualised holistic care with a focus on quality rather than quantity of life, and the involvement of a multidisciplinary team of health professionals (Stayer, 2012).

Paediatric end-of-life care occurs in a variety of contexts, including the acute paediatric setting and the community, in hospice care and in the child's home. The trajectory or path of a child and family's journey from diagnosis to end-of-life care will vary, and for some families this journey may be as short as a few days or weeks, or as long as many years in the case of chronic conditions.

This chapter will provide you with a beginning understanding of some of the common symptoms and concerns for children in end-of-life care and their management, including pain, the management of side-effects of opioids, fatigue, dyspnoea, gastrointestinal disturbances and anxiety. It will also discuss communication with dying children and adolescents, and the importance of family communication and support.

Pain

Pain assessment in children is a complex area requiring keen observation skills and effective, age-appropriate communication. Paediatric pain assessment is discussed in more detail in Chapter 10, and it is recommended that you revise this chapter in relation to the assessment of paediatric pain. In this chapter, paediatric pain management in end-of-life care will be the main focus of discussion. As a foundation for understanding pain management in end-of-life care, it is helpful to review the WHO analgesic ladder.

The WHO analgesic ladder

The WHO first introduced the analgesic ladder in the 1980s as a guide for the management of cancer pain. Previous versions of the analgesic ladder have now been updated and a two-step ladder is now recommended for children (Downing et al., 2015; WHO, 2012). The two-step approach excludes 'weak opioids' such as codeine and tramadol, which did not meet the guidelines for safe use in children (Downing et al., 2015). It retains recognition of the need for a step-up and step-down approach to pain relief. In conjunction with the two-step analgesic ladder for pain management for children, the WHO guidelines recommend using regular dosing schedules by the clock rather than as-needed prescriptions, together with consideration of the individual needs of each child experiencing pain and administering pain relief by the most appropriate route – preferably oral or other non-invasive routes (WHO, 2012).

Non-steroidal anti-inflammatory drugs (NSAIDs), such as paracetamol and ibuprofen, are recommended for mild pain. NSAIDs are frequently used to manage mild pain for children in palliative care due to their effectiveness in inflammatory causes of pain; they are also helpful for pain due caused by bony metastases (Dowden, 2014). The WHO ladder (Figure 13.1) recommends the use of opioids such as morphine for severe pain. Although such opioids remain effective for the management of severe pain, unfortunately they have a variety of side-effects that can increase the suffering of children if not managed promptly and appropriately.

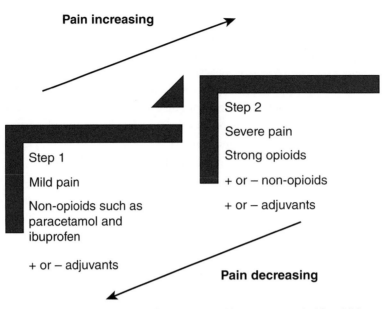

Figure 13.1   The two-step WHO analgesic ladder recommended for children
Source: Adapted from Downing et al. (2015).

Side-effects of opioids

Although opioids such as morphine can provide good pain relief for moderate to severe pain, there are many side-effects related to their use that may need to be addressed. More common side-effects include constipation, pruritus, and nausea and vomiting; less common side-effects are urinary retention, respiratory depression and **myoclonus** (Shaw, 2012). Table 13.1 lists some side-effects of opioid analgesia and strategies that may be used to manage these.

As a beginning clinician working in palliative care, you will need to familiarise yourself with the usual doses of medications commonly prescribed in paediatric palliative care. For further information about commonly used opioids in paediatric palliative care and their recommended dosages, see Shann's (2017) paediatric drug doses formulary and Friedrichsdorf (2019).

Myoclonus – Involuntary twitching that may occur when high doses of opioids are used, due to an accumulation of metabolites, which have neuro-excitory effects.

Non-pharmacological pain relief

In addition to the pharmacological management of pain in paediatric end-of-life care, non-pharmacological strategies have an important complementary role to play. Non-pharmacological pain relief strategies may range from cognitive/behavioural techniques and distraction to strategies involving physical touch, including skin-to-skin contact for infants or massage (Levine et al., 2013).

Cognitive and behavioural techniques encompass a variety of strategies, including guided imagery, hypnosis, relaxation, distraction, storytelling, music and art therapy, and play therapy (Hammond & Gera, 2016; Hyde, Price & Nicholl, 2012; Monterosso & DeGraves, 2012). These approaches acknowledge that pain involves both physical and psychological elements, and although more research evidence is needed regarding

Table 13.1 Side-effects of opioids and strategies to address these

Opioid side-effect and cause	Management
Constipation Decreased intestinal motility due to opioid.	Preventative management with stool-softeners at initiation of opioid treatment.
Pruritus Benign side-effect due to histamine-releasing properties of opioids.	Pruritus will usually resolve within a few days, but antihistamines may need to be prescribed by the medical officer.
Nausea and vomiting An initial side-effect of opioids, but may also be linked to constipation.	Antiemetic therapies such as ondansetron or metoclopramide may need to be prescribed by the medical officer.
Urinary retention An uncommon side-effect of opioids.	Try techniques such as running water and Crede's manoeuvre.
Respiratory depression Very rare when appropriate opioid doses and titration are used. Respiratory depression is usually preceded by a decreased level of consciousness and somnolence.	Accurate assessment is required to distinguish between a reduced respiratory demand and slowing of respirations that may normally accompany a reduction in pain intensity and true respiratory depression. Excessive slowing of respiration rate may be managed by rousing the child, slowing the rate of the opioid infusion or administering oxygen. Reversal agents such as naloxone should be used cautiously, as they rapidly reverse pain relief, which may lead to severe pain and may result in life threatening opioid withdrawal.
Myoclonus Brief involuntary twitching that may occur when high doses of opioids are used, or if they are administered over a long period and are due to an accumulation of metabolites, which have neuro-excitory effects.	Rotating to a different opioid may be a consideration, or the medical officer may need to prescribe benzodiazepines or muscle relaxants.

Source: Adapted from Klick & Hauer (2010); Shaw (2012).

their use in children, many of these cognitive and behavioural strategies may be helpful in targeting perceptions of pain and therefore contribute to overall pain relief.

Massage is commonly used by parents for a variety of health and discomfort-related problems (for example, infant colic, stress reduction, relaxation, sleep problems and musculoskeletal pain), and is also often used in the healthcare setting for relieving discomfort associated with procedures and as a complementary therapy in paediatric cancer (Hughes et al., 2008; Radossi et al., 2018). A systematic review of the use of supportive care interventions, including massage among paediatric patients with cancer, found some evidence for its benefit in cancer on psychosocial outcomes such as anxiety and on other symptoms such as nausea and vomiting, and discomfort and muscle soreness (Radossi et al., 2018). A recent pilot study among children in palliative care in Canada showed a significant reduction in pain and worry following the massage therapy intervention (Genik et al., 2020). Although this study was only a small pilot, its results are promising; however, as with many non-pharmacological approaches, more research is needed to establish its effectiveness, especially in paediatric palliative care (Ernst, 2009; Genik et al., 2020; Schutze et al., 2016).

REFLECTION POINTS 13.1

- Paediatric end-of-life care encompasses the physical, psychosocial and spiritual care of the child, and support for the family leading up to and following the child's death. It may be provided in a hospital or hospice, or at home. How might the setting in which end-of-life care is provided influence your role as a paediatric nurse?
- The two-step WHO analgesic ladder was developed as a guide for the management of pain in children and has a step-up and step-down approach. Why might a step-down approach to pain management be important for paediatric end-of-life care, especially when this care may be delivered over a long period of time, as in the case of life-limiting conditions?
- Opioids such as morphine remain a commonly used analgesic in paediatric end-of-life care; however, they have many side-effects. Why is the ability to assess and manage these side-effects so important for paediatric nurses working in end-of-life care?
- Non-pharmacological pain-relief strategies may also be used to complement pharmacological pain relief in paediatric end-of-life care. Consider some of the non-pharmacological approaches you have seen used in clinical practice. How might these be useful in paediatric end-of-life care? Conduct a database search to find out whether any research been conducted using these approaches in paediatric palliative care.

Dystonia – Involuntary movement with sustained or intermittent muscle contractions resulting in repetitive movements, twisting and unnatural positioning of the limbs, trunk, neck or facial muscles. It may be generalised or focus on one region.

Spasticity – Resistance in muscle tone and hyperreflexia that interferes with mobilising, maintaining a comfortable position and passive movements, and can lead to muscle contractures.

Agitation – Physical and psychological state with physical (restlessness, increased motor activity, disturbed sleep), psychological (anxiety, anger, irritability) and autonomic symptoms (increased heart, respiratory rate and blood pressure, diaphoresis/sweating).

Neurological symptoms

A variety of neurological symptoms can be experienced by paediatric patients at end of life including **dystonia** and **spasticity**, seizures and **agitation**, and they may be challenging to manage. The causative factors associated with these symptoms can be multifaceted, and sometimes myriad symptoms can appear simultaneously. It is therefore important to complete a comprehensive assessment of the presenting symptom/s in order to determine the actual symptom/s present (Rasmussen & Grégoire, 2015).

One approach advocated is to consult with the medical team and consider the following:

- What is the actual symptom you are observing?
- How can you differentiate between this symptom and other possibilities (for example differentiating between spasticity and dystonia)?

- What provoking factors may be occurring – for example, pain?
- Are medications contributing to the symptom? (Rasmussen & Grégoire, 2015)

Once the neurological symptom/s have been identified, an appropriate management approach can be planned. This may be necessitate addressing any causative or provoking factors as well as non-pharmacological and pharmacological strategies.

For further discussion of managing seizure activity in paediatric patients, see Forster and Caughlan (2018) in the Further reading section.

Fatigue

Fatigue is a difficult concept to define, but most agree that it involves both physical and psychological facets. Fatigue remains one of the most common problems experienced by children at end of life (Ullrich et al., 2018; Tomlinson et al., 2011; Ullrich et al., 2010; Wolfe, Grier & Klar, 2000) and has been found to increase as children near death (Tomlinson et al., 2011). Fatigue can comprise both physical and psychological (cognitive and emotional) symptoms, and the descriptions of children and adolescents range from not being able to engage in the activities they enjoy, not being able to participate independently in daily activities, and needing to sleep and rest more often to psychological impacts such as feeling sad, guilty, emotional, annoyed and powerless (Ullrich et al., 2018; Tomlinson et al., 2016). Some examples of children's descriptions of fatigue can be found in Box 13.1.

Fatigue – Feelings of tiredness and lethargy; a multidimensional term that includes physical, psychological, energy and sleep facets.

BOX 13.1 CHILDREN AND ADOLESCENTS' DESCRIPTIONS OF FATIGUE

- Finding it hard to walk, move or run, or participate in sport, physical activities or school
- Feeling like laying around, needing to lie or sit down, or feeling exhausted, drained, weak and tired with no energy and wanting to do nothing
- Feeling sad, upset, irritable, annoyed or mad, or feeling upset when you are emotionally tired
- Feeling not able to play or talk with friends when they visit or call and not wanting to be disturbed by others
- Physical signs such as difficulty keeping eyes open, having a dull face and tired eyes, and feeling dizzy, nauseous or hot and cold flushes
- Feeling sorry for yourself and feeling mentally tired for having to go through so much
- Feeling sleepy or drowsy and falling asleep easily and having disturbed sleep

Source: Adapted from Tomlinson et al. (2016); Hockenberry-Eaton et al. (1998).

Fatigue is a multidimensional problem experienced by dying children, and has been found to be associated with other symptoms such as nausea and vomiting, diarrhoea, nutritional impairment and anaemia, sleep disturbances (especially during hospitalisation) and psychological experiences such as fear, anxiety and sadness (Ullrich et al., 2018; Ullrich et al., 2010). In a recent study among children with advanced cancer fatigue was found to be associated with older age, lower haemoglobin (anaemia) and uncontrolled symptoms such as nausea, coughing, pain and worry (Ullrich et al., 2018). It may also be linked to the side-effects of pain and dyspnoea treatments such as opioids and sedative medications (Ullrich et al., 2010).

Paediatric nurses should use valid and reliable tools/scales to assess for fatigue in children. One assessment scale that has been developed and used to measure fatigue among paediatric cancer patients is the Fatigue Scale – Child for 7–12-year-olds, which was developed by Hockenberry and colleagues (2003). This scale contains 14 items that are completed by the child using a Likert scale format, with total fatigue scores from 0 indicating no fatigue symptoms to 70 indicating high fatigue. More recently, this tool has been reduced to a 10-item scale (Hinds et al., 2010). For children who are able and well enough to self-report, the 18-item PedsQL Multidimensional Fatigue Scale may be used. It measures general, sleep/rest and cognitive fatigue (Colville et al., 2019; Varni et al., 2002).

Fatigue has been described as difficult to treat and manage, although a variety of strategies have been employed in an effort to manage this distressing problem. A small number of studies in paediatric patients undergoing treatment for cancer have investigated exercise for fatigue management; however, the utility of this intervention in end-of-life care is uncertain, due to the child's deteriorating physical condition (Chang et al., 2013). Massage, together with strategies to promote nutrition and energy conservation that have also been used in paediatric cancer studies (Chang et al., 2013), and may be more appropriate for children in end-of-life care. Fatigue among children at end of life may be relieved through the management of sedative effects of opioid medications, reducing anorexia, nausea and vomiting, and improving nutrition, and by addressing sleep disturbances and distressing psychological issues such as sorrow and anxiety (Ullrich et al., 2010). The multifaceted nature of fatigue, and its diverse influencing factors, make it challenging to manage, and further research is needed in paediatric end-of-life care to determine the most effective strategies to combat this problem.

Dyspnoea

Abnormal or difficult breathing is another symptom experienced by children in end-of-life care and is a cause of distress to both the child and the family (Pieper et al., 2018; Pritchard et al., 2008).

In children, **dyspnoea** usually occurs due to a combination of:

Dyspnoea – Abnormal or difficult breathing that may include feelings of tiredness, suffocation, air hunger or panic associated with breathing, awareness of the work of breathing and chest tightness.

- increased work of breathing linked to increased airway resistance, decreased lung compliance or decreased muscle strength or abnormality
- increased ventilation requirements due to metabolic acidosis, hypoxaemia, anaemia or other physiological states (Robinson, 2012).

The management of dyspnoea in paediatric palliative care requires a weighing up or balancing of the burden of treatments, which may be quite aggressive and upsetting for the child, versus the more conservative management of symptoms. This needs to be negotiated constantly between health professionals and the child (if appropriate) and parents (Robinson, 2012). In palliative care, the pathophysiological cause of the dyspnoea may not be pursued, and instead the focus will be on the management of the dyspnoea to ensure the child's comfort.

It is important to acknowledge the psychological relationship with dyspnoea and physiological processes, as this highlights the importance of management strategies that will be targeted towards the child's perceptions, thoughts and feelings about their dyspnoea as well as the underlying physiological processes. The child's psychological state can be linked to and exacerbate feelings of dyspnea and anxiety; feelings of sadness, loneliness and tension can influence perceptions of dyspnea (Pieper et al., 2018). Hallenbeck (2012, p. 849) states that:

> In addressing the suffering associated with dyspnoea we must consider the fact that the mind is not only an agent through which suffering is experienced or perceived, but it also is an active participant in the physiology of dyspnoea.

Parental perceptions are a vital component of the management of dyspnoea in paediatric palliative care, as a child will usually look to their parents to gauge how to interpret most situations. It is very important that parents receive support and education about the possibility that their child may experience breathing difficulties in palliative care, and the importance of remaining calm and reassuring in their child's presence to avoid exacerbating the child's negative perceptions of their dyspnoea, which will in turn worsen their breathing difficulties.

Both non-pharmacological and pharmacological strategies can be used to relieve dyspnoea in children. Non-pharmacological strategies include behavioural interventions such as behaviour modification and techniques to reduce anxiety and controlled breathing techniques. The use of fans to increase circulating air and blow air over a child's face may also be helpful, as some studies using nasal prong flow of air across the nasal passages have achieved relief from dyspnoea in some patients, although the exact mechanism of action is unknown (Abernethy et al., 2010; Craig, Henderson & Bluebond-Langner, 2015; Robinson, 2012; Ullrich & Mayer, 2007). The main pharmacological strategy for the management of dyspnoea in both adult and paediatric patients is the use of opioids such as morphine, fentanyl and oxycodone (Friedrichsdorf, 2019). Opioids work on the mu-receptors in the brainstem and help to lessen the perception of dyspnea the responsiveness to hypercapnia and hypoxia (Friedrichsdorf, 2019). Other strategies may include the use of assisted non-invasive ventilation such as bilevel positive airway pressure (BiPaP) or continuous positive airway pressure (CPAP), but these may not be tolerated well by paediatric patients (Craig, Henderson & Bluebond-Langner, 2015). They may, however, be used at night and during sleep periods to counteract respiratory muscle fatigue, which may enable a child to have more energy to participate in daytime activities (Robinson, 2012). It is important to consider that parents may not want to have their view of their dying child's face obstructed by the masks used in non-invasive ventilation (Ullrich & Mayer, 2007), and this is another example of balancing the need for treatments and their associated burdens for the child and family.

In addition to dyspnoea, paediatric palliative care patients may also experience discomfort relating to frequent coughing, increased secretions and possibly haemoptysis (Craig, Henderson & Bluebond-Langner, 2015). Although more research is needed to determine the best management in children, there are some strategies that can be effective for paediatric patients. Coughing may be linked to impaired swallowing and aspiration or reflux, and in these situations alternative feeding methods may be needed to reduce the risk of aspiration and pharmacological therapies may assist with reflux (Craig, Henderson & Bluebond-Langner, 2015). Physiotherapy and suctioning may also provide some relief from increased secretions. Haemoptysis may occur in some children at end of life, and this is a distressing occurrence for the child and their family, as well as for the healthcare team (Forster, 2012). Efforts are usually made to minimise the visual impact of bleeding through the use of dark-coloured towels, and opioids and anxiolytics such as morphine and midazolam can be used to reduce the child's breathlessness and distress in the event of this occurring (Craig, Henderson & Bluebond-Langner, 2015).

Gastrointestinal disturbances

There are a variety of gastrointestinal (GI) disturbances that may create unnecessary discomfort for children in palliative care, including constipation, nausea and vomiting. These GI disturbances, as mentioned earlier in this chapter, may be linked to opioid administration. Table 13.1 listed some strategies to combat these side-effects of opioid analgesia. In relation to constipation, it is important for paediatric nurses to assess the child's risk as well as stool characteristics. A variety of factors, including the use of opioid medications, limited mobility and a deterioration in both food and fluid intake, can place the child in palliative care at increased risk of constipation. The Bristol Stool Form Scale is a useful visual scale for determining the characteristics of the child's stool, and is easy to use for the child and parents because of its visual depictions (Stewart & McNeilly, 2011).

Nausea and vomiting may also be linked to biochemical and vestibular factors, and disturbances in gastrointestinal motility and function, including decreased motility, malignancies, ascites, adhesions and obstructions, or neurological disturbances resulting in raised intracranial pressure, which may impact on the chemoreceptor trigger zone (CTZ) of the brain and the vomiting centre in the medulla oblongata (Yates, 2012).

Cachexia – The loss of appetite, weight and muscle mass that results from an underlying pathological condition, including those seen in palliative care.

Weight loss and **cachexia** may also occur in paediatric palliative care. Cachexia has its origins in the Greek words *kakos* (bad) and *hexis* (condition), and refers to the loss of appetite, weight and muscle mass that results from an underlying pathological condition, including those seen in palliative care. The physical appearance of their dying child may be distressing for parents (Forster, 2012), and body image and appearance changes that occur as a consequence of treatment may also be a significant concern for children and adolescents with life-limiting illnesses at times throughout their illness trajectory (Choquette, Rennick & Lee, 2016; Lee et al., 2012; Reid, McKeaveney & Martin, 2019).

Nutritional intake may decrease as a child nears end of life, and children will usually be offered small amounts or tastes of foods and fluids as desired, which can be comforting (Crozier & Hancock, 2012). However, sometimes changes such as coughing, gagging and difficulty swallowing may make it difficult and uncomfortable for dying children to eat and drink. Although artificial nutrition and hydration (via nasogastric or parenteral routes) may be considered, these interventions have associated complications, and the palliative care team in partnership with parents will usually weigh up the risks versus the benefits of commencing artificial nutrition

(Rapoport et al., 2013). At this stage, 'although artificial nutrition and hydration may support biological existence and increase weight, there is no evidence that it improves survival or quality of life in dying children or adults' (Rapoport et al., 2013, p. 862). Parents, however, will often feel a strong desire to continue to provide nourishment to their dying child, and may be concerned about their child feeling hunger and thirst, and being uncomfortable if adequate nutrition and hydration are not provided (Pritchard et al., 2008; Rapoport et al., 2013). This is an extremely difficult and emotionally painful time for parents, and any decisions concerning whether to implement or forgo artificial nutrition and hydration need to be supported by the palliative care team. Parents need to be reassured that it is normal for appetite to diminish towards end of life, and that their child will likely not feel the desire to eat or drink.

CASE STUDY 13.1 MATTHEW

Matthew is an 11-year-old boy with acute myeloid leukaemia who is receiving palliative care support after an unsuccessful stem cell transplant. You are visiting Matthew and his family each day at home with the palliative care team. He is surrounded by his parents and younger sister, who is 6 years old. Today you notice that Matthew is struggling to breathe and is quite distressed. Matthew says that he has pain in his stomach and lower back, and can't breathe. He spends some time each day sitting out in the recliner chair in the lounge room, which seems to help with his lower back pain. He has not been eating much in the last few days – just a small amount of milk and cereal each day in the morning and a small taste of whatever the family is eating for dinner.

Anxiety

Children and parents have reported experiencing distressing emotional reactions during their experience of terminal illness, and anxiety is quite prevalent among children in paediatric palliative care (Jacobowski, Radbill & Truba, 2020). Children may feel scared or nervous, and may be dealing with uncertainty and fear of death, thinking about being sick and questioning 'Why me?' (Hildenbrand et al., 2011). The reduction of anxiety for children during end-of-life care is important, as it not only creates distress for the child and parent, but can also have an ongoing impact on parental anxiety and mental health (Jacobowski, et al., 2020; Jalmsell et al., 2010). Children and their parents may utilise a variety of coping strategies, which either avoid or address these distressing emotional issues (Hildenbrand et al., 2011). Music therapy, for example, has been found to promote a sense of calm and relaxation among children in palliative care and their families (Lindenfelser, Hense & McFerran, 2012). Reiki therapy was used on a small sample of children in palliative care in a pilot study in the United States and showed promising effects on pain, anxiety and physiological parameters (Thrane et al., 2017); however, more research is needed on the benefits of complementary therapies in reducing anxiety among children in palliative care.

Communication concerning issues of concern may also be important for reducing anxiety. In a study among adolescents with cancer, participating in a structured, family-centred, advanced care planning program significantly decreased anxiety among adolescents, but unfortunately increased anxiety among family members (Lyon et al., 2014).The program enabled adolescents with cancer and their families to engage in reflection and discussion about their fears, values, spiritual beliefs and preferences in relation to future treatments and care, as well as palliative care (Lyon et al., 2014).

Communication with children and adolescents

Effective end-of-life care for young people increasingly emphasises the importance of engaging in conversations about dying and advanced care planning because adolescents possess growing cognitive and emotional maturity, which means they understand death and want to be involved in decisions concerning their treatment and end-of-life care (Lyon et al., 2014). Sometimes such conversations may be avoided by health professionals, leaving young people struggling to find ways to communicate their thoughts and feelings about the possibility of their own impending death (Forster, 2012).

There are a variety of reasons why such conversations may be avoided or delayed, including health professional discomfort or lack of confidence, uncertainty about the legal competence of a teenager to make decisions regarding their own care and fears about diminishing the adolescent's and/or their family's sense of hope (Wiener et al., 2013). Parents may also not want such conversations to be initiated, as they too may be concerned about leaving the impression with their adolescent that further treatments are unlikely to be successful (Wiener et al., 2013). Whether an adolescent is ready to discuss such issues is currently being researched, and it is important for nurses to recognise that an adolescent's readiness involves a complex interplay of emotional and cognitive preparedness, acceptance and willingness (Bell et al., 2016).

There are a number of paediatric advanced care planning models that have been developed primarily in the United Kingdom and the United States with particular target groups of adolescents, including Footprints (designed for patients with muscular dystrophy), the Family-Centred (FACE) Advanced Care Planning for young people with HIV, and FACE-TC, which adapted this model for teens with cancer (Lyon et al., 2014). In a study of 30 adolescents with cancer, participating in advanced care planning conversations significantly reduced the anxiety of the adolescent (Lyon et al., 2014). These models were delivered by health professionals who undertook specialised training, and the conversations with the adolescent and their family occurred over a number of sessions (Lyon et al., 2009).

There are also models that have been developed for adolescents and young adults such as the Voicing my Choices™ advanced care planning guide (Zadeh, Pao & Wiener, 2015). This guide addresses a variety of areas that may be significant for the adolescent at end of life, including:

- how they would like to be supported so they don't feel alone
- how they want to be comforted in terms of food, readings, music and pain medication
- who they want to make medical treatment decisions for them if they are unable to make these decisions independently
- preferences for life-support treatments
- what they want their friends and family to know about them
- spiritual thoughts and preferences
- how they want to be remembered
- an opportunity to express their own voice through legacy letters to their loved ones.

It is recommended that conversations about advanced care planning with adolescents begin early in their illness trajectory, rather than during a period of deterioration or crisis, and that they then should occur at regular points throughout their treatment and care (Zadeh, Pao & Wiener, 2015). Normally, experienced health professionals who have undertaken specific educational preparation will initiate and facilitate such conversations and you, as a beginning paediatric nurse, may have the opportunity to accompany an experienced colleague during such meetings. It is important to keep in mind that many health professionals experience discomfort with these conversations (Lotz et al., 2015; Zadeh, Pao & Wiener, 2015) and are often not sure about how to initiate such conversations. One approach to initiating such conversations has been developed, and may be a helpful way to broach such discussions (Zadeh, Pao & Wiener, 2015, p. 594):

> Although we are hoping that this next treatment will be helpful, many people your age have told us that they found it helpful to have a say about what they would want or not want if treatment doesn't go as expected. In fact, people your age helped create a guide so that they could put down on paper the things that are important to them.

This approach, from the Voicing my Choices™ advanced care planning guide, recommends using words such as 'in our experience, we have found young people your age often find it important to talk about' or similar as an entrée into discussion of each element of the advanced care plan (Zadeh, Pao & Wiener, 2015).

Younger children may also want to discuss their worries and fears. Play and art therapy are two strategies that may be used to enable younger children to communicate their worries. Play and art therapy can assist paediatric nurses to understand the problems a child is facing, to help the child to verbalise conscious feelings and thoughts, and to act out subconscious feelings and thoughts (Van Breemen, 2009; Walker, 1989). Nurses can also assist parents to engage in play with their child; by doing so, parents may also gain insights into their child's fears and hopes (Van Breemen, 2009).

For the student and beginning nurse, it is important to be aware of the possibility that paediatric patients and their families will want to discuss their thoughts and feelings about death and end-of-life care, and to be alert to possible cues that indicate this need. Your confidence in responding to such cues and engaging in end-of-life conversations will develop through further training and experience. In the meantime, being able to listen to young people and their families, and involving other health professionals when necessary, is important to ensure that any need to discuss these issues is facilitated. By attending family conferences, you will also have the opportunity to observe more experienced health professionals and their communication with children and families in palliative care (Keir & Wilkinson, 2013). This will provide a good opportunity for you to observe body language and the ways in which experienced health professionals express empathy and engage parents – and, if appropriate, the child – in difficult conversations and respond to intense emotions.

Communication and the family in paediatric end-of-life care

Parents of dying children place great emphasis on the communication with health professionals during their child's illness and around the time of their child's death (Meyer et al., 2006). There may be a tendency among health professionals to avoid communication with parents and family members at this time, and to focus on the technical aspects of care (Forster, 2012). However, sensitive and supportive communication is central to the quality of end-of-life care in paediatrics, and can help parents and family members through this overwhelming and devastating time. A recent study in Australia explored discussion prompts that could be used in communication with health professionals and families when a child has a life-limiting illness or during end-of-life care (Ekberg et al., 2020). These researchers acknowledged the daunting nature of communication in these sensitive circumstances and consulted with health professionals and parents to determine the communication prompts that could be used to facilitate communication (Ekberg et al., 2020).

Parents caring for their dying child at home may feel quite uncertain about the physical aspects of their child's care, and may struggle to navigate the emotional aspects of facing their child's impending death. In one Australian study, parents described wanting to talk with health professionals about their feelings, but finding that nurses and doctors did not introduce such topics of conversation (Forster, 2012). Therefore, nurses need to find the time to engage with parents about their thoughts and feelings in order to offer their supportive presence. Parents may feel unable to discuss such feelings with friends and in their social circle, and may feel isolated and alone. In addition, with strain upon both parents simultaneously, they may feel unable to fully support each other while going through their own feelings of grief (Alburquerque, Periera & Narciso, 2016; Moriarty, Carroll & Controneo, 1996).

Although focusing on the parental relationship following the loss of a child, a recent study of bereaved parents in Norway found that while most couples felt they could talk about their feelings with their partners and were satisfied with the support they received, mothers felt less understood than fathers, and fathers felt greater responsibility for caring for their partner following their loss (Dyregrov, Gjestad & Dyregrov, 2020). This highlights that mothers and fathers may respond to and cope with loss differently and need different types of support surrounding the loss of a child (Alburquerque, Periera & Narciso, 2016). Paediatric nurses caring for parents and families in paediatric palliative care need to be sensitive to these parental responses and needs.

It is important that the team of health professionals involved in end-of-life care provides consistent and frequent information to families. The team should also recognise that complex information (even when explained in simple terms) may require repetition, and that parents may need regular meetings in order to be able to make decisions about their child's ongoing care (Crozier & Hancock, 2012).

Grieving parents belong to a minority group in society and are often facing the first loss of their young adult lives and their sense of isolation can make it difficult to seek and receive the support they need (Morris, Fletcher & Goldstein, 2019). Because of the risks for physical and psychological health problems among bereaved parents it is important to ensure parents and families are linked with appropriate support and counselling services and the social work team linked to the hospital, community or hospice team will have the contact details of local support agencies for parents and families.

Further details about information and support agencies for paediatric loss and grief can be found in Forster & Murray (2013); they include the Australian Child and Adolescent Trauma, Loss and Grief Network, the Australian Centre for Grief and Bereavement, and Skylight New Zealand.

Culturally safe end-of-life care

With the diversity of children and families encountered in paediatric end-of-life care, it is important for paediatric nurses to ensure culturally safe care. The concept of cultural safety was first developed by a Māori nurse, Irihapeti Ramsden. The Nursing Council of New Zealand Code of Conduct for nurses defines culture and the delivery of culturally safe care as follows:

> Culture includes, but is not restricted to age or generation; gender; sexual orientation; occupation and socio-economic status; ethnic origin or migrant experience; religious or spiritual beliefs; and disability. The nurse delivering the nursing care will have undertaken a process of reflection on their own cultural identity and will recognise the impact their personal culture has on their professional practice. Unsafe cultural practice comprises any action which diminishes, demeans or disempowers the cultural identity and well-being of an individual. (Nursing Council of New Zealand, 2012, p. 13)

Cultural safety emphasises the need for clinicians to be self-aware of their own culture including the healthcare culture within which they operate, and to be aware of the potential power differentials, impacts of colonialism on Indigenous peoples, and norms, values, beliefs, assumptions and biases, and how these can influence care (Schill & Caxaj, 2019).

By actively involving patients and families in care at end of life and deferring to their preferences, beliefs and values, paediatric nurses can ensure culturally safe care (Schill & Caxaj, 2019). Families may also often appreciate being able to make connections to a broader family network, kin, communities and the land, and there may be personal or cultural rituals that they want practised at end of life (Shahid et al., 2018). Dying at home with support may also be particularly important for some children and families, and can facilitate desired connections with kin and community (Shahid et al., 2018).

REFLECTION POINT 13.2

Communication is sometimes considered challenging for health professionals working with children and families in end-of-life care. What are some techniques you could use to facilitate effective communication in this situation? What are some of the barriers to effective communication in this context?

Siblings

Siblings of the dying child also require support and consideration, as they can be impacted in multiple ways during the course of their brother's or sister's illness and end-of-life care. Their understanding of the situation will be influenced by their age and stage of development, and this will also guide the strategies employed by nurses and the palliative care team in providing effective support.

Often, siblings have had their usual experiences of family life interrupted and changed due to the illness of their sibling. They may have had to experience being cared for by other family members and friends; they may have been required to take on additional responsibilities; and they have, of course, lost time and contact with parents who may have been focused on the care of a sick and dying sibling (Chin, Jaaniste & Trethewie, 2018; Foster et al., 2010). Siblings are also struggling with their own emotional responses to their brother's or sister's illness and impending death, and may experience fear, anger, jealousy, shame and guilt, and feel isolated and forgotten (Chin, Jaaniste & Trethewie, 2018; Foster et al., 2010). Siblings are also often acutely aware of their brother's or sister's condition, and may not reveal this to their parents in order to protect them from the ensuing sadness; similarly, parents may not engage in these discussions with their well children for the same reasons (Malcolm et al., 2014).

In their study of 18 siblings aged 9–22 years in New Zealand, Gaab, Owens and MacLeod (2014) found that siblings wanted to be informed about the impending death of their sibling, and to be included in conversations about symptoms so they could understand what was happening. These preferences were also balanced by the negative aspects of having this knowledge, as siblings then worried more – for example, that their sibling would go to sleep and not awaken, or that conversations about death and dying were then brought up too much, which made it difficult to live as normal a life as possible. Siblings also engaged in helping behaviours and spent time with their sibling, trying to make them smile and stay positive (Gaab, Owens and MacLeod, 2014).

Nurses and the palliative care team can support siblings by:

- involving them in discussions about care and treatment throughout their sibling's illness
- enabling siblings to be involved in caregiving if desired
- assigning a social worker or supporter to specifically work with siblings
- putting families in contact with relevant sibling support groups
- educating the family about the needs of siblings when a child is sick and dying
- encouraging siblings to continue to be involved in their own interests and pursuits

- helping the family to identify a 'safe adult' in the siblings' world to whom they feel they can talk about their feelings and concerns
- providing referrals to psychologists and counsellors when necessary
- asking siblings about their feelings and experiences (Jenholt Nolbris & Nilsson, 2016; Jones, Contro & Koch, 2014).

Grandparents

Grandparents often play a central role in supporting parents and families when a child is ill and dying (Kuhn et al., 2019; Moules et al., 2012), and therefore also need to be supported at this time and following the child's death. Grandparents have been described as experiencing threefold layers of grief when losing a grandchild, as they are grieving the loss of their cherished grandchild, for their son or daughter who is losing/has lost a child and for themselves (Ponzetti & Johnson, 1991). Grandparents may experience disenfranchised grief, where their loss and grief are not recognised or acknowledged by others (Tatterton & Walshe, 2018). Grandparents may not discuss their own emotions and inner turmoil because of a need to be strong for their adult child and other grandchildren, and they may prioritise the needs of these family members above their own (Kuhn et al., 2019; Moules et al., 2012; Youngblut et al., 2010; Youngblut et al., 2015). It is important for nurses to be aware of grandparents' feelings, and to provide opportunities for them to talk about their feelings and concerns and to access support services (Youngblut et al., 2010; Youngblut et al., 2015). In addition, because grandparents are often not directly involved in parent and palliative care team meetings, they may have questions about their grandchild's condition and management (Wakefield et al., 2016); with parental consent, paediatric nurses are well positioned to provide this informational support to grandparents.

Self-care and professional boundaries

Caring for children and families at end of life can affect paediatric nurses and the multidisciplinary team, and it is crucial to be mindful of your own wellbeing when encountering paediatric end-of-life care. Many clinical settings offer debriefing and one-to-one counselling for clinicians who want to talk through their feelings. Health professionals use a variety of self-care strategies to assist their coping, and it may be helpful to talk with your experienced colleagues to learn about the effective coping strategies they use. Seeking support from colleagues has been identified as a strategy that many health professionals use in paediatric end-of-life care (Forster & Hafiz, 2015; Zander & Hutton, 2010).

Providing care at end of life occurs within an intimate family circle, and parents have commented on how much they appreciate the 'humanity' of health professionals at this time and their ability to provide support, one human being to another (Forster, 2012). However, it is also important to be aware of professional boundaries as well so you can behave professionally but still connect with families on a personal level (Erikson & Davies, 2017). Paediatric nurses need to reflect on how they can navigate these boundaries, and be empathetic and offer support without becoming over-involved to the detriment of their own wellbeing and the therapeutic relationship (Erikson & Davies, 2017). For example, while parents may appreciate the expressions of sadness from health professionals (Forster & Windsor, 2014), if nurses become too distraught and cannot function in their caring role, then they need to take some time out and ask another person to take their place so as not to shift the focus from the dying child and family to the health professional. They will also need to seek some support to work through their own feelings of distress and grief.

Paediatric nurses and the multidisciplinary team sometimes feel uncertain about whether or not to attend funeral services when a child dies, and this can also be considered a tension between personal and professional boundaries (Erikson & Davies, 2017). Attending funeral services may be considered an important part of the bereavement support extended to families who have lost a child, and this is often the case when health professionals have come to know a child and family over many years during the trajectory of the child's illness. Grieving parents often value this expression of support from clinicians during their time of loss (Erikson & Davies, 2017). Parents sometimes feel that their relationship with health professionals ends too abruptly following the loss of their child, and some ongoing support will often be needed from a designated support person or team (Butler, Hall & Copnell, 2018). Paediatric tertiary hospitals and palliative care teams often hold memorial/remembrance services for families who have lost a child, and this is an opportunity for both families and staff to reconnect, share memories and express support.

SUMMARY

- For some families, the death of a child remains a sad reality. The leading causes of paediatric death include medical conditions, injury, cancer and nervous system diseases. These children and their families require specialised end-of-life care that recognises and supports the unique needs of the dying child and their family. Paediatric nurses play a central role in the coordination and provision of this care.
- Paediatric palliative or end-of-life care involves the physical, psychosocial and spiritual care of the child and their family. Its commencement and duration may vary depending on the child's illness and trajectory, and it may be provided in a variety of settings, including hospitals, community care, hospices and the child's home.
- Children may experience a variety of problems at end of life, including pain, side-effects of opioid medications, fatigue, dyspnoea, gastrointestinal problems and anxiety. Nurses caring for children at end of life need to be able to assess and identify these physical and psychological concerns, and collaborate with the multidisciplinary team to alleviate these. Research into the effectiveness of management strategies is still needed in paediatric end-of-life care.
- Depending on their development and understanding, children and young people may wish to discuss their fears and worries about dying, and adolescents may like to be involved in advance care planning conversations. The skills to facilitate such conversations will develop with further specialised preparation and experience, and beginning paediatric nurses can observe more experienced colleagues and increase their

awareness of the communication skills used. Being a supportive presence and having a willingness to listen are valuable skills.

- Communication with the dying child's family should be informative and sensitive, and provide family members with the opportunity to ask questions, be involved in planning care and management decisions, and disclose fears, concerns and emotions arising from caring for their dying child and their impending loss. Parents may feel isolated and unable to share their feelings with family, friends and even with each other as they struggle with their own feelings of grief. Siblings and grandparents will also need special attention and support as they face the loss of their loved one.

- Paediatric nurses and health professionals who care for children and families at end of life need to be conscious of their own self-care and develop coping strategies to manage the physical and psychological impacts of caregiving. Over time, clinicians learn to appropriately navigate the personal and professional boundary tensions that exist in supporting children and families in this intimate context of paediatric end-of-life care.

LEARNING ACTIVITIES

13.1 Based on your reading in this chapter, what do you think are the main problems being experienced by our case study patient, Matthew? For each problem you identify, write down why this may be occurring for Matthew.

13.2 What strategies could you use to alleviate these problems for Matthew?

13.3 How would you involve Matthew and his family in your plan of care?

FURTHER READING

Erikson, A & Davies, B 2017, Maintaining integrity: How nurses navigate boundaries in pediatric palliative care, *Journal of Pediatric Nursing*, 35, pp. 42–9.

Forster, EM and Caughlan, M 2018, Neurological nursing skills, in E Forster & JA Fraser (eds), *Paediatric nursing skills for Australian nurses*. Cambridge University Press, Melbourne, pp. 169–83.

Forster, EM & Hafiz, AH 2015, Paediatric death and dying: Exploring coping strategies of health professionals and perceptions of support provision, *International Journal of Palliative Nursing*, 21(6), pp. 294–301.

Forster E & Murray J 2013, Loss and grief. In M Barnes & J Rowe (eds), *Child, youth and family health: Strengthening communities*, Elsevier, New York, pp. 260–78.

Twycross, A & Stinson, J 2014, Physical and psychological pain relief methods in children, in A Twycross, S Dowden & J Stinson (eds), *Managing pain in children: A clinical guide for nurses and health professionals*, John Wiley & Sons, Chichester, pp. 86–99. This reading provides an overview of a variety of physical and psychological pain-relief strategies and current research evidence concerning their use in paediatric patients. It will provide you with a beginning understanding of pain-relief strategies and how they have been used effectively for children experiencing pain.

REFERENCES

Abernethy, AP et al. 2010, Effect of palliative oxygen versus medical (room) air in relieving breathlessness in patients with refractory dyspnoea: A double-blind randomized controlled trial, *The Lancet*, 376(9743), pp. 784–93.

Albuquerque, S, Pereira, M & Narciso, I 2016 Couple's relationship after the death of a child: A systematic review. *Journal of Child and Family Studies*, 25(1), pp. 30–53.

Australian Institute of Health and Welfare (AIHW) 2020, *Australia's children*, cat. no. CWS 69, AIHW, Canberra.

Bell, CJ, Smythe, E, Diver, J, Dickens, D & Hinds, PS 2016, Exploring readiness to engage in difficult discussions with adolescents living with advanced cancer, *Biology of Blood and Marrow Transplantation*, 22(3), pp. S115–S116.

Butler, AE, Hall, H & Copnell, B 2018, The changing nature of relationships between parents and healthcare providers when a child dies in the paediatric intensive care unit, *Journal of Advanced Nursing*, 74(1), pp. 89–99.

Chang, C, Mu, P, Jou, S, Wong, T & Chen, Y 2013, Systematic review and meta-analysis of non-pharmacological interventions for fatigue in children and adolescents with cancer, *Worldviews on Evidence-based Nursing*, 10(4), pp. 208–17.

Child and Youth Mortality Review Committee (CYMC) 2019, *14th data report: 2013–17*, Health Quality & Safety Commission, Wellington.

Chin, WL, Jaaniste, T & Trethewie, S 2018, The role of resilience in the sibling experience of pediatric palliative care: What is the theory and evidence?, *Children*, 5, p. 97.

Choquette, A, Rennick, JE & Lee, V 2016, Back to school after cancer treatment: Making sense of the adolescent experience, *Cancer Nursing*, 39(5), pp. 393–401.

Colville, GA, Pierce, CM & Peters, MJ 2019, Self-reported fatigue in children following intensive care treatment, *Pediatric Critical Care Medicine*, 20(2), e98–e101.

Craig, F, Henderson, EM & Bluebond-Langner, M 2015, Management of respiratory symptoms in paediatric palliative care, *Current Opinion in Supportive and Palliative Care*, 9(3), pp. 217–26.

Crozier, F & Hancock, LE 2012, Pediatric palliative care: Beyond the end of life, *Pediatric Nursing*, 38(4), pp. 198–227.

Dowden, S 2014, Pharmacology of analgesic drugs, in A Twycross, SJ Dowden & J Stinson (eds), *Managing pain in children: A medical guide for nurses and health professionals*, John Wiley & Sons, Chichester.

Downing, J, Jassal, SS, Mathews, L, Brits, H & Friedrichsdorf, SJ 2015, Pediatric pain management in palliative care, *Pain Management*, 5(1), pp. 23–5.

Dyregrov, A, Gjestad, R & Dyregrov, K 2020, Parental relationships following the loss of a child, *Journal of Loss & Trauma*, 25(3), pp. 224–44.

Ekberg, S et al. 2020, Finding a way with words: Delphi study to develop a discussion prompt list for paediatric palliative care, *Palliative Medicine*, 34(3), pp. 291–9.

Erikson, A & Davies, B 2017, Maintaining integrity: How nurses navigate boundaries in pediatric palliative care, *Journal of Pediatric Nursing*, 35, pp. 42–9.

Ernst, E 2009, Massage therapy for cancer palliation and supportive care: A systematic review of randomised clinical trials, *Supportive Care in Cancer*, 17(4), pp. 333–7.

Forster, EM 2012, Parent and staff perceptions of bereavement support surrounding loss of a child, PhD thesis, University of Queensland.

Forster, EM & Hafiz, AH 2015, Paediatric death and dying: Exploring coping strategies of health professionals and perceptions of support provision, *International Journal of Palliative Nursing,* 21(6), pp. 294–301.

Forster EM & Murray J 2013, Loss and grief, in M Barnes & J Rowe (eds), *Child, youth and family health: Strengthening communities*, Elsevier, New York, pp. 260–78.

Forster, EM & Windsor, C 2014, Speaking to the deceased child: Australian health professional perspectives in paediatric end of life care, *International Journal of Palliative Nursing*, 20(10), pp. 502–8.

Foster, TL, Lafond, DA, Reggio, C & Hinds, PS 2010, Pediatric palliative care in childhood cancer nursing: From diagnosis to cure or end of life, *Seminars in Oncology Nursing*, 26(4), pp. 205–21.

Friedrichsdorf, S 2019, From tramadol to methadone: Opioids in the treatment of pain and dyspnea in pediatric palliative care, *The Clinical Journal of Pain*, 35(6), pp. 501–8.

Gaab, EM, Owens, GR & MacLeod, RD 2014, Siblings caring for and about pediatric palliative care patients, *Journal of Palliative Medicine*, 17(1), pp. 62–7.

Genik, LM, McMurty, M, Marshall, S, Rapoport, A & Stinson, J 2020, Massage therapy for symptom reduction and improved quality of life in children with cancer in palliative care: A pilot study, *Complementary Therapies in Medicine*, 48, p. 102263.

Hallenbeck, J 2012, Pathophysiologies of dyspnoea explained: Why might opioids relieve dyspnoea and not hasten death?, *Journal of Palliative Medicine*, 15(8), pp. 848–53.

Hammond, SS & Gera, R 2016, Oncologic pain in pediatrics, *Journal of Pain Management*, 9(2), pp. 165–75.

Hildenbrand, AK, Clawson, KJ, Alderfer, MA & Marsac, ML 2011, Coping with pediatric cancer strategies employed by children and their parents to manage cancer-related stressors during treatment, *Journal of Pediatric Oncology Nursing*, 28(6), pp. 344–54.

Hinds, PS et al. 2010, Psychometric and clinical assessment of the 10-item reduced version of the fatigue scale-child instrument, *Journal of Pain and Symptom Management*, 39(3), pp. 572–8.

Hockenberry, MJ et al. 2003, Three instruments to assess fatigue in children with cancer: The child, parent and staff perspectives, *Journal of Pain and Symptom Management*, 25, pp. 319–28.

Hockenberry-Eaton, M et al. 1998, Fatigue in children and adolescents with cancer, *Journal of Pediatric Oncology Nursing*, 15(3), pp. 172–82.

Hughes, D, Ladas, E, Rooney, D & Kelly, K 2008, Massage therapy as a supportive care intervention for children with cancer, *Oncology Nursing Forum*, 35(3), pp. 431–42.

Hyde, C, Price, J & Nicholl, H 2012, Neuropathic pain management in children, *International Journal of Palliative Nursing*, 18(10), pp. 476–82.

Jacobowski, N, Radbill, L & Truba, N 2020 Beyond the SSRI: Assessment and Treatment of Depression and Anxiety in Pediatric Palliative Care, *Journal of Pain and Symptom Management*, 59(2), pp. 494–5.

Jalmsell, L, Kreicbergs, U, Onelov, E, Steineck, G & Henter, J 2010, Anxiety is contagious: Symptoms of anxiety in the terminally ill child affect long-term psychological wellbeing in bereaved parents, *Pediatric Blood & Cancer*, 54(5), pp. 751–7.

Jenholt Nolbris, M & Nilsson, S 2016, Sibling supporters' experiences of giving support to siblings who have a brother or a sister with cancer, *Journal of Pediatric Oncology Nursing*, 34(2), pp. 83–9.

Jones, BL, Contro, N & Koch, KD 2014, The duty of the physician to care for the family in pediatric palliative care: Context, communication, and caring, *Pediatrics*, 133 (Supp. 1), pp. S8–S15.

Keir, A & Wilkinson, D 2013, Communication skills training in paediatrics, *Journal of Paediatrics and Child Health*, 49(8), pp. 624–8.

Klick, JC & Hauer, J 2010, Pediatric palliative care, *Current Problems in Pediatric and Adolescent Health Care*, 40(6), pp. 120–51.

Kuhn, E, Schalley, S, Potthoff, M & Weaver, MS 2019, The arc of generational care: A case series considering grandparent roles and care needs in pediatric palliative care, *Journal of Social Work in End-of-life & Palliative Care*, 15(2–3), pp. 99–110.

Lee, M, Mu, P, Tsay, S, Chou, S, Chen, Y & Wong, T 2012, Body image of children and adolescents with cancer: A metasynthesis on qualitative research findings, *Nursing & Health Sciences*, 14(3), 381–90.

Levine, D et al. 2013, Best practices for pediatric palliative cancer care: A primer for clinical providers, *Journal of Supportive Oncology*, 11(3), pp. 114–25.

Lindenfelser, KJ, Hense, C & McFerran, K 2012, Music therapy in pediatric palliative care: Family-centered care to enhance quality of life, *American Journal of Hospice & Palliative Medicine*, 29(3), pp. 219–26.

Lotz, J, Jox, RJ, Borasio, GD & Fuhrer, M 2015 Pediatric advance care planning from the perspective of health care professionals: A qualitative interview study, *Palliative Medicine*, 29(3), pp. 212–22.

Lyon, ME et al. 2009, Who will speak for me? Improving end-of-life decision-making for adolescents with HIV and their families, *Pediatrics*, 123(2), pp. e199–e206.

Lyon, ME, Jacobs, S, Briggs, L, Cheng, YI & Wang, J 2014, A longitudinal, randomized, controlled trial of advance care planning for teens with cancer: Anxiety, depression, quality of life, advance directives, spirituality, *Journal of Adolescent Health*, 54(6), pp. 710–17.

Malcolm, C, Gibson, F, Adams, S, Anderson, G & Forbat, L 2014, A relational understanding of sibling experiences of children with rare life-limiting conditions: Findings from a qualitative study, *Journal of Child Health Care*, 18(3), pp. 230–40.

Meyer, EC, Ritholz, MD, Burns, JP & Truog, RD 2006, Improving quality of end-of-life care in the pediatric intensive care unit: Parents' priorities and recommendations, *Pediatrics*, 117(3), pp. 649–57.

Monterosso, L & DeGraves, S 2012, Paediatric palliative care, in M O'Connor, S Lee & S Aranda (eds), *Palliative care nursing: A guide to practice* (3rd ed.), Ausmed, Melbourne.

Moriarty, HJ, Carroll, R & Controneo, M 1996, Differences in bereavement reactions within couples following death of a child, *Research in Nursing & Health*, 9(6), pp. 461–9.

Morris, S, Fletcher, K & Goldstein, R 2019, The grief of parents after the death of a young child, *Journal of Clinical Psychology in Medical Settings* 26(3), pp. 321–38.

Moules, NJ, Laing, CM, McCaffery, G, Tapp, DM & Strother, D 2012, Grandparents' experiences of childhood cancer, Part 1: Doubled and silenced, *Journal of Pediatric Oncology Nursing*, 29(3), pp. 119–32.

Nursing Council of New Zealand, 2012, *Code of conduct for nurses*, Nursing Council of New Zealand, Wellington, viewed 29 March 2021, www.nursingcouncil.org.nz/ Public/Nursing/Standards_and_guidelines/NCNZ/nursing-section/Standards_and_ guidelines_for_nurses.aspx

Pieper, L, Zernikow, B, Drake, R, Frosch, M, Printz, M & Wager, J 2018, Dyspnea in children with life-threatening and life-limiting complex chronic conditions, *Journal of Palliative Medicine*, 21(4), pp. 552–64.

Ponzetti, JJ & Johnson, MA 1991, The forgotten grievers: Grandparents' reactions to the death of grandchildren, *Death Studies*, 15(2), pp. 157–67.

Pritchard, M et al. 2008, Cancer-related symptoms most concerning to parents during the last week and last day of their child's life, *Pediatrics*, 121(5), pp. e1301–e1309.

Queensland Family and Child Commission (QFCC) 2019, *Australian and New Zealand child death statistics 2017 and annual report deaths of children and young people Queensland 2018–2019*, Queensland Family and Child Commission, Brisbane.

Radossi, AL et al. 2018, A systematic review of integrative clinical trials for supportive care in pediatric oncology: A report from the International Society of Pediatric Oncology, T&CM collaborative, *Support Care in Cancer,* 26, pp. 375–91.

Rapoport, A, Shaheed, J, Newman, C, Rugg, M & Steel, R 2013, Parental perceptions of forgoing artificial nutrition and hydration during end-of-life care, *Pediatrics*, 131(5), pp. 861–9.

Rasmussen, LA & Grégoire, M 2015, Challenging neurological symptoms in paediatric palliative care: An approach to symptom evaluation and management in children with neurological impairment, *Paediatrics & Child Health*, 20(3), pp. 159–65.

Reid, J, McKeaveney, C & Martin, P 2019 Communicating with adolescents and young adults about cancer-associated weight loss, *Current Oncology Reports*, 21(2), p. 15.

Robinson, WM 2012, Palliation of dyspnoea in paediatrics, *Chronic Respiratory Disease*, 9(4), pp. 251–6.

Schill, K & Caxaj, S 2019, Cultural safety strategies for rural Indigenous palliative care: A scoping review, *BMC Palliative Care*, 18, p. 21.

Schutze, T, Langler, A, Zuzak, TJ, Schmidt, P & Zernikow, B 2016, Use of complementary and alternative medicine by pediatric oncology patients during palliative care, *Supportive Care in Cancer*, 24, pp. 2869–75.

Shahid, S, Taylor, EV, Cheetham, S, Woods, JA, Aoun, SM & Thompson, SC 2018, Key features of palliative care service delivery to Indigenous peoples in Australia, New Zealand, Canada and the United States: A comprehensive review, *BMC Palliative Care*, 17, p. 72.

Shann, F 2017, *Drug doses RCH Intensive Care Unit* (16th ed.), Royal Children's Hospital, Melbourne.

Shaw, TM 2012, Pediatric palliative pain and symptom management, *Pediatric Annals*, 41(8), pp. 329–34.

Stayer, D 2012, Pediatric palliative care: A conceptual analysis for pediatric nursing practice, *Journal of Pediatric Nursing*, 27, pp. 350–6.

Stewart, G & McNeilly, P 2011, Opioid-induced constipation in children's palliative care, *Nursing Children and Young People*, 23(8), pp. 31–4.

Tatterton, MJ &Walshe, C 2018 Understanding the bereavement experience of grandparents following the death of a grandchild from a life-limiting condition: A meta-ethnography, *Journal of Advanced Nursing*, 75, pp. 1406–17.

Thrane, SE, Maurer, SH, Ren, D, Danford, CA & Cohen, SM 2017, Reiki therapy for symptom management in children receiving palliative care: A pilot study, *American Journal of Hospice and Palliative Medicine*, 34(4), pp. 373–9.

Tomlinson, D et al. 2011, Chemotherapy versus supportive care alone in pediatric palliative care for cancer: Comparing the preferences of parents and health care professionals, *Canadian Medical Association Journal*, 183(17), pp. 1252–8.

Tomlinson, D, Zupanec, S, Jones, H, O'Sullivan, C, Hesser, T & Sung, L 2016, The lived experience of fatigue in children and adolescents with cancer: A systematic review, *Support Care Cancer*, 24, pp. 3623–31.

Ullrich, CK, Dussel, V, Orellana, L, Kang, TI, Rosenberg, AR, Feudtner, C & Wolfe, J 2018, Self-reported fatigue in children with advanced cancer: Results of the PediQUEST study, *Cancer*, 124, pp. 3776–83.

Ullrich, CK & Mayer, O 2007, Assessment and management of fatigue and dyspnoea in pediatric palliative care, *The Pediatric Clinics of North America*, 54(5), p. 735.

Ullrich, CK et al. 2010, Fatigue in children with cancer at the end of life, *Journal of Pain and Symptom Management*, 40(4), pp. 483–94.

Van Breemen, C 2009, Using play therapy in paediatric palliative care: Listening to the story and caring for the body, *International Journal of Palliative Nursing*, 15(10), pp. 510–14.

Varni, JW, Burwinkle, TM, Katz, ER, Meeske, K & Dickinson, P 2002, The PedsQL in pediatric cancer: Reliability and validity of the Pediatric Quality of Life Inventory Generic Core Scales, Multidimensional Fatigue Scale, and cancer module, *Cancer*, 94, pp. 2090–2106.

Wakefield, C, Lin, S, Drew, D, McLoone, J, Doolan, E, Young, A, Fardell, J & Cohn, R 2016, Development and evaluation of an information booklet for grandparents of children with cancer, *Journal of Pediatric Oncology Nursing*, 33(5), pp. 361–9.

Walker, C 1989, Use of art and play therapy in pediatric oncology, *Journal of Pediatric Oncology Nursing*, 6, pp. 121–6.

Wiener, L, Zadeh, S, Wexler, LH & Pao, M 2013, When silence is not golden: Engaging adolescents and young adults in discussions around end of life care choices, *Pediatric Blood Cancer*, 60(5), pp. 715–18.

Wolfe, J, Grier, HE & Klar, N 2000, Symptoms and suffering at the end of life in children with cancer, *New England Journal of Medicine*, 342, pp. 326–33.

World Health Organization (WHO) 1998, WHO definition of palliative care for children, viewed 21 January 2014, www.who.int/cancer/palliative/definition/en

—— 2012, *WHO guidelines on the pharmacological treatment of persisting pain in children with medical illnesses*, WHO, Geneva.

Yates, P 2012, Nausea and vomiting in palliative care nursing, in M O'Connor, S Lee & S Aranda (eds), *Palliative care nursing: A guide to practice*, 3rd ed., Ausmed, Melbourne, pp. 167–77.

Youngblut, JM, Brooten, D, Blais, K, Hannan, J & Niyonsenga, T 2010, Grandparents' health and functioning after a grandchild's death, *Journal of Pediatric Nursing*, 25(5), pp. 352–9.

Youngblut, JM, Brooten, D, Blais, K, Kilgore C & Yoo, C 2015, Health and functioning in grandparents after a young grandchild's death, *Journal of Community Health*, 40, pp. 956–66.

Zadeh, S, Pao, M & Wiener, L 2015, Opening end-of-life discussions: How to introduce Voicing My CHOiCES™, an advance care planning guide for adolescents and young adults, *Palliative and Supportive Care*, 13(3), pp. 591–9.

Zander, M & Hutton, A 2010 Coping and resilience factors in pediatric oncology nurses, *Journal of Pediatric and Oncology Nursing*, 27(2), pp. 94–108.

Index